Hitesh Chopra
Vinod Kumar Gauttam
Ajmer Singh Grewal
Kavita Munjal
Editors

Phyto-Nanomedicine

Advancements and Development in Drug Discovery and Delivery Systems

nova
Medicine & Health
New York

DOI: https://doi.org/10.52305/FTHM2247

Library of Congress Cataloging-in-Publication Data

ISBN: 979-8-89530-317-7 (Hardcover)
ISBN: 979-8-89530-356-6 (e-Book)

Published by Nova Science Publishers, Inc. † New York

Contents

Preface

The integration of traditional herbal medicine with advanced nanotechnology is revolutionizing drug discovery and therapeutic delivery. "Phyto-Nanomedicine: Advancements and Development in Drug Discovery and Delivery Systems" is designed to illuminate this dynamic intersection, offering a comprehensive resource for researchers, clinicians, and pharmaceutical scientists. Herbal medicine has been a cornerstone of healthcare across cultures, leveraging the therapeutic potential of phytochemicals derived from plants. Despite their historical efficacy, many phytochemicals face challenges such as poor solubility, limited bioavailability, and stability issues in modern therapeutic contexts. Nanotechnology offers innovative solutions to these challenges, improving the delivery and efficacy of herbal remedies by manipulating materials at the molecular scale. This book explores how nanotechnology can enhance the development of phytomedicines, bridging the gap between ancient practices and contemporary medical innovations.

The book begins with an exploration of how nanotechnology enhances the delivery systems for phytoherbals. It discusses how nanomaterials can improve the solubility and stability of herbal compounds, addressing issues such as poor absorption and enabling the treatment of various conditions more effectively. The transformative role of nanoparticles in drug discovery and delivery is also examined, with a focus on how nanomaterials can enhance drug specificity, repurpose conventional drugs, and boost the efficacy of natural immunomodulators. This section underscores the potential of nanoparticles to advance therapeutic strategies. Further, the application of nanotechnology to achieve targeted drug delivery for phytoherbals is discussed. By leveraging nanoscale materials, this approach addresses challenges such as poor solubility, bioavailability, and first-pass metabolism, offering benefits like reduced side effects, controlled release, and improved biocompatibility. The book explores the application of nanotechnology-enhanced phytoherbals in treating neurodegenerative diseases like Alzheimer's and Parkinson's. These sections highlight the potential of nanomedicines to improve treatment outcomes by enhancing the solubility, bioavailability, and delivery of herbal compounds across the blood-brain barrier. In cardiovascular therapy, the book examines how nanophytoherbals can improve treatment efficacy by targeting inflammation and oxidative stress. It discusses both the benefits and potential risks, exploring how these advanced formulations could be integrated with conventional drugs for optimized treatment. The use of nanophytoherbals in managing diabetes is also covered, with a focus on how nanotechnology enhances the synthesis, characterization, and application of these formulations. The book reviews how encapsulated anti-diabetic phytochemicals improve therapeutic outcomes. In wound care, the book highlights how nanomedicine addresses challenges in tissue regeneration, inflammation control, and targeted drug delivery. It explores advancements in scar prevention and tissue remodeling, aiming to improve treatment outcomes through nanotechnology. The book further explores the application of nanophytoherbals in skin care, obesity therapy, and immune-boosting treatments.

It discusses how nanotechnology can enhance the efficacy of phytocompounds in these areas, addressing challenges such as poor penetration, stability, and targeted delivery. The potential of nanophytochemicals in cancer therapy is examined, with a focus on how nanocarriers can improve drug delivery and overcome challenges like multidrug resistance. The book aims to enhance the effectiveness of plant-derived anticancer treatments through advanced nanomedicines. Finally, the book provides a global perspective on the impact of nanophytoherbals in various fields, including cosmetics, respiratory diseases, and clinical applications. It offers a comprehensive overview of the latest advancements, safety considerations, and regulatory challenges, emphasizing the need for standardized safety assessments and regulatory harmonization.

This book aims to advance the field of nanophytoherbals by integrating traditional herbal knowledge with modern technology. It serves as a valuable resource for understanding the transformative impact of nanotechnology on herbal medicine, fostering innovation, and improving healthcare outcomes across diverse medical conditions. We invite all those passionate about healthcare, research, and herbal medicine to explore this transformative work, blending ancient remedies with modern advancements. Our hope is that this book equips and inspires readers to leverage nature's powerful healing resources for a healthier future.

Hitesh Chopra, PhD
Department of Biosciences, Saveetha School of Engineering, Saveetha Institute of Medical and Technical Sciences, Chennai, Tamil Nadu, India

Vinod Kumar Gauttam, PhD
Shiva Institute of Pharmacy, Bilaspur, Himachal Pradesh, India

Ajmer Singh Grewal, PhD
Guru Gobind Singh College of Pharmacy, Yamuna Nagar, Haryana, India

Kavita Munjal, PhD
Amity Institute of Pharmacy, Amity University, Noida, Uttar Pradesh, India

Chapter 1

Nanotechnology-Enhanced Delivery Systems for Phytoherbals: Bridging Ancient Remedies and Modern Therapeutics

Anshika Chaudhary
Rohan Nagpal
Somia Chauhan
and Shreya Kaul*
Amity Institute of Pharmacy, Amity University, Noida, Uttar Pradesh, India

Abstract

Herbal remedies, rooted in ancient practices, have gained widespread use across the globe. Advances in phytochemical and phytopharmacological sciences have clarified the composition and biological properties of numerous products derived from medicinal plants. The efficacy of many medicinal plants depends on the presence of active compounds. However, several biologically active constituents encounter challenges in cellular absorption due to factors such as large molecular size, poor lipid membrane permeability, inadequate solubility, and susceptibility to instability in biological environments, along with extensive first-pass metabolism. These limitations result in diminished bioavailability and therapeutic effectiveness, rendering some extracts clinically underutilized. To address these challenges, nanotechnology emerges as a promising solution by attaching or encapsulating herbal therapeutic molecules with appropriate nanomaterials, including polymeric nanoparticles (NPs), metallic NPs, lipid-based NPs, ceramic NPs, magnetic NPs, protein-based NPs, carbon nanotubes, quantum dots, dendrimers, and hybrid NPs. The convergence of phytoherbals and nanotechnology creates opportunities for addressing a wide range of health conditions, from bacterial infections to chronic diseases such as cancer and wound healing.

Keywords: nanophytomedicine, phytochemical bioenhancement, phytochemical nanoformulations, target-specific delivery

* Corresponding Author's Email: skaul@amity.edu.

In: Phyto-Nanomedicine
Editors: Hitesh Chopra, Vinod Kumar Gauttam, Ajmer Singh Grewal et al.
ISBN: 979-8-89530-317-7

Abbreviations

ALGD	Anionic linear globular dendrimer
AN	Apigenin
BA	Boswellic acid
BBR	Berberine
CBE	Coffee berry extract
CM	Chamomile oil
CUR	Curcumin
CQDs	Carbon quantum dots
DD	Dendrimer
DDS	Drug delivery systems
DO-ptGQD	Donepezil hydrochloride-conjugated graphene quantum dots
EE	Entrapment efficiency
GA	Gallic acid
GB	Ginkgolide B
MNPs	Metallic nanoparticles
NeO	Neem oil
NLC	Nanostructured lipid carriers
PAMAM	Polymer-conjugated polyamidoamine
PD	Parkinson's disease
PEG	Polyethylene glycol
PLA	Polylactic acid
PLGA	Poly(lactic-co-glycolic) acid
PVA	Polyvinyl alcohol
QDs	Quantum dots
siRNA	Small interfering RNA
SJW	St. John's wort
SLN	Solid lipid nanoparticles
SM	Silymarin
Trl-GNPs	Trl-polyphenol-coated gold nanoparticles

Introduction

Across centuries and continents, traditional medicinal systems such as Siddha and Ayurveda in India have leveraged the therapeutic properties of bioactive plants. Today, herbal medicines occupy a prominent position in the pharmaceutical landscape, celebrated for their efficacy and minimal adverse effects. Despite the vast diversity of plant species, only a small fraction exhibits pharmacological effects, with merely 5–15% considered medicinally relevant (Elkordy et al., 2021). Today, despite advancements in modern medicine, 80% of the world still relies on indigenous healing practices. The demand for herbal remedies is increasing globally, driving the mass production of herbal medicinal products available in various forms, including powders, capsules, creams, and, more recently, nanoparticulate formulations. Natural drug formulations encompass a range of dosage forms derived from herbs or their derivatives, obtained through processes such as extraction and distillation (Ambwani et al., 2019). Herbal medicines are widely utilized for their affordability and perceived safety; however, they face several challenges that hinder their effectiveness and safety. One significant issue is the rapid release of herbal drugs, which may be accompanied by potential unknown toxicity and limited oral absorption. Herbal drugs often suffer from insolubility, leading to reduced bioavailability and increased systemic clearance. As a result, higher doses or repeated administration may be necessary to achieve adequate efficacy (Ahmed & Kumar, 2020). This challenge highlights the importance of developing improved delivery systems to sustain release and target delivery, thereby enhancing patient compliance. Traditional medicines often struggle to reach their intended target sites adequately, dispersing throughout the body due to the physicochemical properties of the medication, which can lead to diminished therapeutic effectiveness (Elkordy et al., 2021). This dispersion underscores the need for targeted delivery methods. The presence of various phytoconstituents in herbal plants contributes to formulation instability, posing significant challenges in delivering these medicines to their intended sites. Compounds such as flavonoids, tannins, and terpenoids, while water-soluble, encounter difficulties in crossing biological membranes, resulting in limited absorption and effectiveness. Additionally, their larger molecular size further reduces bioavailability (Kumari et al., 2022). To address these limitations, advancements in drug delivery systems (DDS) specifically tailored for plant-based medicines have been developed. Nanotechnology-based delivery systems act as drug carriers capable of overcoming various challenges faced by herbal medicines. This field, which focuses on functional art and technology, plays a crucial role in refining strategies and dosage methods within the 1 to 100 nm range. Developing novel drug delivery systems for herbal products is essential, as it offers several advantages, such as reducing the need for repeated dosing, enhancing therapeutic effectiveness by minimizing toxicity, and increasing bioavailability (Sabuj & Islam, 2020). Integrating herbal extracts into innovative formulation systems provides additional benefits, including improved bulk administration, reduced preoccupation, enhanced bioavailability, improved pharmacological activity, stabilized formulations, enhanced tissue macrophage distribution, sustained delivery, and protection against physicochemical deterioration (Riaz et al., 2023). This book chapter offers an overview of nanotechnology and explores its intersection with delivery systems for herbal drugs, incorporating relevant research studies. Additionally, this compilation details various nano-carriers used in herbal DDS and analyzes associated research findings in depth.

Phytoherbals as Therapeutic Agents

Phytoherbals, derived from plants, have been used for centuries across various cultures as remedies for ailments and to promote wellness. Rooted in traditional medicine, they provide a diverse array of bioactive substances with medicinal benefits. Due to their varied chemical compositions, phytoherbals offer a rich source of therapeutic agents that continue to captivate the interest of modern medicine. Their superior safety profiles and lower toxicity compared to synthetic drugs make them appealing therapeutic interventions. Phytoherbals encompass a wide range of chemical constituents, including alkaloids, flavonoids, terpenoids, phenolic compounds, essential oils, saponins, lignans, tannins, glycosides, and polysaccharides, as listed in Table 1.

Table 1. Phytoherbal groups with their active compounds and therapeutic effects

Phytoherbal Group	Active Compounds	Therapeutic Effects	Example Plants	Reference
Alkaloids	Morphine, Codeine, Quinine	Analgesic, anti-inflammatory, antimalarial	Opium Poppy, Cinchona Bark	(Riaz et al., 2023)
Flavonoids	Catechins, Quercetin	Antioxidant, anti-inflammatory, anticancer	Green Tea, Citrus Fruits	(Oluwole et al., 2022)
Terpenoids	Curcumin (CUR), Cannabinoids	Anti-inflammatory, antimicrobial	Turmeric, Cannabis	(Masyita et al., 2022)
Phenolic Compounds	Resveratrol, Oleuropein	Antioxidant, cardioprotective, anticancer	Berries, Olive Oil	(Sun & Shahrajabian, 2023)
Essential Oils	Linalool, Eucalyptol	Antibacterial, calming	Lavender, Eucalyptus	(Ramdani et al., 2023)
Saponins	Ginsenosides, Dioscin	Cholesterol reduction, anticancer	Ginseng, Dioscorea	(Ramdani et al., 2023)
Lignans	Secoisolariciresinol, Podophyllotoxin	Hormone-balancing, cardiovascular support	Flaxseeds, Sesame Seeds	(Oluwole et al., 2022)
Tannins	Hamamelitannin, Ellagitannins	Antioxidant, antimicrobial	Witch Hazel, Oak Bark	(Oluwole et al., 2022)
Glycosides	Digoxin, Anthraquinone	Cardiac benefits, laxative	Foxglove, Rhubarb	(Li et al., 2021)
Polysaccharides	Beta-glucans, Ganoderic acids	Immunomodulatory, anti-inflammatory	Reishi Mushroom, Turkey Tail Mushroom	(Li et al., 2021)

Table 2. Phytoherbals challenges and their nanotechnology-based solutions

Phytoherbals Challenges	Nanotechnology Solutions	Explanation
Poor Bioavailability	Nanoencapsulation	Enhances absorption and bioavailability of phytoherbal compounds by protecting them from degradation and enhancing solubility.
Instability	Liposomal Encapsulation	Protects sensitive bioactive compounds from environmental degradation (e.g., light, heat, and oxidation), improving stability.
Low Solubility	Nanoemulsions	Improves the solubility of hydrophobic phytoherbal compounds, allowing for better absorption and bioavailability.
Rapid Metabolism and Elimination	Solid Lipid Nanoparticles (SLNs)	Provides controlled and sustained release of phytoherbals, reducing rapid metabolism and elimination.
Poor Targeting	Polymeric NPs	Enhances targeted delivery of phytoherbal compounds to specific tissues or cells, increasing therapeutic efficacy and reducing side effects.
Toxicity of Active Components	Gold and Silver NPs	Reduces the required dose of toxic phytoherbal components by enhancing their therapeutic effects, thus minimizing toxicity.
Inconsistent Dosage	Nanofibers	Allows for controlled and uniform release of phytoherbal compounds, ensuring consistent and accurate dosage.
Short Half-Life	Nanocarriers	Extends the half-life of phytoherbal compounds in the bloodstream, enhancing their therapeutic duration.
Limited Penetration	Nanoformulations	Enhances the penetration of phytoherbal compounds through biological barriers (e.g., skin, mucosa), improving efficacy.
Taste and Odor Issues	Encapsulation in NPs	Masks unpleasant taste and odor of phytoherbal compounds, improving patient compliance.

These compounds exhibit a broad spectrum of pharmacological activities, including anti-inflammatory, antioxidant, antimicrobial, and immunomodulatory effects (Tanaka & Kashiwada, 2021).

Integrating Nanotechnology and Phytoherbals

The integration of nanotechnology with phytoherbals represents a promising frontier in medicine, merging the ancient wisdom of herbal remedies with nanoscale innovations. Nanotechnology enhances the therapeutic potential of phytoherbals by overcoming biological barriers and improving cellular uptake. Nanocarriers can navigate obstacles such as the blood-brain barrier and the gastrointestinal epithelium, enabling phytochemicals to reach previously inaccessible targets. Furthermore, nanoparticles (NPs) can be designed to target specific tissues or cells, thereby reducing off-target effects and increasing therapeutic efficacy. This is achieved by functionalizing NPs with ligands or antibodies for precise delivery (Ahmed & Kumar, 2020). NPs protect phytochemicals from degradation and enzymatic metabolism, thereby improving their stability and prolonging circulation time in the bloodstream. They also enhance the solubility and bioavailability of poorly water-soluble phytochemicals. Moreover, nanotechnology facilitates combination therapies by co-encapsulating multiple phytochemicals or integrating them with conventional drugs, potentially enhancing therapeutic outcomes and overcoming drug resistance (Dewi et al., 2022). Additionally, nanocarriers can incorporate targeting ligands, imaging agents, or stimuli-responsive elements for real-time monitoring and precise control of drug delivery. This approach not only enhances the stability and shelf life of phytoherbal products but also addresses challenges related to storage and transportation (Sabuj & Islam, 2020). Table 2 depicts the challenges associated with phytoherbals and the corresponding nanotechnology-based solutions (Dewi et al., 2022).

Diverse Nanocarriers for Phytoherbal Delivery

Polymeric NPs

Are microscopic entities composed of biocompatible polymeric materials, extensively utilized in DDS. Common natural polymers used in the formulation of polymeric NPs include chitosan, alginate, gelatin, hyaluronic acid, and dextran. In contrast, synthetic polymers encompass poly(lactic-co-glycolic acid) (PLGA), polyethylene glycol (PEG), polyvinyl alcohol (PVA), and polylactic acid (PLA). The composition of polymeric NPs can be customized by varying the type of polymer, molecular weight, and, when applicable, the ratio of co-polymers (Azadpour et al., 2021). Ginkgolide B (GB), a compound derived from Ginkgo biloba known for its neuroprotective properties, faces challenges in oral administration due to poor bioavailability. Zhao et al. (2020) aimed to enhance its effectiveness in the treatment of Parkinson's disease (PD). The use of GB nanoparticles (GB-NPs) facilitated sustained release of GB, increasing its potential to reach the brain and effectively manage PD. Experiments conducted on Madin-Darby canine kidney cells revealed multiple entry mechanisms for these NPs, leading to their accumulation in endoplasmic organelles and lysosomal vesicles. Studies in zebrafish demonstrated that GB-NPs were able to cross various barriers, including the blood-brain barrier and blood-retinal barrier. In models of MPP+-induced neuronal damage, GB-NPs exhibited notable neuroprotective effects (Zhao et al., 2020). Silymarin (SM), a potent antioxidant, faces solubility challenges that hinder its therapeutic application. Azadpour et al. developed PLGA NPs loaded with SM, enhancing its anti-inflammatory efficacy against sepsis and septic shock (Azadpour et al., 2021). In another investigation, starch was utilized to improve the solubility and effectiveness of *Triphala Churna*, a formulation rich in polyphenols and vitamin C (Nallasamy et al., 2020). Natural compounds present a promising avenue for breast cancer treatment due to their lower toxicity compared to synthetic drugs. To illustrate this, Zafar et al. (2022) developed hybrid NPs containing apigenin (AN), a naturally occurring flavonoid found in chamomile, artichokes, parsley, and vine spinach. The NPs demonstrated enhanced penetration and antioxidant activity compared to pure AN. Optimized AN-NPs reduced cell viability to 31.98% in MCF-7 cells after 24 hours, compared to 49.39% with pure AN, resulting in a lower IC_{50} value (Zafar et al., 2022). Similarly, AN-PLGA NPs exhibited significantly lower IC_{50} values, being 7.8 and 10.8 times less than that of pure AN, when targeting pulmonary carcinoma cells (B16F10 and A549) (Sen et al., 2021). In another related study, AN-NPs demonstrated nearly five-fold lower IC_{50} values against HepG2 and MCF-7 cell lines compared to pure AN (Zhai et al., 2013).

Lipid-Based NPs

Lipid-based NPs are innovative DDS that utilize lipids as their primary building blocks. These NPs are designed to encapsulate drugs or therapeutic agents within a lipid matrix, providing numerous advantages in targeted drug delivery. Types of lipid-based NPs include liposomes, SLNs, and nanostructured lipid carriers (NLCs). These NPs incorporate phospholipids for structural integrity, fatty acids for stabilization, and triglycerides as core materials. Cholesterol enhances membrane stability and drug entrapment efficiency (EE), while surfactants assist in stabilization. Together, these components ensure that NPs are stable, biocompatible, biodegradable, and capable of controlled drug release (Kumar, 2018). To address the challenges of poor tissue permeability and degradation of chamomile oil (CM) while enhancing its wound regenerative capabilities, SLNs were developed. In vivo experiments demonstrated that CM-SLNs exhibited promising effects on wound regeneration, improving skin structure, contraction, growth factor levels, and reducing inflammation and metalloproteinase ratios (Gad et al., 2019) Nemati and colleagues formulated SLNs containing neem oil (NeO) and evaluated their efficacy against Toxoplasma infection by assessing morphology, size, and toxicity. NeO-SLNs exhibited concentration-dependent toxicity, effectively killing over 70% of tachyzoites at all concentrations, indicating their potential for targeting cysts (Nemati et al., 2022). In another study, SLNs were developed for the topical application of safranal, leading to the formulation of a polyherbal sunscreen cream that offers broad-spectrum protection (Sanju et al., 2022). In a study, quercetin was encapsulated within PEG liposomes to enhance its anticancer effects. This formulation significantly improved the solubility and bioavailability of quercetin. The findings suggest that PEG-quercetin liposomes have the potential to target tumors, provide sustained drug release, and enhance quercetin's solubility, offering a promising strategy for addressing malignancies (Li et al., 2021). A study found that liposomes containing coffee berry extract (CBE) improved stability and anti-aging effects on the skin compared to free CBE. These liposomal formulations demonstrated lower toxicity in human dermal fibroblasts and exhibited enhanced anti-aging properties. Clinical trials revealed that the application of liposomes significantly improved skin elasticity and reduced melanin levels (Saewan et al., 2023). In a recent study, researchers formulated NLCs loaded with St. John's wort (SJW) extract and assessed their wound-healing potential. The optimized formulation demonstrated remarkable wound-healing effects in vivo, underscoring its potential for effective wound treatment (Sotirova et al., 2023). NLCs demonstrated prolonged release of thymol and exhibited high retention in the skin, particularly within the epithelial and dermal layers. Antibacterial analysis revealed that thymol-NLC gels effectively reduced the viability of C. acnes while preserving the balance of the skin microbiota (Folle et al., 2024).

Vesicular NPs

Vesicular NPs are hollow, spherical structures utilized in DDS to encapsulate drugs or active compounds. The various types of vesicular NPs include liposomes, niosomes, transfersomes, ethosomes, and transethosomes. These structures offer enhanced drug stability, prolonged circulation, and targeted delivery. Liposomes are composed of phospholipid bilayers, making them compatible with both hydrophilic and hydrophobic drugs. Niosomes, which are made from non-ionic surfactants, improve stability and bioavailability. Transfersomes are deformable liposomes enhanced with edge activators, enabling them to penetrate pores and narrow channels in the skin for improved transdermal drug delivery. The stability and drug release kinetics of these vesicular systems are determined by the components used, such as lipids and surfactants (Al-Enazi et al., 2023). *Lycium barbarum,* commonly known as goji or wolfberry, is renowned for its immune-modulating, antioxidative, antidiabetic, anti-aging, anti-carcinoma, and antihypertensive properties. However, its efficacy is hindered by limited solubility, potential toxic effects, and gut disintegration. To address these challenges, Pavaloiu et al. encapsulated polyphenols extracted from *Lycium barbarum* leaves within liposomes. In tests conducted on L-929 mouse fibroblasts, the liposomes demonstrated a protective effect against H_2O_2-induced cell damage after 24 hours (Păvăloiu et al., 2021). The primary challenge associated with essential oils is their susceptibility to light and high volatility, which limits their clinical utility. To enhance their biopharmaceutical properties, researchers developed liposomes loaded with essential oils derived from *Salvia triloba* and *Rosmarinus officinalis*. These liposomes exhibited favorable characteristics and maintained stability over time. Additionally, they demonstrated significant antibacterial activity against various strains, including *Klebsiella pneumoniae* (Risaliti et al., 2019). Castangia and her team formulated transferosomes that encapsulate Jabuticaba (*Myrciaria jaboticaba*) extract, which contains flavonoids. This formulation demonstrated enhanced regenerative abilities in human keratinocytes (Castangia et al., 2021). Boswellic acid (BA), derived from *Boswellia serrata*, encounters challenges in oral administration due to poor absorption and extensive metabolism. To address these issues, transferosomes for transdermal BA delivery were developed. These transferosomes, optimized for size and drug entrapment, demonstrated effective permeation through the skin, providing sustained release over 24 hours. The formulation shows promising potential for enhancing BA delivery to deeper skin layers, thereby improving therapeutic outcomes (Varia et al., 2022). Researchers have shown that niosomes enhance solubility and minimize side effects when used with herbal products, addressing challenges typically associated with whole plant extracts. In a study by Imtiaz et al. (2023), a niosomal formulation of *Tradescantia pallida* leaf extract was developed for diabetes treatment. This formulation exhibited controlled drug release and significant antidiabetic activity in vitro, as evidenced by alpha-amylase inhibition and non-enzymatic glycosylation assays. Binding studies indicated that the niosomes altered the protein structure, contributing to the observed antidiabetic effects (Imtiaz et al., 2023). A recent study investigated the use of niosomes to enhance the anti-neoplastic and bactericidal properties of Pistacia atlantica. The findings demonstrated that niosomes exhibited significantly increased cytotoxic activity against BT-20 and MCF-10 carcinoma cells, as well as enhanced bactericidal effects against *Pseudomonas aeruginosa*, *Staphylococcus epidermidis*, and *Candida albicans*, compared to the extract alone (Al-Enazi et al., 2023).

Metallic NPs

Metallic NPs (MNPs) serve as effective carriers for delivering a variety of therapeutic agents. Metals such as iron, zinc, titanium, gold, silver, palladium, and copper exhibit enhanced and customizable optical properties. Their surfaces can be easily modified to attach targeting agents and active biomolecules, allowing for tailored delivery systems. Moreover, MNPs can accommodate the loading of multiple drugs, which can significantly enhance therapeutic efficacy (Chandrakala et al., 2022). In this study, silver NPs (DH-AgNPs) and gold NPs (DH-AuNPs) were synthesized using extracts from *Angelicae Pubescentis* Radix. Both types of NPs demonstrated promising antioxidative properties against DPPH radicals. DH-AgNPs exhibited antimicrobial efficacy against *E. coli, S. aureus, P. aeruginosa*, and *S. enterica*. Additionally, the cytotoxicity observed in RAW264.7 macrophages suggests their potential for targeted treatment of inflammation (Markus et al., 2017). Nirmala et al. aimed to create and analyze Trl-polyphenol-coated gold NPs (Trl-GNPs) derived from *Triphala*, known for their potential anticancer properties. The study assessed cellular viability in MDA-MB-231 triple-negative mammary carcinoma cells and examined the interactions of Trl-GNPs with tubulin. The results revealed that Trl-GNPs inhibited cell proliferation by disrupting the tubulin structure, leading to abnormalities in the microtubule network and subsequent cell cycle arrest (Nirmala et al., 2021). El-Zayat et al. focused on utilizing the concentrate of *Ephedra aphylla* to synthesize selenium and zinc NPs and evaluate their biological traits, including antioxidant, anticancer, and antimicrobial properties. The synthesized NPs exhibited high antioxidant activity as determined by the DPPH assay. Notably, selenium NPs demonstrated strong cytotoxic effects against various cancer cell lines, including MCF-7, HepG2, Hep2, HCT-116, PC3, and HeLa. Additionally, these NPs displayed significant microbicidal potency against both bacterial and fungal strains (El-Zayat et al., 2021). Another investigation aimed to create copper NPs (CuNPs) using the extract of *Allium saralicum* R.M. Fritsch (CuNPs@Allium). In antibacterial and antifungal tests, CuNPs@Allium outperformed standard antibiotics. Furthermore, *in vivo* studies conducted on rats with cutaneous wounds demonstrated significant wound healing effects when treated with CuNPs@Allium ointment, as evidenced by a reduction in wound area and enhanced tissue regeneration (Tahvilian et al., 2019). A research investigation assessed the impact of various extraction methodologies and concentrations on the characteristics and biological properties of silver NPs synthesized using *Echinacea purpurea* L. extracts. These NPs exhibited enhanced antioxidant activity, as measured by DPPH activity, and demonstrated bacteriostatic efficacy against *E. coli* and *C. albicans*, surpassing the effectiveness of the original extracts (Fierascu et al., 2022).

Quantum Dots

Quantum dots (QDs) are semiconductor NPs made from materials such as cadmium selenide, cadmium sulfide, or lead sulfide. They exhibit size-dependent optical properties due to quantum confinement effects, allowing for tunable emission wavelengths. This characteristic makes QDs valuable for fluorescence-based imaging and labeling in biological systems. Additionally, their small dimensions enable efficient penetration across biological barriers. QDs also demonstrate excellent photostability and resistance to photobleaching. In targeted drug delivery, QDs can transport therapeutic agents to specific tissues or cells. By modifying their surface with targeting moieties, QDs can selectively interact with receptors that are overexpressed on diseased cells, facilitating precise delivery of therapeutic payloads while minimizing off-target effects (Agarwal et al., 2023). Dermatologists are increasingly favoring *Aloe vera* gel for wound healing due to its ability to boost collagen levels and enhance cross-linking. The combination of carbon QDs (CQDs) with *Aloe vera* may further enhance cellular stimulation, improving penetration and therapeutic effects. Curcumin (CUR), a potent naturally derived anticancer agent, often faces challenges such as low solubility and a short half-life, which limit its effectiveness in DDS. To address these challenges, Karami et al. developed a novel hydrogel nanocarrier using chitosan, alumina, and CQDs through a specialized double nanoemulsion method. This formulation demonstrated controlled and pH-sensitive release of CUR. Cellular studies on breast cancer cells indicated slow and programmed cell death, highlighting the nanocarrier's effectiveness in delivering curcumin for tumor treatment (Karami et al., 2023). *Polygala tenuifolia*, an herb known for its rich neuroprotective and anti-inflammatory compounds, is commonly used to enhance memory, cognitive function, and alleviate symptoms of depression. To harness its potential for Alzheimer's disease treatment, Tak et al. synthesized donepezil hydrochloride-conjugated graphene QDs (DO-ptGQDs) using a one-pot hydrothermal method with *Polygala tenuifolia* root extract. Behavioral tests indicated that DO-ptGQDs significantly improved learning and memory abilities within just 7 days. The formulation exhibited a higher inhibition of acetylcholinesterase activity, increased levels of protein and glutathione, and reduced levels of nitric oxide and lipid peroxides. Histological analysis demonstrated better preservation of cellular organization with DO-ptGQDs compared to other formulations (Tak et al., 2022).

Dendrimers

A dendrimer (DD) is a nanoscale, star-like polymer nanocarrier characterized by a tree-like structure with multiple branching arms extending from a central core. These branches provide a unique surface with heterogeneous functional units, allowing for the simultaneous delivery of multiple drugs. The functional units on the dendrimer's surface can be tailored to enable targeted drug delivery to specific sites. Dendrimer nanocarriers possess tunable surface functionality, facilitating precise control over their interactions with biological molecules and tissues. Their distinct characteristics—such as precise nanoscale size, extensive branching, polyvalency, aqueous solubility, and inner cavities—render dendrimers promising candidates for various biological applications and drug delivery systems (Xiong et al., 2018). Berberine (BBR), a natural alkaloid recognized for its potential anti-cancer properties, faces challenges in pharmacokinetics that limit its therapeutic efficacy. To enhance its delivery, dendrimers such as polymer-conjugated polyamidoamine (PAMAM) have been utilized. An investigation examined the delivery of BBR using PAMAM dendrimers through two methods: conjugation (BPC) and encapsulation (BPE). The results indicated that BPC exhibited significantly higher antitumorigenic effects on MCF-7 and MDA-MB-468 mammary carcinoma cells compared to BPE. Both formulations demonstrated minimal hemolytic toxicity, with BPC showing superior pharmacokinetic profiles (Gupta et al., 2017). DDs hold significant promise in cancer management due to their ability to effectively transport medications directly to tumor sites while minimizing systemic toxicity. In a recent study, nanovehicles were developed to deliver therapeutic agents alongside small interfering RNA (siRNA). Curcumin (CUR) was encapsulated within PAMAM dendrimers, and the surface amino groups of the dendrimers were utilized to attach Bcl-2 siRNA, resulting in the formation of PAMAM-Cur/Bcl-2 siRNA NPs. This innovative formulation demonstrated improved cellular internalization, enhanced solubility and stability of CUR, and synergistically induced apoptosis in HeLa carcinoma cells (Ghaffari et al., 2020). In a related study, researchers formulated a delivery system combining celastrol with EpCAM aptamer and DDs to target EpCAM-rich tumors. This system was tested in SW620 colon carcinoma cells using cell culture and murine models, focusing on cancer cell targeting, apoptosis induction, and biosafety in both mice and zebrafish models. The results indicated that the biomolecular conjugates-maintained stability under physiological conditions and significantly induced apoptosis in SW620 cells (Ge et al., 2020). Mehrizi et al. investigated Anionic Linear Globular Dendrimers (ALGD) as a carrier for betulinic acid (BTA) to address its low solubility and high toxicity in the treatment of leishmaniasis. The encapsulation of BTA within ALGD nanoparticles resulted in a remarkable 700-fold increase in solubility and eliminated toxicity *in vivo.* Administering BTA at a dosage of 40 mg/kg significantly reduced the Leishmania major parasite count both *in vitro* and *in vivo*, suggesting a safer and more effective treatment approach for leishmaniasis (Mehrizi et al., 2021).

Conclusion

The convergence of herbal medicine and nanotechnology represents a promising frontier in medical research, combining the rich therapeutic heritage of herbal remedies with the precision and efficacy of nanoscale DDS. Herbal medicines, rooted in centuries-old traditional knowledge, offer a diverse array of natural compounds with therapeutic benefits. However, challenges such as inadequate bioavailability, limited solubility, and non-specific targeting have hindered their widespread application. The integration of nanotechnology into herbal DDS addresses these challenges by providing innovative solutions for enhanced drug delivery. Various NPs serve as effective vehicles for encapsulating herbal extracts, boosting solubility and bioavailability while allowing for controlled release and targeted delivery to specific regions. Additionally, the utilization of nanotechnology in herbal DDS has the potential to mitigate toxicity concerns associated with conventional formulations, thereby enhancing the safety profile of herbal medicines. Despite these advancements, the collaborative efforts of researchers in unraveling the intricacies of herbal nano DDS hold significant promise for personalized medicine and improved patient outcomes.

References

Agarwal, K., Rai, H., & Mondal, S. (2023). Quantum dots: an overview of synthesis, properties, and applications. *Materials Research Express* 10 (6): 062001.

Ahmed, S., & Kumar, S. (2020). Application of Nanotechnology on Herbal Drug formulation: A Review. *J Adv Res NanoSci NanoTech* 2(1): 16-20.

Al-Enazi, N. M., Alsamhary, K., Ameen, F., & Nobre, M. A. L. (2023). Novel Vesicular Formulation Based on a Herbal Extract Loaded with Niosomes and Evaluation of Its Antimicrobial and Anticancer Potential. *Microbiology Research* 14(4): 2133–2147.

Ambwani, S., Tandon, R., & Ambwani, T. K. (2019). Metal Nanodelivery Systems for Improved Efficacy of Herbal Drugs. *Biosciences, Biotechnology Research Asia* 16(2): 251–261.

Azadpour, M., Farajollahi, M. M., Dariushnejad, H., Varzi, A. M., Varezardi, A., & Barati, M. (2021). Effects of synthetic silymarin-PLGA nanoparticles on M2 polarization and inflammatory cytokines in LPS-treated murine peritoneal macrophages. *Iranian Journal of Basic Medical Sciences* 24(10).

Castangia, I., Manca, M. L., Allaw, M., Hellström, J., Granato, D., & Manconi, M. (2021). Jabuticaba (Myrciaria jaboticaba) peel as a sustainable source of anthocyanins and ellagitannins delivered by phospholipid vesicles for alleviating oxidative stress in human keratinocytes. *Molecules* 26(21).

Chandrakala, V., Aruna, V., & Angajala, G. (2022). Review on metal nanoparticles as nanocarriers: current challenges and perspectives in drug delivery systems. *Emergent Materials* 5 (6): 1593–1615).

Dewi, M. K., Chaerunisaa, A. Y., Muhaimin, M., & Joni, I. M. (2022). Improved Activity of Herbal Medicines through Nanotechnology. *Nanomaterials* 2022, 12(22): 4073.

Elkordy, A. A., Haj-Ahmad, R. R., Awaad, A. S., & Zaki, R. M. (2021). An overview on natural product drug formulations from conventional medicines to nanomedicines: Past, present and future. *Journal of Drug Delivery Science and Technology* 63 (1): 102459.

El-Zayat, M. M., Eraqi, M. M., Alrefai, H., El-Khateeb, A. Y., Ibrahim, M. A., Aljohani, H. M., Aljohani, M. M., & Elshaer, M. M. (2021). The Antimicrobial, Antioxidant, and Anticancer Activity of Greenly Synthesized Selenium and Zinc Composite Nanoparticles Using Ephedra aphylla Extract. *Biomolecules* 11(3): 470.

Fierascu, I. C., Fierascu, I., Baroi, A. M., Ungureanu, C., Ortan, A., Avramescu, S. M., Somoghi, R., Fierascu, R. C., & Dinu-Parvu, C. E. (2022). Phytosynthesis of Biological Active Silver Nanoparticles Using Echinacea purpurea L. Extracts. *Materials* 15(20): 7327.

Folle, C., Marqués, A., Díaz Garrido, N., Carvajal Vidal, P., Sánchez López, E., Suñer Carbó, J., Halbaut, L., Mallandrich, M., Espina, M., Badia, J., Baldoma, L., García, M. L., & Calpena, A. C. (2024). Gel-Dispersed Nanostructured Lipid Carriers Loading Thymol Designed for Dermal Pathologies. *International Journal of Nanomedicine* 19: 1225–1248.

Gad, H. A., Abd El-Rahman, F. A. A., & Hamdy, G. M. (2019). Chamomile oil loaded solid lipid nanoparticles: A naturally formulated remedy to enhance the wound healing. *Journal of Drug Delivery Science and Technology* 50: 329–338.

Ge, P., Niu, B., Wu, Y., Xu, W., Li, M., Sun, H., Zhou, H., Zhang, X., & Xie, J. (2020). Enhanced cancer therapy of celastrol *in vitro* and *in vivo* by smart dendrimers delivery with specificity and biosafety. *Chemical Engineering Journal* 383: 123228.

Ghaffari, M., Dehghan, G., Baradaran, B., Zarebkohan, A., Mansoori, B., Soleymani, J., Ezzati Nazhad Dolatabadi, J., & Hamblin, M. R. (2020). Co-delivery of curcumin and Bcl-2 siRNA by PAMAM dendrimers for enhancement of the therapeutic efficacy in HeLa cancer cells. *Colloids and Surfaces B: Biointerfaces*, 188: 110762.

Gupta, L., Sharma, A. K., Gothwal, A., Khan, M. S., Khinchi, M. P., Qayum, A., Singh, S. K., & Gupta, U. (2017). Dendrimer encapsulated and conjugated delivery of berberine: A novel approach mitigating toxicity and improving *in vivo* pharmacokinetics. *International Journal of Pharmaceutics*, 528(1–2): 88–99.

Imtiaz, F., Islam, M., Saeed, H., Ahmed, A., Asghar, M., Saleem, B., Farooq, M. A., Khan, D. H., & Peltonen, L. (2023). Novel phytoniosomes formulation of Tradescantia pallida leaves attenuates diabetes more effectively than pure extract. *Journal of Drug Delivery Science and Technology*, 83: 104399.

Karami, M. H., Pourmadadi, M., Abdouss, M., Kalaee, M. R., Moradi, O., Rahdar, A., & Díez-Pascual, A. M. (2023). Novel chitosan/γ-alumina/carbon quantum dot hydrogel nanocarrier for targeted drug delivery. *International Journal of Biological Macromolecules*, 251: 126280.

Kumar, R. (2019). Lipid-Based Nanoparticles for Drug-Delivery Systems. *Nanocarriers for Drug Delivery: Nanoscience and Nanotechnology in Drug Delivery*. 249-284.

Kumari, S., Goyal, A., Gürer, E. S., Yapar, E. A., Garg, M., Sood, M., & Sindhu, R. K. (2022). Bioactive Loaded Novel Nano-Formulations for Targeted Drug Delivery and Their Therapeutic Potential. In Pharmaceutics. *MDPI* 14(5): 1091.

Li, J., Li, Z., Gao, Y., Liu, S., Li, K., Wang, S., Gao, L., Shi, M., Liu, Z., Han, Z., & Qiu, Y. (2021). Effect of a Drug Delivery System Made of Quercetin Formulated into PEGylation Liposomes on Cervical Carcinoma *In Vitro* and *In Vivo*. *Journal of Nanomaterials*. 389934.

Li, Y., Dai, M., Wang, L., & Wang, G. (2021). Polysaccharides and glycosides from Aralia echinocaulis protect rats from arthritis by modulating the gut microbiota composition. *Journal of Ethnopharmacology*, 269: 113749.

Markus, J., Wang, D., Kim, Y. J., Ahn, S., Mathiyalagan, R., Wang, C., & Yang, D. C. (2017). Biosynthesis, Characterization, and Bioactivities Evaluation of Silver and Gold Nanoparticles Mediated by the Roots of Chinese Herbal Angelica pubescens Maxim. *Nanoscale Research Letters* 12(1): 1–12.

Masyita, A., Mustika Sari, R., Dwi Astuti, A., Yasir, B., Rahma Rumata, N., Emran, T. Bin, Nainu, F., & Simal-Gandara, J. (2022). Terpenes and terpenoids as main bioactive compounds of essential oils, their roles in human health and potential application as natural food preservatives. *Food Chemistry: X* 13: 100217.

Mehrizi, T. Z., Mosaffa, N., Khamesipour, A., Hoseini, M. H. M., Shahmabadi, H. E., Ardestani, M. S., & Ramezani, A. (2021). A Novel Nanoformulation for Reducing the Toxicity and Increasing the Efficacy of Betulinic Acid Using Anionic Linear Globular Dendrimer. *Journal of Nanostructures* 11(1): 143–152.

Nallasamy, P., Ramalingam, T., Nooruddin, T., Shanmuganathan, R., Arivalagan, P., & Natarajan, S. (2020). Polyherbal drug loaded starch nanoparticles as promising drug delivery system: Antimicrobial, antibiofilm and neuroprotective studies. *Process Biochemistry* 92: 355–364.

Nemati, S., Mohammad Rahimi, H., Hesari, Z., Sharifdini, M., Jalilzadeh Aghdam, N., Mirjalali, H., & Zali, M. R. (2022). Formulation of Neem oil-loaded solid lipid nanoparticles and evaluation of its anti-Toxoplasma activity. *BMC Complementary Medicine and Therapies*, 22: 122.

Nirmala, J. G., Rachineni, K., Choudhary, S., Hosur, R. V., & Lopus, M. (2021). Triphala polyphenols-functionalized gold nanoparticles impair cancer cell survival through induction of tubulin dysfunction. *Journal of Drug Delivery Science and Technology* 61; 102167.

Oluwole, O., Fernando, W. B., Lumanlan, J., Ademuyiwa, O., & Jayasena, V. (2022). Role of phenolic acid, tannins, stilbenes, lignans and flavonoids in human health – a review. *International Journal of Food Science and Technology* 57 (10).

Păvăloiu, R. D., Sha'at, F., Neagu, G., Deaconu, M., Bubueanu, C., Albulescu, A., Sha'at, M., & Hlevca, C. (2021). Encapsulation of polyphenols from lycium barbarum leaves into liposomes as a strategy to improve their delivery. *Nanomaterials* 11(8): 1938.

Ramdani, D., Yuniarti, E., Jayanegara, A., & Chaudhry, A. S. (2023). Roles of Essential Oils, Polyphenols, and Saponins of Medicinal Plants as Natural Additives and Anthelmintics in Ruminant Diets: A Systematic Review. *Animals* 13 (4): 767.

Riaz, M., Khalid, R., Afzal, M., Anjum, F., Fatima, H., Zia, S., Rasool, G., Egbuna, C., Mtewa, A. G., Uche, C. Z., & Aslam, M. A. (2023). Phytobioactive compounds as therapeutic agents for human diseases: A review. *Food Science and Nutrition* 11(6): 2500-2529.

Risaliti, L., Kehagia, A., Daoultzi, E., Lazari, D., Bergonzi, M. C., Vergkizi-Nikolakaki, S., Hadjipavlou-Litina, D., & Bilia, A. R. (2019). Liposomes loaded with Salvia triloba and Rosmarinus officinalis essential oils: *In vitro* assessment of antioxidant, antiinflammatory and antibacterial activities. *Journal of Drug Delivery Science and Technology* 51: 493–498.

Sabuj, M. Z. R., & Islam, N. (2020). Nanophytomedicine: An Effective Way for Improving Drug Delivery and Bioavailability of Herbal Medicines. *Nanophytomedicine*, 55–70.

Saewan, N., Jimtaisong, A., Panyachariwat, N., & Chaiwut, P. (2023). *In Vitro* and *In Vivo* Anti-Aging Effect of Coffee Berry Nanoliposomes. *Molecules*, 28(19).

Sanju, N., Vineet, M., & Kumud, M. (2022). Development and Evaluation of a Broad spectrum Polyherbal Sunscreen formulation using Solid Lipid Nanoparticles of Safranal. *Journal of Cosmetic Dermatology* 21(10): 4433–4446.

Sen, R., Ganguly, S., Ganguly, S., Debnath, M. C., Chakraborty, S., Mukherjee, B., & Chattopadhyay, D. (2021). Apigenin-Loaded PLGA-DMSA Nanoparticles: A Novel Strategy to Treat Melanoma Lung Metastasis. *Molecular Pharmaceutics* 18(5): 1920-1938.

Sotirova, Y., Gugleva, V., Stoeva, S., Kolev, I., Nikolova, R., Marudova, M., Nikolova, K., Kiselova-Kaneva, Y., Hristova, M., & Andonova, V. (2023). Bigel Formulations of Nanoencapsulated St. John's Wort Extract—An Approach for Enhanced Wound Healing. *Gels* 9(5):360.

Sun, W., & Shahrajabian, M. H. (2023). Therapeutic Potential of Phenolic Compounds in Medicinal Plants—Natural Health Products for Human Health. *Molecules* 28 (4): 1845.

Tahvilian, R., Zangeneh, M. M., Falahi, H., Sadrjavadi, K., Jalalvand, A. R., & Zangeneh, A. (2019). Green synthesis and chemical characterization of copper nanoparticles using Allium saralicum leaves and assessment of their cytotoxicity, antioxidant, antimicrobial, and cutaneous wound healing properties. *Applied Organometallic Chemistry* 33(12).

Tak, K., Sharma, P., Sharma, R., Dave, V., Jain, S., & Sharma, S. (2022). One-pot hydrothermal green synthesis of Polygala tenuifolia mediated graphene quantum dots for acetylcholine esterase inhibitory activity. *Journal of Drug Delivery Science and Technology* 73: 103486.

Tanaka, N., & Kashiwada, Y. (2021). Phytochemical studies on traditional herbal medicines based on the ethnopharmacological information obtained by field studies. *Journal of Natural Medicines* 75(4): 762-783.

Varia, U., Joshi, D., Jadeja, M., Katariya, H., Detholia, K., & Soni, V. (2022). Development and evaluation of ultradeformable vesicles loaded transdermal film of boswellic acid. *Future Journal of Pharmaceutical Sciences* 8(1).

Xiong, Z., Shen, M., & Shi, X. (2018). Dendrimer-based strategies for cancer therapy: Recent advances and future perspectives. *Science China Materials* 61(11): 1387-1403.

Zafar, A., Alruwaili, N. K., Imam, S. S., Alsaidan, O. A., Ahmed, M. M., Yasir, M., Warsi, M. H., Alquraini, A., Ghoneim, M. M., & Alshehri, S. (2022). Development and Optimization of Hybrid Polymeric Nanoparticles of Apigenin: Physicochemical Characterization, Antioxidant Activity and Cytotoxicity Evaluation. *Sensors* 22(4): 1346.

Zhai, Y., Guo, S., Liu, C., Yang, C., Dou, J., Li, L., & Zhai, G. (2013). Preparation and *in vitro* evaluation of apigenin-loaded polymeric micelles. *Colloids and Surfaces A: Physicochemical and Engineering Aspects*, 429: 24-30.

Zhao, Y., Xiong, S., Liu, P., Liu, W., Wang, Q., Liu, Y., Tan, H., Chen, X., Shi, X., Wang, Q., & Chen, T. (2020). Polymeric nanoparticles-based brain delivery with improved therapeutic efficacy of ginkgolide b in Parkinson's disease. *International Journal of Nanomedicine* 15: 10453–10467.

Chapter 2

Nanoparticles in Phyto-Nanomedicine: Innovations in Drug Discovery and Delivery Systems

Jyotiram Arjun Sawale[1,*]
Vinod Kumar Gauttam[2]
Vivek Chourasia[3]
Suhas P. Padmane[4]
Dhrubajyoti Sarkar[5]
Kavita Munjal[6]
and Teena Vishwakarma[3]

[1]Krishna Institute of Pharmacy, Krishna Vishwa Vidyapeeth (Deemed to be University), Karad, Maharashtra, India
[2]Shiva Institute of Pharmacy, Bilaspur, Himachal Pradesh, India
[3]I.E.S. Institute of Pharmacy, I.E.S. University, Bhopal, Madhya Pradesh, India
[4]Gurunanak College of Pharmacy, Mauza-Nari, Nagpur, Maharashtra, India
[5]Faculty of Pharmaceutical Science, Assam Down Town University Sankar Madhab Path, Gandhinagar, Panikhaiti, Guwahati, Assam, India
[6]Amity Institute of Pharmacy, Amity University, Noida, Uttar Pradesh, India

Abstract

Nanotechnology, operating at the nanoscale, is reshaping medical interventions by harnessing the unique properties of nanoparticles. These minute structures effectively distribute drugs, overcome biological barriers, and selectively target disease sites. Their larger surface area-to-volume ratio allows nanomaterials to efficiently load multiple molecules, making them particularly valuable in cancer treatment for enhancing drug specificity and improving patient outcomes. The use of nanomaterials as drug delivery vehicles is a cornerstone of nanomedicine, which not only enhances drug efficacy but also facilitates the repurposing of conventional drugs. The immune system protects against pathogens, with compromised immunity increasing susceptibility to various diseases. Continuous exposure to external factors can disrupt homeostasis, resulting in a rise in diseases, emphasizing the importance of maintaining a balanced immune response. Natural

[*] Corresponding Author's Email: jyotisawale@gmail.com.

In: Phyto-Nanomedicine
Editors: Hitesh Chopra, Vinod Kumar Gauttam, Ajmer Singh Grewal et al.
ISBN: 979-8-89530-317-7

substances with immunomodulating effects, such as medicinal plants, probiotics, prebiotics, melatonin, vitamins, and minerals, are gaining attention for their cost-effectiveness and fewer adverse effects. Nanotechnology is revolutionizing pharmaceutical sciences, with herbal nano-formulations emerging for their diverse applications and enhanced efficacy at reduced dosages. These advancements highlight nanotechnology's transformative potential in advancing therapeutic strategies for medical progress.

Keywords: nanotechnology, phytomedicine, COVID 19, nanoparticles, targeted drug delivery

Abbreviations

AD	Alzheimer's disease
CN	Carbon nanotubes
GA G	lycyrrhizic acid
GPx	Glutathione peroxidase
GANP	Glycyrrhizic acid nanoparticles
MN	Metal nanoparticles
MNP	Magnetic nanoparticles
NPs	Nanoparticles
NS	Nanostructures
PIP	Piperine
PNPs	Phyto-nanoparticles
PtdIns3K	Phosphatidylinositol 3-kinase
QD	Quantum dots
Se	Selenium
SLBN	Solid lipid nanoparticles
SN	Semiconductor nanoparticles

Introduction

Proposed by Professor N. Taniguchi in 1974, nanotechnology has brought revolutionary changes to drug delivery and general medical care. This field involves the creation of nanoscale materials measuring billionths of a meter. Nanoparticles (NPs) are clusters of atoms ranging from 1 to 100 nm, possessing specific structures and sizes that confer unique and enhanced properties. They can be classified into organic (e.g., carbon-based) and inorganic (e.g., semiconductors, metals, and magnetic NPs) categories. Recently, inorganic NPs, particularly metallic ones like gold and silver, have garnered significant attention for their superior material properties and functional adaptability, positioning them as promising agents in biomedicine. Nanotechnology has seamlessly integrated into modern tools, driving technological advancements in everyday applications. The emphasis on small-sized NPs, typically ranging from 1 to 100 nanometers, has gained global recognition due to their remarkable applications across physical, chemical, and biological sciences. Research efforts in nanotechnology have democratized its features, making these advancements accessible to the general population, as illustrated in Figure 1.

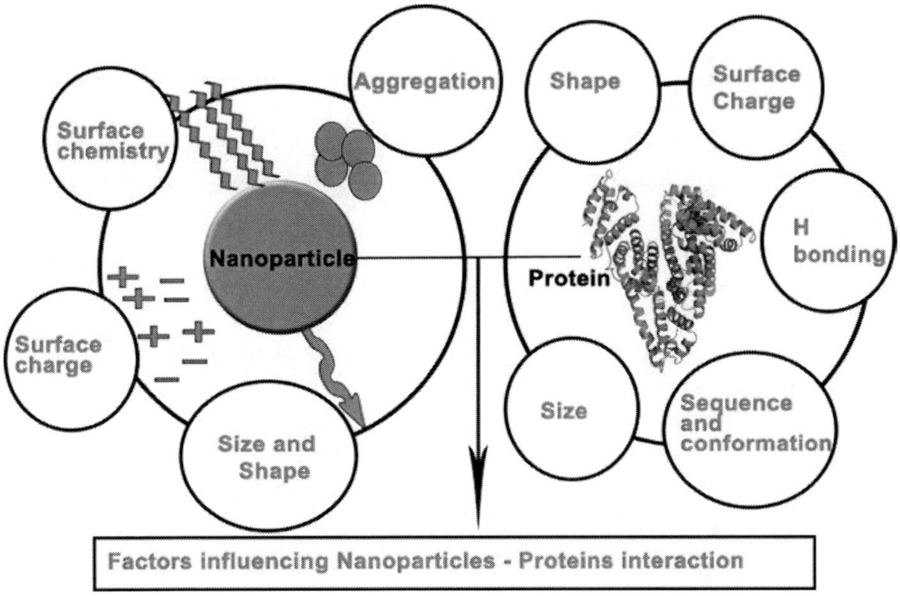

Figure 1. Schematic representation of factors influencing NP-protein interactions.

Nobel laureate Richard P. Feynman's visionary statement, "There's Plenty of Room at the Bottom," fueled interest and paved the way for revolutionary developments in nanotechnology. Manipulating materials at the nanoscale induces changes in their properties, resulting in extraordinary optical, magnetic, and electrical characteristics. These unique nanoscale properties can be applied across various fields, including electronics, batteries, fuel additives, solar cells, catalysts, the electrochemical industry, defense, cosmetics, medicine, food and beverage additives and packaging, agriculture, biosensors, detection, vaccines, antibiotics, and pharmaceutical delivery. NPs play a crucial role in the production of various nanomaterials, including carbon nanotubes (CNTs), metal NPs (MNPs), ceramic NPs (CNPs), and semiconductor NPs (SNPs) (Patil & Chandrasekaran, 2020). Alternatively, stable silver NPs can be synthesized using plant extracts through a process known as green synthesis. Plant extracts, rich in secondary metabolites, contain various functional groups that facilitate the reduction and stabilization of NPs. This approach eliminates the need for commonly used chemical agents. Nanotechnology in cancer treatment offers effective solutions to challenges such as drug solubility and stability. Silver nanomaterials, when used as carriers for therapeutic molecules, can enhance the potency and activity of anti-inflammatory drugs. Studies have demonstrated that silver NPs exhibit cytotoxic effects on cancer cells by altering cell morphology, reducing cell viability, and triggering oxidative stress. Additionally, research has shown that they can induce autophagy by activating the class III phosphatidylinositol 3-kinase (PtdIns3K) pathway, leading to anti-inflammatory effects. Various mechanisms, including cell cycle arrest, cytotoxicity, apoptosis, oxidative stress, and DNA damage, contribute to their effectiveness in cancer treatment (Salih et al., 2023).

Nanotechnology in Drug Discovery and Delivery

In South India, traditional healers draw upon ancient texts by figures such as Bohar and Saint Agasthiar to employ herbo-mineral preparations as therapies for contemporary illnesses. This practice involves synthesizing metal-based medicine in nanoformulations through herbal treatments, a tradition that dates back thousands of years. The Siddha system of medicine utilizes various herbal-mineral formulations, including Chenduram (sulfide form), Parpam (oxide form), Pathangam (sublimation product), and Chunnam (caustic oxide preparation). Highly effective formulations like Parpam and Chenduram have impressive shelf lives, exceeding 100 and 75 years, respectively. Despite the significant role of metals in Siddha medicine, concerns about their potential toxicity limit public acceptance and clinical use. Additionally, there is a lack of comprehensive scientific validation for these formulations, which further complicates their acceptance in modern medical practice (Kahsay et al., 2019). Simultaneously, nanotechnology, which focuses on nanometer-sized objects, has made significant advancements across various domains, including materials, medical devices, and systems. Synthesized silver NPs, ranging from tens to hundreds of nanometers in size, are finding applications in nanomedicine, promising enhanced specificity and reduced dosage requirements. However, concerns regarding environmental and occupational impacts have emerged due to the lack of comprehensive toxicity studies. Gold, historically utilized in Chrysotherapy for various diseases, is now being explored in organo-gold complexes, which exhibit potential antitumor and antimicrobial properties (Al-Ansari et al., 2021). Contemporary research in nanomedicine focuses on developing novel nanomaterials with intrinsic potential, along with green-synthesized nanocarriers for targeted drug delivery that minimizes harm to normal cells. The high surface area-to-volume ratio, stability, and enhanced performance of nanotechnology drive the advancement of nanomedicines for various medical applications. There is a growing demand for plant-mediated natural nanomedicines for chemopreventive purposes, and the production of nanocarrier drugs through green synthesis methods is viewed as a sustainable initiative that can reduce side effects while increasing treatment efficacy (Nassar et al., 2016). In the context of cancer, lung cancer is the leading cause globally, followed closely by breast cancer. While radiotherapy and chemotherapy are established treatment options, they often come with a range of side effects. The development of green-synthesized zero-valent colloidal nano-silver as an anticancer agent offers a promising alternative for precise nano-delivery, potentially minimizing adverse effects (Jha & Shimpi, 2018).

The Intersection of Nanotechnology and Phyto-Medicine for Enhanced Therapeutic Outcomes

Although the field of nanomedicine and nanotechnology is relatively new, it has made significant strides in the treatment of burns in recent years. Nanostructures (NSs) serve as vital delivery vehicles in various therapeutic applications, including cell therapy, tissue growth, disease treatment, advanced antibiotics, and wound healing. This progress showcases a range of innovative platforms, such as films, 3D scaffolds, and NPs, that respond to stimuli like light, enzymes, pH, and ultrasound activation. These advancements indicate the potential for large-scale NSs, including nanofibers, NPs, films, and 3D scaffolds, to play a critical role in wound healing and burn regeneration. Such innovative approaches promise more effective and targeted treatments in burn care and infection management.

Wound Healing and Burn Infections

The treatment of burns and skin reconstruction is complex and is being investigated across multiple areas. The emergence of antibiotic-resistant pathogens in recent years has intensified the challenge of addressing topical antimicrobial resistance in burn injuries, posing a significant threat to public health. As a result, there is an increasing imperative to develop more effective antimicrobial agents. New therapeutic approaches based on nanoscale structures have emerged, particularly in the context of burn wounds and infections, offering promising advancements in therapy and skin regeneration in the post-antibiotic era. NSs have demonstrated remarkable antimicrobial activity against resistant strains while also facilitating the regeneration of burn-injured skin. These NPs can be categorized into two main groups: inorganic and organic NPs. Organic NPs encompass nano-emulsions, polymer NPs, micelles, liposomes, nanogels, and solid lipid NPs (SLNPs). In contrast, inorganic NPs include carbon-based NPs (such as fullerenes, carbon nanotubes, graphene, and nanodiamonds), gold NPs, copper NPs, titanium dioxide NPs, silver NPs, magnetic NPs (MNPs), and quantum dots (QDs). The exploration of these nanoscale structures holds great promise for revolutionizing burn wound care and effectively addressing the challenges posed by antibiotic-resistant microorganisms (Jahromi et al., 2018).

Antiviral

NPs play a crucial role in cancer treatment and enhance the efficacy of drugs against bacteria, fungi, and viruses. The application of nanotechnology in medicine relies on the minuscule size of NPs, which range from 1 to 100 nm, allowing them to penetrate living cells, particularly human cells. Nanomaterials possess protective characteristics that prevent the enclosed drug or anti-infective agent from degrading. The rapid dissemination and adaptability to genetic mutations make viral infections a significant threat to human health. Effective management of infectious diseases requires appropriate strategies, largely dependent on the severity of the illness and the mode of transmission. In recent years, the emergence of new viruses such as Zika, Ebola, Nipah, and various coronaviruses has resulted in substantial mortality. Among these, coronaviruses, including MERS-CoV and SARS, are particularly dangerous. The application of nanotechnology in combating viral infections presents a promising avenue, offering potential solutions to enhance antiviral treatments and improve overall disease management (Sarkar et al., 2022).

COVID 19 Infection

Curcumin, a pharmacological compound derived from turmeric, exhibits antiviral properties against various viruses, indicating its potential for treating COVID-19 infections. Research has focused on curcumin in a nanomicelle form, with an average size of 10 nm, to enhance the oral absorption of curcuminoids. Curcumin encounters challenges in traditional formulations due to its lipophilicity and gastrointestinal malabsorption. Nanomicelles, such as sinacurcumin, significantly improve water solubility by encapsulating curcuminoids within their lipophilic structures, leading to enhanced absorption. Warm Curcumin Soft Gel dissolves in the acidic environment of the stomach, allowing the micromicelles to remain stable for up to six hours. In a mouse model simulating COVID-19, glycyrrhizic acid (GA) NPs (GANP) selectively target affected tissues, particularly in the lungs. GANP exhibits anti-inflammatory properties, reducing organ damage and increasing survival rates in afflicted mice. Furthermore, GANP nanocomposites enhance the biocompatibility of GA, providing a foundation for its broader application. These GANPs may target inflammatory regions through the enhanced permeability and retention (EPR) effect in the surrogate mouse model of COVID-19, thereby boosting treatment efficacy and potentially serving as therapeutic agents for COVID-19 (Dubey et al., 2022). In the field of nanoparticle-based medication development, copper NPs (Cu-NPs), cobalt NPs (Co-NPs), silver NPs (Ag-NPs), and zinc oxide NPs (ZnO-NPs) are garnering attention due to their unique physico-chemical properties. However, challenges related to nano-biofortification processes—particularly concerning the human health implications of nano-nutrients—raise significant questions. The transformation of nutrients into nanoparticles, along with the feasibility and cost implications of this process, are pressing concerns, especially for developing nations amidst the global impact of COVID-19. Moreover, the use of nanoparticles has the potential to address treatment challenges associated with COVID-19. For instance, when bacteria are diluted and mixed, the efficacy of active ingredients can be compromised. NPs can help halt the spread of bacteria by inducing long-term damage, offering a promising avenue for mitigating the virus's reproductive cycle (Gupta et al., 2022).

Cancer

In recent years, numerous studies have highlighted the potent anti-inflammatory properties of flavonoids, particularly the subclass Aβ. This subclass possesses a unique molecular structure that targets breast cancer, making it a promising candidate for both the prevention and treatment of this cancer type. Apigenin (AP) demonstrated unique physicochemical and biological properties that are crucial for effective cancer treatment. Its stability and reactivity allow it to interact with various stages of cancer development, including key enzymes and molecules. One of the significant challenges with AP is its limited bioavailability. However, NPs have emerged as a promising solution for enhancing AP's delivery and interaction within cancer cells. Research shows that encapsulating or conjugating NPs with AP can substantially improve its absorption, solubility, bioavailability, and biodegradation. These enhancements contribute to increased chemo-preventive and chemotherapeutic efficacy, making NPs a valuable tool in optimizing AP's therapeutic potential in cancer treatment (Adel et al., 2022).

Alzheimer's Disease

Extensive research has focused on the protective effects of selenium (Se) against neurodegenerative diseases, particularly Alzheimer's disease (AD). Selenium has been shown to inhibit the formation of Aβ fibrils, aid in the breakdown of existing fibrils, and exhibit potent antioxidant activity, all of which are crucial mechanisms in combating the progression of AD. Despite these benefits, conventional selenium supplements face challenges, including limited absorption and potential toxicity, underscoring the need for novel carriers that can increase its bioavailability and provide controlled release. Moderate consumption of organic selenium offers numerous health benefits. Studies have demonstrated that yeast-derived selenium can improve learning and memory, enhance neuronal activity, promote synaptic protection, and reduce protein synthesis and hyperphosphorylation, making it a promising candidate for slowing AD progression. Beyond its role in neurodegenerative diseases, selenium has also shown efficacy in combating other conditions, including cancer, due to its antioxidant properties mediated by enzymes such as glutathione peroxidase (GPx). Selenium's ability to chelate biometals, such as copper (Cu), zinc (Zn), and iron (Fe), is particularly important in AD, as these metals are involved in oxidative stress and AD pathology. Moreover, selenium can effectively neutralize toxic metals like cadmium (Cd), mercury (Hg), and aluminum (Al) by forming inert complexes, thus reducing their toxicity. This multifaceted action highlights selenium's potential in mitigating both neurodegenerative and other systemic diseases (Vicente-Zurdo et al., 2023).

Phyto-Nanomedicine as a Solution to Challenges in Traditional Drug Delivery Systems

Nanotechnology has emerged as one of the most fascinating and intricate areas of research due to its distinctive electronic properties, which have a profound impact on fields such as biomedical engineering, modern information science, water purification, and medicine. Among the various nanomaterials, metal nanoparticles—particularly silver NPs (AgNPs)—stand out for their broad range of applications. These include antioxidant and anti-inflammatory activities, incorporation into food products, cancer research, cosmetics, medical treatments, DNA testing, and cell imaging. The synthesis of silver nanoparticles has been widely studied, with silver nitrate solutions being a common starting material. Various methods, including electromagnetic radiation, microwave radiation, chemical agents, and biotechnology, have been explored for this purpose. While these conventional techniques can produce pure, well-shaped, and well-dispersed AgNPs, they come with several limitations. The high costs, reliance on physical and chemical processes, and the use of strong reducing agents pose potential risks to both human health and the environment. These challenges have driven the search for more sustainable, eco-friendly alternatives for nanoparticle synthesis (Wang et al., 2018).

Phytochemicals refer to the diverse range of bioactive compounds derived from plants, known for their medicinal properties. These compounds hold significant potential for treating various conditions, including neurodegenerative diseases, inflammation, aging, diabetes, and pain. In recent years, nanotechnology has been integrated into the field of phytochemistry to enhance the bioavailability and efficacy of phytonutrients. This technological advancement helps minimize toxicity and allows for sustained performance, particularly for targeted therapeutic applications. Phytochemicals can be categorized into six groups based on their chemical structures and properties: carbohydrates, lipids, phenols, terpenes, nitrogen-containing compounds, and alkaloids. Among these, alkaloids—organic compounds present in foods like honey and black pepper—have garnered considerable attention as promising candidates for therapeutic use, owing to their bioactive potential in disease management. The application of nanotechnology to these compounds further enhances their therapeutic effectiveness (Munjal et al., 2020). Piperine (PIP), a natural alkaloid found in *Piper nigrum* (black pepper) and Indian long pepper, is recognized for its wide range of pharmacological benefits, making it significant on a global scale (Munjal et al., 2023). Despite its therapeutic potential, PIP faces challenges related to poor solubility and bioavailability, which limit its effectiveness in pre-clinical and clinical development. This places PIP in the Biopharmaceutics Classification System (BCS) class II, known for compounds with low solubility but high permeability. To address these limitations and enhance its medicinal value, advanced preparation techniques and nanotechnology-based approaches have been explored. The US Food and Drug Administration (FDA) has classified PIP and its derivatives as generally safe for use in foods and for medical purposes, underscoring its therapeutic importance (Arora et al., 2023).

Targeted Drug Delivery

The integration of nanostructures and nanophases into various disciplines, particularly in nanomedicine and drug delivery systems, has significantly advanced both biological and physical research. Nanotechnology's applications in diagnostics, treatment, regenerative medicine, gene therapy, oncology, and therapeutics have been transformative. Nanomaterials' unique properties, including their customizable size, dimensions, and material composition, have paved the way for the development of specialized NPs in diverse fields. One of the most promising advancements in this area is biogenic synthesis, a process that uses natural active molecules, such as plant or cell extracts, to manufacture NPs. This eco-friendly method, often referred to as "green synthesis," involves the reduction of dissolved metals into NPs, leading to the development of novel materials with applications in cancer therapy, tissue regeneration, sustainable energy, and chemical catalysis. Green nanotechnology, in particular, combines sustainable engineering practices with green medicine, promoting the creation of non-toxic, environmentally friendly nanomaterials that can be synthesized at low temperatures with minimal environmental impact. Life cycle assessments help ensure the sustainability of these processes throughout their design and development phases. Among the most promising advancements in green nanotechnology are phyto-NPs (PNPs), which are synthesized using biogenic methods. These NPs, produced from plant extracts, offer unique properties and site-specific action, which enhances drug efficiency, especially in anticancer applications. Plants play a key role in this green NP production due to their non-pathogenic nature and the regulated assembly of NPs enabled by plant-based phytoconstituents. Phytochemicals, including phenolics, aid in the chelation of metal ions, allowing for the synthesis of metal NPs (MNPs) such as silver, selenium, iron, gold, silicon, cerium, titanium, and zinc. These MNPs have significant therapeutic potential, and their synthesis is streamlined by the phytochemicals' ability to reduce metal ions to their base metal forms. The one-step biosynthetic approach to producing PNPs has become a focal point in nanotechnology, offering a simplified method of creating plant-based NPs with diverse biological functions. This innovation is especially critical for improving drug delivery systems, where sophisticated carriers are essential for protecting drugs from degradation and ensuring their targeted, site-specific release. These advancements in nanoparticle synthesis and green nanotechnology have the potential to revolutionize diagnostics and therapeutics, providing more effective and environmentally sustainable solutions (Puri et al., 2024).

Challenges and Future Perspectives

The European Union has acknowledged several key social challenges, including those related to health, demographic change, wellbeing, energy, food security, sustainable agriculture, and environmental sustainability. To address these concerns, flagship projects such as Graphene and the Human Brain Project have received substantial funding. These initiatives have already made notable progress, particularly in the fields of healthcare, diagnostics, nano-delivery systems, and the development of artificial organs. The next significant phase involves translating these scientific advancements into clinical applications to address broader global challenges such as disease management, poverty alleviation, water scarcity, and other socio-economic issues. Nanotechnology is positioned at the forefront of these efforts, offering numerous advantages in various domains. For instance, nano-systems have demonstrated immense potential in tissue reconstruction, imaging, biological sensing, drug delivery, and precision medical interventions. However, significant challenges remain, especially regarding the safe commercialization of nanomaterials. This includes issues related to rigorous testing and the establishment of comprehensive regulatory frameworks to ensure that nanomaterials are both safe for consumers and environmentally friendly. Additionally, opportunities for nanotechnology applications are expanding in fields such as food production, sustainable agriculture, eco-safety, and microbiome research. There is also growing interest in developing alternatives to antibiotics to combat antimicrobial resistance. Globally, researchers and policymakers are striving to overcome both intellectual and existential challenges using the power of nanoscience and nanotechnology. By addressing the testing, regulatory, and ethical challenges associated with nanomaterials, these efforts aim to maximize the positive impact of nanotechnology on society while minimizing risks (Feng et al., 2014; Gu et al., 2013; Rakovich et al., 2014). In anticancer research, the extensive use of phytochemicals has been hindered by poor solubility and retention in clinical applications. Phyto-nanomedicine, which utilizes NPs, addresses these limitations and enhances therapeutic efficacy by modulating pharmacokinetics and pharmacodynamics. Passive targeting through enhanced permeability and retention effects allows nanoparticle-based drugs to target tumors. Active targeting ligands are conjugated to nano-formulations to improve tumor specificity. Site-specific drug delivery minimizes nonspecific delivery and reduces toxicity. PEGylation, the addition of polyethylene glycol, extends the half-life of phyto-nanomedicines in circulation. Combining immunomodulatory phyto-nanomedicines with current immunotherapies or employing DNA-encapsulated nano-formulations for CAR-T therapy could enhance immuno-oncological interventions. Phytochemicals exhibit anti-cancer stem cell properties, suggesting that combining conventional chemotherapeutics with phytochemicals could target both cancer stem cells and cancer cells. Additionally, combining phytochemicals with miRNA or siRNA via nanomedicine can control cancer cells, tumor cells, and their microenvironment. Novel combinatory nanoformulations, integrating phytochemicals with fluorescent dyes and targeting agents, hold promise for both clinical and diagnostic applications. Challenges in clinical translation include cost, safety, toxicity, mass production, and product variability. Further research is needed to improve the design, production, and interaction of plant-based nanomedicines. Collaboration among academics, researchers, physicians, pharmaceutical companies, and regulatory agencies is essential for translating plant nanomedicine into clinical practice and making it suitable for cancer treatment (Jiang et al., 2015; Mitragotri et al., 2015; Thomas et al., 2011; Zhang et al., 2013). Nanomedicine offers a promising future for developing personalized medicine, advancing disease diagnosis and treatment, and promoting tissue regeneration and healing. A significant approach in nanomedicine involves the development of nanorobots and nano-sensors that can perform complex tasks within the body, including drug delivery, disease diagnosis, and tissue repair. Additionally, NPs enhance the treatment of complex diseases by enabling the simultaneous delivery of multiple therapies. NPs can also serve as non-diagnostic tools for early diagnosis. The integration of artificial intelligence and nanomedicine promises to enable accurate disease detection and diagnosis, as well as more efficient and effective drug delivery. However, several issues need to be addressed, including safety and chemical concerns, regulatory considerations, and budget constraints. Continued investment and collaboration among researchers, clinicians, and industry partners will be crucial to overcoming these challenges and unlocking the full potential of nanomedicine (Giri et al., 2021; Lu et al., 2021; Patil et al., 2008).

Conclusion

Nanomedicine is an emerging field that holds great promise for applications such as drug delivery, disease diagnosis, and tissue engineering. Treatment plans utilizing NPs have demonstrated potential in improving patient outcomes and enhancing overall quality of life. However, issues such as safety concerns, chemical implications, regulatory considerations, and costs need to be addressed. Despite these challenges, the future of nanomedicine appears bright, and continued investment and collaboration among researchers, clinicians, and industry partners can help overcome these obstacles and unlock the potential of this powerful field. The integration of nanotechnology with herbal medicine emerges as a crucial tool, contributing to advancements in herbal medicine research by enhancing bioavailability and reducing toxicities. While there are safety and efficacy challenges associated with traditional medicine, there is significant potential for nanotechnology-based herbal medicines. In summary, herbal nanomedicines are recognized for their safety, improved bioavailability, and heightened therapeutic efficacy compared to conventional herbal and synthetic drugs.

References

Adel, M., Zahmatkeshan, M., Akbarzadeh, A., Rabiee, N., Ahmadi, S., Keyhanvar, P., Rezayat, S. M., & Seifalian, A. M. (2022). Chemotherapeutic effects of Apigenin in breast cancer: Preclinical evidence and molecular mechanisms; enhanced bioavailability by nanoparticles. *Biotechnology Reports*, *34*, e00730.

Al-Ansari, M. M., Al-Dahmash, N. D., & Ranjitsingh, A. (2021). Synthesis of silver nanoparticles using gum Arabic: Evaluation of its inhibitory action on Streptococcus mutans causing dental caries and endocarditis. *Journal of Infection and Public Health*, *14*(3), 324-330.

Arora, S., Singh, B., Kumar, S., Kumar, A., Singh, A., & Singh, C. (2023). Piperine Loaded Drug Delivery Systems for Improved Biomedical Applications: Current Status and Future Directions. *Health Sciences Review*, 100138.

Dubey, A. K., Chaudhry, S. K., Singh, H. B., Gupta, V. K., & Kaushik, A. (2022). Perspectives on nano-nutraceuticals to manage pre and post COVID-19 infections. *Biotechnology Reports*, *33*, e00712.

Feng, S., Caire, R., Cortazar, B., Turan, M., Wong, A., & Ozcan, A. (2014). Immunochromatographic diagnostic test analysis using Google Glass. *ACS nano*, *8*(3), 3069-3079.

Giri, G., Maddahi, Y., & Zareinia, K. (2021). A brief review on challenges in design and development of nanorobots for medical applications. *Applied Sciences*, *11*(21), 10385.

Gu, Z., Aimetti, A. A., Wang, Q., Dang, T. T., Zhang, Y., Veiseh, O., Cheng, H., Langer, R. S., & Anderson, D. G. (2013). Injectable nano-network for glucose-mediated insulin delivery. *ACS nano*, *7*(5), 4194-4201.

Gupta, A., Kumar, A., & Dubey, B. (2022). Complex dynamics of Leslie–Gower prey–predator model with fear, refuge and additional food under multiple delays. *International Journal of Biomathematics*, *15*(08), 2250060.

Jahromi, M. A. M., Zangabad, P. S., Basri, S. M. M., Zangabad, K. S., Ghamarypour, A., Aref, A. R., Karimi, M., & Hamblin, M. R. (2018). Nanomedicine and advanced technologies for burns: Preventing infection and facilitating wound healing. *Advanced drug delivery reviews*, *123*, 33-64.

Jha, M., & Shimpi, N. G. (2018). Green synthesis of zero valent colloidal nanosilver targeting A549 lung cancer cell: *in vitro* cytotoxicity. *Journal of Genetic Engineering and Biotechnology*, *16*(1), 115-124.

Jiang, X., Valdeperez, D., Nazarenus, M., Wang, Z., Stellacci, F., Parak, W. J., & Del Pino, P. (2015). Future perspectives towards the use of nanomaterials for smart food packaging and quality control. *Particle & Particle Systems Characterization*, *32*(4), 408-416.

Kahsay, M. H., Tadesse, A., RamaDevi, D., Belachew, N., & Basavaiah, K. (2019). Green synthesis of zinc oxide nanostructures and investigation of their photocatalytic and bactericidal applications. *RSC advances*, *9*(63), 36967-36981.

Lu, W., Yao, J., Zhu, X., & Qi, Y. (2021). Nanomedicines: redefining traditional medicine. *Biomedicine & Pharmacotherapy*, *134*, 111103.

Mitragotri, S., Anderson, D. G., Chen, X., Chow, E. K., Ho, D., Kabanov, A. V., Karp, J. M., Kataoka, K., Mirkin, C. A., & Petrosko, S. H. (2015). Accelerating the translation of nanomaterials in biomedicine. *ACS nano*, *9*(7), 6644-6654.

Munjal, K., Ahmad, S., Gupta, A., Haye, A., Amin, S., & Mir, S. R. (2020). Polyphenol-enriched fraction and the compounds isolated from *Garcinia indica* fruits ameliorate obesity through suppression of digestive enzymes and oxidative stress. *Pharmacognosy Magazine* 16(70), S236-S245.

Munjal K., Gautam, V. K., Goel, Y., Ahamad, J., & Mir, S. R. (2023). 'Qualitative Diagnostic Features of Alkaloidal Spices.' In *Analysis of Food Spices* (pp. 135-150): CRC Press.

Nassar, W., El-Ansary, M., Sabry, D., Mostafa, M. A., Fayad, T., Kotb, E., Temraz, M., Saad, A. N., Essa, W., & Adel, H. (2016). Umbilical cord mesenchymal stem cells derived extracellular vesicles can safely ameliorate the progression of chronic kidney diseases. *Biomaterials research*, *20*(1), 1-11.

Patil, M., Mehta, D. S., & Guvva, S. (2008). Future impact of nanotechnology on medicine and dentistry. *Journal of Indian society of periodontology*, *12*(2), 34.

Patil, S., & Chandrasekaran, R. (2020). Biogenic nanoparticles: A comprehensive perspective in synthesis, characterization, application and its challenges. *Journal of Genetic Engineering and Biotechnology*, *18*, 1-23.

Puri, A., Mohite, P., Maitra, S., Subramaniyan, V., Kumarasamy, V., Uti, D. E., Sayed, A. A., El-Demerdash, F. M., Algahtani, M., & El-Kott, A. F. (2024). From nature to nanotechnology: The interplay of traditional medicine, green chemistry, and biogenic metallic phytonanoparticles in modern healthcare innovation and sustainability. *Biomedicine & Pharmacotherapy*, *170*, 116083.

Rakovich, T. Y., Mahfoud, O. K., Mohamed, B. M., Prina-Mello, A., Crosbie-Staunton, K., Van Den Broeck, T., De Kimpe, L., Sukhanova, A., Baty, D., & Rakovich, A. (2014). Highly sensitive single domain antibody–quantum dot conjugates for detection of HER2 biomarker in lung and breast cancer cells. *ACS nano*, *8*(6), 5682-5695.

Salih, R., Bajou, K., Shaker, B., & Elgamouz, A. (2023). Antitumor effect of algae silver nanoparticles on human triple negative breast cancer cells. *Biomedicine & Pharmacotherapy*, *168*, 115532.

Sarkar, J., Das, S., Aich, S., Bhattacharyya, P., & Acharya, K. (2022). Antiviral potential of nanoparticles for the treatment of Coronavirus infections. *Journal of Trace Elements in Medicine and Biology*, *72*, 126977.

Thomas, C. R., George, S., Horst, A. M., Ji, Z., Miller, R. J., Peralta-Videa, J. R., Xia, T., Pokhrel, S., Mädler, L., & Gardea-Torresdey, J. L. (2011). Nanomaterials in the environment: from materials to high-throughput screening to organisms. *ACS nano*, *5*(1), 13-20.

Vicente-Zurdo, D., Rosales-Conrado, N., & León-González, M. E. (2023). Unravelling the *in vitro* and *in vivo* potential of selenium nanoparticles in Alzheimer's disease: A bioanalytical review. *Talanta*, 269, 125519.

Wang, L., Wu, Y., Xie, J., Wu, S., & Wu, Z. (2018). Characterization, antioxidant and antimicrobial activities of green synthesized silver nanoparticles from Psidium guajava L. leaf aqueous extracts. *Materials Science and Engineering: C*, *86*, 1-8.

Zhang, C., Yin, A. X., Jiang, R., Rong, J., Dong, L., Zhao, T., Sun, L. D., Wang, J., Chen, X., & Yan, C. H. (2013). Time–Temperature indicator for perishable products based on kinetically programmable Ag overgrowth on Au nanorods. *ACS nano*, *7*(5), 4561-4568.

Chapter 3

The Role of Nanotechnology in Delivering Phytoherbals as Targeted Drug Delivery Systems

Himanshi Tanwar[1,2,*]
Manu Sharma[1]
Munish Ahuja[2]
and Ravi Berwal[2]
[1]Department of Pharmacy, Banasthali Vidyapith, Banasthali, Jaipur, Rajasthan, India
[2]Department of Pharmaceutical Sciences, Guru Jambheshwar University of Science and Technology, Hisar, Haryana, India

Abstract

Nanotechnology has emerged as a promising field in drug delivery systems, and when combined with phytochemicals or herbal extracts, it opens up new possibilities for targeted and efficient drug delivery. Compared to traditional drug delivery systems, it offers several advantages, such as requiring smaller quantities of the drug. The use of lower doses results in fewer side effects, and nanotechnology allows the drug to target specific areas, from organs down to the gene level, without exposing other parts of the body. Herbal medicines have their own advantages over synthetic drugs, as numerous scientific studies report that herbal-based treatments typically have fewer side effects and can be used safely for long-term treatment of chronic diseases. However, due to first-pass metabolism, higher doses of herbal medicines may sometimes be necessary, which can increase the risk of unwanted side effects. By combining nanotechnology with targeted drug delivery systems, herbal medicines can become even more beneficial. Nanotechnology in delivering phytoherbals as targeted drug delivery systems involves the use of nanoscale materials and structures to enhance the therapeutic potential of herbal compounds. Key advantages include improved solubility, bioavailability, targeted delivery, controlled release, protection of phytochemicals, and biocompatibility. This chapter focuses on phytoherbal formulations in achieving targeted drug delivery using nanotechnology, highlighting the critical role of nanotechnology in improving these aspects of drug delivery.

[*] Corresponding Author's Email: tanwarhimanshi@gmail.com.

In: Phyto-Nanomedicine
Editors: Hitesh Chopra, Vinod Kumar Gauttam, Ajmer Singh Grewal et al.
ISBN: 979-8-89530-317-7

Keywords: phytoherbals, nanotechnology, side effects, drug, drug delivery systems

Abbreviations

HIV	Human Immunodeficiency Virus
SLNs	Silver Nano Particles
G. biloba	*Ginkgo biloba*
TCH	Traditional Chinese Herbs and Spices

Introduction

Nanotechnology is a field of science and engineering focused on the design, creation, and utilization of structures, devices, and systems through precise manipulation of atoms and molecules at the nanoscale (Forokhzad et al., 2009). Phytomedicine has long been a crucial source of medicinal compounds, playing a pivotal role in healthcare since ancient times. Today, approximately 50% of effective drugs are derived from natural sources (Kingston et al., 2011). The increasing use of phytomedicine is attributed to its superior therapeutic efficacy and reduced side effects compared to allopathic medicines. Extensive research in phytochemicals and pharmacology has already been conducted and is well-documented (Jia et al., 2009). However, despite their promising *in-vitro* activity, the *in-vivo* efficacy of phytomedicines is often limited by challenges such as poor water solubility, lipophilicity, and inappropriate molecular size, which result in suboptimal absorption and reduced systemic availability. A deeper understanding of the biopharmaceutics and pharmacokinetics of phytomedicine is essential for developing rational dosage regimens that optimize their therapeutic potential (Gunasekaran et al., 2014). A medicinal plant refers to any plant containing substances in one or more of its organs that can be used for therapeutic purposes or serve as precursors for the synthesis of beneficial drugs. The therapeutic potential of herbal bioactives has been extensively documented in various traditional medicine systems, including Unani, Siddha, Ayurveda, and Traditional Chinese Medicine. Today, approximately one-third of the most widely used pharmaceuticals are derived from plants or other natural sources (Abayomi et al., 2013; Teja et al., 2022). Medicinal plants play a vital role in more than 90% of traditional medicine formulations and preventive therapies. The global trade in medicinal herbs has grown significantly, surpassing an annual value of USD 100 billion (Sofowora et al., 2013).

Nanotechnology in Drug Delivery Systems

Nanotechnology has emerged as a promising field in drug delivery systems, offering new possibilities for precise and efficient drug delivery when combined with phytochemicals or herbal extracts. Through methods like sonication, chemotherapeutic drugs or phytochemicals can be incorporated into nanostructures formed from naturally sourced lipids. These lipid nanoparticles represent a unique, organic drug delivery technology, characterized by easy biodegradability and an absence of environmental hazards. Plant-derived lipid nanoparticles offer a targeted approach to delivering drugs directly to specific sites within the body (Afroj et al., 2021; Chavda et al., 2023). By manipulating the size, surface properties, and material composition, nanoparticles can be designed as intelligent systems capable of encapsulating both therapeutic and imaging agents, while also exhibiting stealth properties. These systems can target specific tissues and enable controlled-release therapy, reducing drug-related toxicity and improving patient compliance through less frequent dosing (Rizvi and Saleh, 2018). Nanotechnology enhances drug efficacy, safety, and patient adherence, thus improving overall dosage form performance and contributing to lower healthcare costs. It also increases the success of drugs that may otherwise struggle to pass clinical trials. Nanotechnology shows great potential as a preferred drug delivery carrier, particularly for conventional drugs used in the treatment and management of severe diseases such as cancer, asthma, hypertension, HIV, and diabetes (Emeje et al., 2012).

Traditional Drug Delivery System vs Nanotechnology in Drug Delivery Systems

Compared to traditional drug delivery systems, nanotechnology offers several advantages, such as requiring smaller drug quantities, which results in fewer side effects. It enables the precise targeting of specific areas, from organs down to the gene level, without exposing other parts of the body to the drug. Conventional formulations like syrups, capsules, tablets, and decoctions often struggle to overcome the limitations associated with herbal drugs. However, the application of nanotechnology in herbal medicine has proven to be highly effective (Ali et al., 2015). Herbal drugs possess inherent advantages over synthetic drugs, as numerous scientific studies have shown. These medications typically cause fewer side effects and can be used over extended periods for the treatment of chronic diseases. Despite this, challenges such as first-pass metabolism can necessitate higher dosages, potentially leading to unwanted effects. By integrating nanotechnology with targeted drug delivery systems, the therapeutic benefits of herbal medicines can be significantly enhanced (Karimi et al., 2015).

Potential of Phytoherbals as Novel Drug Delivery

While our nation has a rich heritage of Ayurvedic exploration, its full potential has only recently gained broader recognition. With the promising prospects of herbal-based novel drug delivery systems, many researchers are now focused on developing advanced formulations such as controlled and sustained-release systems, transdermal and mucoadhesive systems, nanoparticles, microcapsules, microparticles, and implants. These innovations aim to maximize the therapeutic potential of herbs. However, the effectiveness of these medicines is often hindered by the use of outdated and conventional administration methods. Many concentrated herbal formulations are susceptible to damage in the highly acidic environment of the stomach. Furthermore, certain compounds may be altered by the liver before they can enter the bloodstream, leading to poor absorption. If the drug is not absorbed into the circulation at an adequate concentration, its therapeutic efficacy is compromised, and undesirable side effects may occur (Sterer et al., 2008). Phytopharmaceuticals refer to drugs derived from plants, in contrast to those synthesized from chemicals. The body generally utilizes these plant-based supplements more effectively when taken regularly. As a result, they tend to produce fewer or no adverse effects and offer better retention in the circulatory system, allowing for the development of more comprehensive and effective medicines. Synthetic drugs, on the other hand, are more likely to cause unwanted reactions, as certain artificial compounds, not found in nature, are sometimes rejected by the body. These reactions vary: some may be mild and cause minor discomfort, while others can be severe and even life-threatening. It is important to note that while adverse effects from phytopharmaceuticals are rare, interactions with other medications are still possible. Because phytopharmaceuticals are single, sterile compounds that can be easily adjusted, they are more readily incorporated into modern drug delivery systems, making them more accessible than raw plant materials or spices (Verma et al., 2007). Numerous studies have investigated lipid-based drug delivery systems and found them effective for the regulated and targeted distribution of medications. Pharmacosomes are amphiphilic entities that contain active hydrogen and are bound to phospholipids, enhancing the biopharmaceutical properties of the drug and increasing its bioavailability. Phytosomes, derived from plants such as Silybum marianum, Ginkgo biloba, and ginseng, consist of a unique combination of phospholipids and lipophilic structures. These formulations are highly lipophilic, exhibiting greater bioavailability and efficacy in treating diseases. The findings from these studies can be applied to treat severe liver disorders arising from metabolic dysfunction or viral processes, using locally manufactured medicines that possess superior pharmacokinetic and pharmacological characteristics. Phytosomes are formed when certain components of natural concentrates, such as flavonolignans and terpenoids, are sub-atomically connected to phospholipids like phosphatidylcholine through a polar end, facilitating their delivery (Chung et al., 2001). Phytosomes have a wide range of medical and cosmetic applications. While many potential medical uses for phytosomes remain to be discovered, ongoing research is expected to reveal more opportunities in the future (Kumar et al., 2020). By utilizing novel drug delivery technologies that combine authentic herbs with refined phytopharmaceuticals or phytosomes, we can harness the benefits of both. Integrating modern pharmaceutical delivery mechanisms into Indian Ayurvedic medicine is crucial for effectively combating serious ailments (Ma et al., 2001).

Role of Nanotechnology in Delivering Phytoherbals as Targeted Drug Delivery Systems

The role of nanotechnology in delivering phytoherbals as targeted drug delivery systems involves leveraging nanoscale materials and structures to enhance the therapeutic effectiveness of herbal compounds. Key aspects of this approach include improved solubility, bioavailability, targeted delivery, controlled release, protection of phytochemicals, and biocompatibility (Gabriel, 2004). The emergence of nanotechnology has led to promising advancements in drug delivery systems, particularly when combined with phytochemicals or herbal extracts, creating numerous possibilities for efficient and targeted delivery. Solid lipid nanoparticles (SLNs) are emerging as effective colloidal delivery systems, enabling the transport of herbal compounds to various organs, including the brain, through oral administration. Research has shown that the concentration of drugs within phytocompounds encapsulated in SLNs can be approximately 5–10 times higher than that of their native counterparts. Additionally, modifying the surface of

SLNs facilitates the controlled release of bioactive compounds from herbs during oral delivery. This innovation opens new avenues for enhancing the effectiveness of various phytocompounds loaded into SLNs for managing diverse chronic ailments (Ganesan et al., 2018; Zhao et al., 2002).

Nanotechnology as Targeted Drug Delivery Systems

Enhanced Solubility and Bioavailability

Many phytochemicals derived from herbal extracts exhibit poor solubility and low bioavailability. Nanotechnology can be employed to encapsulate these phytochemicals in nanoparticles, significantly improving their solubility and enhancing bioavailability. This approach ensures that a greater proportion of the drug reaches the target site. By encapsulating phytochemicals in nanocarriers, a higher concentration can be delivered to specific areas, such as within the nail (Prabha et al., 2024).

Targeted Drug Delivery

Nanoparticles can be formulated to target specific tissues or cells, allowing for the direct delivery of phytoherbals to the site of action. By functionalizing nanoparticles with ligands that bind to specific receptors on target cells, the selectivity of drug delivery is enhanced, minimizing potential side effects. This targeted approach ensures that phytoherbals are specifically directed to the nail bed and surrounding tissues, reducing systemic exposure and improving treatment effectiveness (Ambwani et al., 2018).

Controlled Release

Nanoparticles facilitate the controlled and sustained release of phytochemicals, providing a prolonged therapeutic effect. This controlled release optimizes the pharmacokinetics of herbal compounds, resulting in a more effective and sustained therapeutic outcome for the treatment of severe diseases affecting the nails (Flores et al., 2013).

Protection of Herbal Extracts

Herbal compounds can be sensitive to environmental factors. Nanoparticles serve as protective carriers, shielding phytoherbals from degradation caused by light, oxygen, and moisture, thereby ensuring the stability of the active ingredients. Additionally, they form a protective layer over the nail, preventing drug degradation under various environmental conditions (Kavya et al., 2022).

Combination Therapy

Nanotechnology enables the combination of various phytochemicals or herbal extracts within a single nanoparticle system. This approach allows for synergistic effects, where the combined action of multiple compounds enhances therapeutic efficacy and targets multiple pathways (Kumar et al., 2018).

Diagnosis and Imaging

Nanoparticles can serve dual purposes by incorporating diagnostic and imaging agents. This dual functionality facilitates targeted drug delivery while enabling real-time monitoring of drug distribution. Such capabilities allow for adjustments in treatment plans based on individual patient responses (Korac and Kambholja, 2011).

Reduced Side Effects

Targeted delivery minimizes the exposure of healthy tissues to phytochemicals, thereby reducing the likelihood of side effects. This is especially important for herbal compounds, which typically have fewer side effects compared to synthetic drugs; targeted delivery further enhances their safety profile (Salunkhe et al., 2020).

Biocompatibility

The use of biocompatible materials in nanocarriers ensures minimal toxicity and immunogenicity, promoting their acceptance in the human body. This enhances the safety profile of the drug delivery system, making it suitable for clinical applications (Barot et al., 2012).

Improved Penetration Through the Nail Plate

The nanoscale size of carriers, such as nanoparticles or nanoemulsions, facilitates their penetration through the dense structure of the nail plate. This enhancement improves the delivery of phytoherbals to the underlying tissues, where they can exert therapeutic effects against fungal infections and other nail-related conditions (Ullah et al., 2022).

Personalized Medicine

The flexibility of nanotechnology enables the design of personalized drug delivery systems tailored to individual patient characteristics, optimizing treatment outcomes. This versatility allows for the customization of transungual delivery systems, aligning them with specific herbal formulations and supporting personalized treatment approaches for improved clinical results (Kusuma et al., 2022). The integration of nanotechnology with phytoherbals in drug delivery systems demonstrates significant potential to enhance the safety, effectiveness, and specificity of herbal therapies (Aggarwal et al., 2023).

The Role of Nano Carriers in Topical/Transungual Delivery

In recent years, there has been significant interest in the use of nanoparticles for topical and transungual drug delivery. When utilized for topical delivery, nanoparticles can be easily applied over the nail, effectively circumventing the side effects associated with oral medications. The incorporation of nanoparticles not only enhances drug targeting but also improves drug profiles and permeation (Bhattacharjee et al., 2021). Nanoemulsions, composed of droplets made from lipid and surfactant blends, typically range in size from 10 to 500 nm. They possess essential attributes for treating fungal infections, enhancing solubilization, stability, and permeation potential. Nanoemulsions serve as an excellent alternative to less stable liposomes. Considerable research has focused on nanoemulsion therapy for onychomycosis, often formulated as gels, commonly referred to as "nanoemulgels" (Abd Elsalam and Abouelatta, 2023). Liposomes are double-layered vesicles composed of phospholipids, featuring an aqueous core and an outer phospholipid membrane. They are suitable for drug delivery in both hydrophobic and hydrophilic environments. Due to their advantageous properties—including enhanced skin penetration, biocompatibility, robustness, reduced toxicity, and sustained release—liposomes have found widespread application in topical and transungual drug delivery. Along with ethosomes, liposomes are believed to exploit specific lipophilic pathways in the nail, making them promising options for drug delivery to the nails. Both liposomes and ethosomes have been successfully utilized to incorporate certain antifungal medications for topical antifungal treatment (Alexander et al., 2016).

Challenges in the Development of Phytomedicine

Typically, phytomedicines are characterized as secondary metabolites, and the chemical isolation and identification of these compounds present significant challenges (Egert et al., 2011). The production of active components in phytomedicine encounters numerous hurdles. Generally, the levels of these secondary metabolites in plants are low, and their composition can vary based on factors such as botanical species, specific chemotypes, the anatomical part of the plant used (e.g., flowers, leaves, seeds, roots), and environmental conditions including storage, sunlight exposure, humidity, soil type, time of harvest, and geographic location (Qureshi et al., 2013). Screening phytomedicines from plants introduces an additional set of challenges. Although high-throughput methods are commonly employed in pharmaceutical drug screening, they are not well-suited for phytomedicine due to the presence of numerous drug compounds in crude extracts. Moreover, certain active constituents in plants can yield misleading results when screened using high-throughput techniques. The processes of identifying and isolating active constituents, as well as fractionation, are also time-consuming, often requiring weeks or even months. Additionally, the supply of active ingredients poses another challenge, as substantial quantities; often several hundreds of grams are required for preclinical development, contingent on the intended application (Kingston et al., 2011).

Herbal Phytoconstituents Integrated into Nano Formulations

Puerarin, the primary active component derived from the roots of Pueraria lobata (Willd.) Ohwi, exhibits extensive pharmacological effects. Various nanotechnological approaches have been explored to enhance the bioavailability of puerarin, with one notable method being the use of a SLN carrier system. Compared to a puerarin suspension, the absorption of SLN-puerarin is significantly faster, as indicated by a shorter Tmax. Additionally, SLN-puerarin demonstrates over threefold higher bioavailability than the puerarin suspension (Luo et al., 2021). Ginkgo biloba extract is widely used for its antioxidant and anti-aging properties, including topical applications. Studies comparing standard Ginkgo biloba extract with the extract complexed with phospholipids indicate that topical application of the latter enhances peripheral circulation due to its anti-inflammatory activity, with greater efficacy observed when formulated as phytosomes. The bioavailability and pharmacokinetic profiles of the conventional Ginkgo biloba extract and its phytosomal form reveal a significant increase in bioavailability for the phytosomal complex (Alharbi et al., 2021). Nanotechnology has facilitated the development of nanocarriers incorporating herbal antioxidants, notably Salvia miltiorrhiza Bunge (Danshen), known for its ability to enhance blood circulation and exhibit valuable antioxidant effects. Formulations created using nanotechnology demonstrate superior antioxidant bioactivities compared to traditional herbal plant-based formulations made using grinding methods. This highlights that active constituents in nanotechnology formulations are released more rapidly than those prepared through conventional powdering techniques (Liu et al., 2007). An environmentally sustainable bottom-up approach was utilized to create silver bio-nanostructures from Salvia officinalis L. (sage) leaf extract. The sage exhibited bioreduction properties during silver nanoparticle synthesis. To enhance biocompatibility and stability, the sage silver nanoparticles were encapsulated within two types of liposomes: Chla-DPPC- and soybean lecithin lipid vesicles. These innovative, environmentally friendly silver phytonanostructures, crafted with sage extract, demonstrated substantial antioxidant activities ranging from 86.5% to 98.6% (Mishra et al., 2022). Numerous plants are currently under investigation for their potential in nanoparticle synthesis. Gold nanoparticles, within the size range of 2–20 nm, have been successfully produced using live Medicago sativa (Alfalfa). Alfalfa, a perennial flowering plant from the legume family Fabaceae, is widely cultivated as a vital forage crop globally, serving various purposes including grazing, hay production, silage, and acting as green manure (Rajasekaran et al., 2024). Nanoparticles of Ni, Zn, Ag, Co, and Cu have been synthesized from living plants such as Brassica juncea (Indian mustard), Medicago sativa (Alfalfa), and Helianthus annuus (common sunflower). The latter, an annual forb of the genus Helianthus, is grown for its fruits and edible oil, serving various purposes in agriculture and industry. Brassica juncea is also known for its nanoparticle properties, recognized by names such as Chinese mustard and brown mustard (Gharehyakheh, 2024). Cinnamomum camphora, known as the camphor tree or camphor laurel, is an evergreen tree from which extracts are utilized for nanoparticle synthesis, offering advantages over microbial synthesis due to the ease of culturing and maintaining plant cells. Many plants actively absorb and detoxify metal ions from soils and solutions, leading to the formation of insoluble complexes with the metal ions in the form of nanoparticles (Nair et al., 2022). Plant leaf extracts have been employed in the synthesis of silver and gold nanoparticles, producing pure metallic nanoparticles of both types. Euphorbia hirta, also known as asthma-plant, is a pantropical weed native to the tropical Americas. This hairy herb thrives in open grasslands, roadsides, and pathways in warmer regions, having been introduced in India and Australia. It is utilized in traditional herbal medicine. Nerium indicum Linn., belonging to the Apocynaceae family, is toxic in all parts and has various medicinal uses, including anti-helminthic, diaphoretic, carminative, febrifuge, and repellent properties (Li et al., 2024). A patent describes an oral preparation based on herbs designed for regular retention in the buccal cavity. The formula includes herbs such as *Radix polygoni multiflori, Rhizoma ligustici chuanxiong, Rhizoma drynariae, Calculus bovis, Herba ecliptae, Indigo naturalis, Pericarpium trichosanthis, Radix sophorae flavescentis, Spina gleditsia,* and *Radix sophorae flavescentis*. For convenient portability, chewing gum, pastes, and gels were identified as the most effective formulations for oral retention. Regular use of this herbal combination has been shown to prevent hair loss, promote new hair growth, and gradually darken hair on the scalp and face (Borodina et al., 2008). Clinical research indicates that gugulipid, a standardized extract derived from the oleo gum pitch of Commiphora wightii, can lower harmful serum lipid levels in the bloodstream. The development of gugulipid microparticles utilized a range of ingredients, including chitosan, egg whites, sodium alginate, ethyl cellulose, cellulose acetate, gelatin, and beeswax. The physicochemical characteristics of these microparticles were thoroughly examined, and verification of the captured gugulipid within the organized microparticles was conducted through HPLC profiling, revealing distinct detachment of Guggulsterone-E and -Z (Shen et al., 2008).

Herbal Phytoconstituents Used as Therapeutics

The utilization of nanoparticles significantly enhances the absorption and distribution of Traditional Chinese Herbs and spices (TCH) within the body. A combination of peach seeds, safflowers, angelica roots, Szechwan lovage rhizomes, Rehmannia roots, red peony roots, syphons, gadflies, night crawlers, and ground bugs underwent a process that involved drying, chopping, extracting, pulverizing into fluid particles using ultrasonic waves, separating, and ultimately nanometerizing into nanoparticles, resulting in a liquid with nanometer colliders. The thrombolytic activities of TCH nanoparticles contribute to a rapid reduction in emboli within blood vessels, facilitating the restoration of blood flow. Compared to non-nanoparticle TCHs, the thrombolytic effects of nanoparticles exhibit significant amplification (Palanivel et al., 2018; Ochubiojo et al., 2012). Rheumatoid arthritis is typically managed through various therapies, including anti-inflammatory and disease-modifying antirheumatic drugs. However, the severe side effects associated with these treatments have led to the exploration of alternative approaches, with phytotherapy emerging as a promising option (Sarah and Rimbach, 2011). The therapeutic potential of phytotherapy lies in its ability to target multiple inflammatory mediators, such as cytokines, nitric oxide, adhesion molecules, chemokines, arachidonic acid, lipoxygenase, and nuclear factor kappa B. Furthermore, nanomedicine presents a notable formulation strategy to address challenges linked to phytoconstituents, including poor bioavailability, high first-pass metabolism, and low stability. Various phytoconstituents, including curcumin, resveratrol, thymoquinone, berberine, celastrol, hesperidin, sinomenine, triptolide, quercetin, and ferulic acid, have been successfully formulated in nanoparticulate form and utilized in the management of rheumatoid arthritis (Prabha et al., 2024; Joshi et al., 2022).

Conclusion

Nanotechnology significantly enhances the efficacy of phytoherbals in drug delivery systems by improving solubility, bioavailability, and targeted delivery while minimizing side effects. Nanocarriers, such as solid lipid nanoparticles and liposomes, effectively protect and deliver herbal compounds, offering controlled release and reduced degradation. This innovative approach not only augments therapeutic effectiveness but also supports personalized medicine by tailoring treatments to individual needs. Despite the challenges associated with phytomedicine, including variability in active components and complex isolation processes, nanotechnology presents a promising avenue for optimizing herbal therapies and advancing their clinical applications.

References

Abayomi, S., Ogunbodede, E., & Onayade, A. (2013). The role and place of medicinal plants in the strategies for disease prevention. *African Journal of Traditional, Complementary and Alternative Medicines*, 10(5), 210-229.

Abd-Elsalam, W. H., & Abouelatta, S. M. (2023). Contemporary techniques and potential transungual drug delivery nanosystems for the treatment of onychomycosis. AAPS *Pharm Sci Tech* 24(6), 150.

Afroj, S. C., Anand, S. B., Lalita, K. D., & Santosh, A. P. (2021). Recent advances in herbal nano technology. *International Journal of Creative Research Thoughts* 9: d321-d325.

Agrawal, V., Patel, R., & Patel, M. (2023). Design, characterization, and evaluation of efinaconazole loaded poly (D, L-lactide-co-glycolide) nanocapsules for targeted treatment of onychomycosis. *Journal of Drug Delivery Science and Technology,* 80, 104157.

Alexander, A., Patel, J. R., & Saraf, S. (2016). Recent expansion of pharmaceutical nanotechnologies and targeting strategies in the field of phytopharmaceuticals for the delivery of herbal extracts and bioactives. *Journal of Controlled Release,* 241, 110-124.

Alharbi, W. S., Fahad A., Almughem, Alshaimaa M., Almehmady, S. J. Jarallah, Wijdan, K., Alsharif, N. M., Alzahrani., & Alshehri, A. A. (2021). Phytosomes as an emerging nanotechnology platform for the topical delivery of bioactive phytochemicals. *Pharmaceutics,* 13(9), 1-20.

Ali, K., Majlesi, M., & Mahmoud, R. (2015). Herbal versus synthetic drugs; beliefs and facts. *Journal of Nephropharmacology,* 4(1), 1-27.

Ambwani, S., Tandon, R., Ambwani, T. K., & Malik, Y. S. (2018). Current knowledge on nano delivery systems and their beneficial applications in enhancing the efficacy of herbal drugs. *Journal of Experimental Biology and Agricultural Sciences*, 6(1), 87-107.

Barot, B. S., Parejiya, P. B., Patel, H. K., Mehta, M. D., & Shelat, P. K. (2012). Microemulsion-based antifungal gel delivery to nail for the treatment of onychomycosis: Formulation, optimization, and efficacy studies. *Drug Delivery and Translational Research,* 2, 463-476.

Bhattacharjee, B., Nikita, D., Dhunusmita, B., Arka, K., & Nasima, A. (2021). Understanding the drug delivery through nails: a comprehensive review. *Journal of Drug Delivery and Therapeutics,* 11(4), 116-131.

Borodina, T. N., Rumsh, L. D., Kunizhev, S. M., Sukhorukov, G. B., Vorozhtsov, G. N., Feldman, B. M., Rusanova, A. V., Vasil'eva, T. V., Strukova, S. M., & Markvicheva, E. A. (2008). Entrapment of herbal extracts into biodegradable microcapsules. *Biochemistry (Moscow) Supplement Series B: Biomedical Chemistry*, 2, 176-182.

Chavda, V. P., Nalla, L. V., Balar, P., Bezbaruah, R., Apostolopoulos, V., Singla, K. R., Khadela, A., Vora, L., & Uversky, V. N. (2023). Advanced phytochemical-based nanocarrier systems for the treatment of breast cancer. *Cancers*, 15(4), 1023-1030.

Chung, H., Burk, H., & Shu, K. (2001). Herbal-based oral composition and process for producing the same. *European Patent EP0862446.*

Emeje, M. O., Obidike, I. C., Akpabio, E. I., & Ofoefule, S. I. (2012). Nanotechnology in drug delivery. *Recent Advances in Novel Drug Carrier Systems*, 1, 1-22.

Flores, F. C., De Lima, J. A., Ribeiro, R. F., Alves, S. H., Rolim, C. M. B., Ruy Carlos R., Beck, & Da Silva, B. C. (2013). Antifungal activity of nanocapsule suspensions containing tea tree oil on the growth of Trichophyton rubrum. *Mycopathologia*, 175, 281-286.

Forokhzad, O. C., & Langer, R. (2009). Impact of nanotechnology on drug delivery. *American Chemical Society*, 3, 16-20.

Gabriel, S. A. (2004). Introduction to nanotechnology and its applications to medicine. *Surgical Neurology*, 61(3), 216-220.

Ganesan, P., Ramalingam, P., Karthivashan, G., Ko, Y. T., & Choi, D. K. (2018). Recent developments in solid lipid nanoparticle and surface-modified solid lipid nanoparticle delivery systems for oral delivery of phyto-bioactive compounds in various chronic diseases. *International Journal of Nanomedicine*, 13, 1569-1583.

Gharehyakheh, S. (2024). Unlocking the power of nature: Safeguarding refrigerated camel meat with herb-extracted (Anethum graveolens leaves) zinc nanoparticles. *Applied Organometallic Chemistry*, 38, e7267.

Gunasekaran, T., Haile, T., Nigusse, T., & Dhanaraju, M. D. (2014). Nanotechnology: An effective tool for enhancing bioavailability and bioactivity of phytomedicine. *Asian Pacific Journal of Tropical Biomedicine*, 4, S1-S7.

Jia, L., & Zhao, Y. (2009). Current evaluation of the millennium phytomedicine-ginseng (I): etymology, pharmacognosy, phytochemistry market and regulations. *Current Medicinal Chemistry,* 16, 2475-2484.

Joshi, M., Pathak, K., & Dhaneshwar, S. (2022). Nanotechnology-based strategies for effective delivery of phytoconstituents for the management of rheumatoid arthritis. *Pharmacological Research-Modern Chinese Medicine*, 2, 100061.

Karimi, A., Majlesi, M., & Rafieian-Kopaei, M. (2015). Herbal versus synthetic drugs; beliefs and facts. *Journal of Nephropharmacology*, 4(1), 1-27.

Kavya, T. P., Mithiya, J., Kate, A. S., Bairwa, K., & Siddheshwar, K. (2022). Herbal nanomedicines: Recent advancements, challenges, opportunities and regulatory overview. *Phytomedicine*, 96, 1538-1550.

Kingston, D. G. I. (2011). Modern natural products drug discovery and its relevance to biodiversity conservation. *Journal of Natural Products*, 74, 496-511.

Korac, R. R., & Khambholja, K. M. (2011). Potential of herbs in skin protection from ultraviolet radiation. *Pharmacognosy Reviews*, 5(10), 164.

Kumar, D., Vats, N., Saroha, K., & Rana, A. C. (2020). Phytosomes as emerging nanotechnology for herbal drug delivery. *Sustainable Agriculture Reviews*, 43, 217-237.

Kumar, P. J., Das, G., Fraceto, L. F., Campos, E. V. R., Rodriguez-Torres, M. D. P., Acosta-Torres, L. S., & Diaz-Torres, L. A. (2018). Nano based drug delivery systems: Recent developments and future prospects. *Journal of Nanobiotechnology*, 16(1), 1-33.

Kusuma, D. M., Chaerunisaa, A. Y., Muhaimin, M., & Joni, I. M. (2022). Improved activity of herbal medicines through nanotechnology. *Nanomaterials*, 12(22), 4073.

Li, G., Xiaoman, Q., Jingtao, W., Xuan, W., Tianyu, W., Ying, L., Yuwei, C., & Yonghui, X. (2024). Highly stable electrochemical sensing platform for the selective determination of pefloxacin in food samples based on a molecularly imprinted-polymer-coated gold nanoparticle/black phosphorus nanocomposite. *Food Chemistry*, 436, 137753.

Liu, J. R., Chen, G. F., Shih, H. N., & Kuo, P. C. (2008). Enhanced antioxidant bioactivity of Salvia miltiorrhiza (Danshen) products prepared using nanotechnology. *Phytomedicine*, 15(1-2), 23-30.

Luo, M. X., Hua, S., & Shang, Q. Y. (2021). Application of nanotechnology in drug delivery systems for respiratory diseases. *Molecular Medicine Reports*, 23(5), 1-17.

Ma, B., Duan, X., & Wang, Z. (2000). Clinical and experimental study on Shuanghua aerosol in treating infantile upper respiratory tract infection. *Chinese Journal of Integrated Traditional and Western Medicine*, 20(9), 653-655.

Mishra, Y., Ibrahim, H., Amin, M., Mishra, V., Vyas, M., Kumar, P. P., Gupta, M., & Kanday, R. (2022). Application of nanotechnology to herbal antioxidants as improved phytomedicine: An expanding horizon. *Biomedicine and Pharmacotherapy*, 153, 113413.

Nair, A., Mallya, R., Suvarna, V., Khan, A. T., Momin, M., & Omri, A. (2022). Nanoparticles—Attractive carriers of antimicrobial essential oils. *Antibiotics*, 11(1), 108.

Ochubiojo, E. M., Obidike, C. I., Akpabio, E. I., & Ofoefule, I. S. (2012). Nanotechnology in drug delivery. *Recent Advances in Novel Drug Carrier Systems*, 1, 1-145).

Palanivel, G., Ramalingam, P., Karthivashan, P., Tag Ko, Y., & Choi, D. (2018). Recent developments in solid lipid nanoparticle and surface-modified solid lipid nanoparticle delivery systems for oral delivery of phyto-bioactive compounds in various chronic diseases. *International Journal of Nanomedicine*, 13, 1569-1583.

Prabha, J., Kumar, M., Kumar, D., Chopra, S., & Bhatia, A. (2024). Nano-platform strategies of herbal components for the management of rheumatoid arthritis: A review on the battle for next-generation formulations. *Current Drug Delivery*, 21(8), 1082-1105.

Qureshi, A. N., & Mohammed, A. (2013). Mood disorders and complementary and alternative medicine: A literature review. *Neuropsychiatric Disease and Treatment*, 1, 639-658.

Rajasekaran, M., Krishnamoorthi, S., & Vijayaragavan, M. (2024). An experimental investigation of the effects of blending camphor oil infused with jack fruit biodiesel and nanoparticles on the performance, combustion, and exhaust emissions of a compression ignition engine. *Proceedings of the Institution of Mechanical Engineers, Part E: Journal of Process Mechanical Engineering*, 1, 09544-09556.

Rizvi, S. A. A., & Saleh, A. M. (2018). Applications of nanoparticle systems in drug delivery technology. *Saudi Pharmaceutical Journal*, 26(1), 64-70.

Salunkhe, P., Bhoyar, P., Gode, A., & Shewale, S. P. (2020). Application of nanotechnology to the extraction of herbal components for medicinal uses. *Current Nanomaterials*, 5(1), 4-11.

Sarah, E., & Rimbach, G. (2011). Which sources of flavonoids: complex diets or dietary supplements. *Advances in Nutrition*, 2(1), 8-14.

Shen, Y. J., Zhang, Z. W., Luo, G. X., Wang, X., & Wang, F. H. (2008). Nanoparticles of traditional Chinese herbs inhibit thrombosis *in vivo*. *British Journal of Hematology*, 93, J1457.

Sofowora, A., Ogunbodede, E., & Onayade, A. (2013). The role and place of medicinal plants in the strategies for disease prevention. *African Journal of Traditional, Complementary and Alternative Medicines*, 10(5), 210-229.

Sterer, N., Nuas, S., Mizrahi, B., Goldenberg, C., Weiss, E. I., Domb, A., & Perez Davidi, M. (2008). Oral malodor reduction by a palatal mucoadhesive tablet containing herbal formulation. *Journal of Dentistry*, 36(7), 535-539.

Teja, P. K., Mithiya, J., Kate, A. S., Bairwa, K., & Chauthe, S. K. (2022). Herbal nanomedicines: Recent advancements, challenges, opportunities and regulatory overview. *Phytomedicine*, 96, 1538-1590.

Ullah, K. H., Rasheed, F., Naz, I., Haq, N. U., Fatima, H., Kanwal, N., & Ur-Rehman, T. (2022). Chitosan nanoparticles loaded Poloxamer 407 gel for transungual delivery of terbinafine HCl. *Pharmaceutics*, 14(11), 23-53.

Verma, M., Gupta, P. K., Varsha, B. P., & Purohit, A. P. (2007). Development of transdermal drug dosage formulation for the anti-rheumatic ayurvedic medicinal plants. *Ancient Science of Life*, 1, 66-69.

Zhao, H., Wang, K., Zhao, Y., & Pan, L. (2002). Novel sustained-release implant of herb extract using chitosan. *Biomaterials,* 23, 4459-4462.

Chapter 4

Applications of Nanophytoherbals in Alzheimer's Therapy

Parul Sood*
Gagandeep Kaur
and Nitin Jangra
Chitkara University School of Pharmacy, Chitkara University, Himachal Pradesh, India

Abstract

The incidence of neurodegenerative disorders is rising with the aging population, with Alzheimer's disease (AD) being the most common among the elderly. AD is a progressive neurodegenerative illness that impairs nerve cell regeneration, significantly affecting brain and neuronal function. Cognitive impairment and dementia are highly prevalent among AD patients worldwide. Current medications for AD offer only symptomatic relief without preventing or reversing disease progression and often come with considerable side effects. This has prompted researchers to explore new therapeutic targets, focusing on natural sources due to their reduced side effects and cost-effectiveness. Medicinal herbs, known for their multi-compound nature, offer advantages over single-target drugs for treating complex diseases. However, challenges such as poor solubility, low bioavailability, and limited ability to cross the blood–cerebrospinal fluid (CSF) and blood–brain barrier (BBB) restrict the effectiveness of herbal extracts and active phytoconstituents. Nanomedicine, a product of nanotechnology, has emerged as a promising strategy for both AD diagnosis and treatment. Nanomedicines can facilitate the delivery of therapeutic compounds across BBB and CSF due to their small size, while improving stability, pharmacokinetics, and biocompatibility of herbal medications. This chapter explores various nano-herbal formulations designed for identifying and managing AD, offering significant promise for advancing research and clinical applications in the field.

Keywords: Alzheimer's disease, blood brain barrier, nanophytoherbals, nanotechnology

---

* Corresponding Author's Email: parul.sood@chitkarauniversity.edu.in.

In: Phyto-Nanomedicine
Editors: Hitesh Chopra, Vinod Kumar Gauttam, Ajmer Singh Grewal et al.
ISBN: 979-8-89530-317-7

Abbreviations

AD	Alzheimer's disease
AG	Andrographolides
AuNPs	Gold nanoparticles
BBB	Blood Brain Barrier
BRB	Berberine
CA	Caffeic Acid
CD	Carbon dots
CSF	Cerebrospinal fluid
EGCG	Epigallocatechin gallate
LPs	Liposomes
NEs	Nanoemulsions
NGs	Nanogels
NRG	Naringenin
PIP	Piperine
QC	Quercetin
RSV	Resveratrol
SeNPs	Selenium nanoparticles
SLNPs	Solid Lipid nanoparticles

Introduction

Alzheimer's disease (AD) is the most prevalent form of dementia, characterized by a progressively declining central nervous system. The World Health Organization estimates that around 50 million people worldwide have dementia, of which AD is the most common form of the disease, potentially contributing to 60-70% of all cases. The estimated global burden of dementia is projected to be 82 million people by 2030 and 152 million by 2050 (Vaiserman et al., 2020). Elderly individuals with AD often exhibit a range of symptoms, most notably memory impairment, which severely impacts their overall well-being and quality of life. Several factors contribute to the development of AD, including reduced physical activity, infections, smoking, and coexisting conditions such as obesity and diabetes (Pugazhenthi et al., 2017). The exact etiology of AD remains uncertain, but key pathogenic features include the accumulation of amyloid-β (Aβ) plaques and the hyperphosphorylation of tau proteins in nerve fibers (Sood et al., 2023a). Other potential mechanisms contributing to AD development include reduced brain metabolism (Xu et al., 2023), disruption of the blood-brain barrier (BBB), impaired cellular autophagy, disrupted calcium homeostasis, increased oxidative stress, neuroinflammation, and heightened neuronal death (Yarns et al., 2022). Current treatment options are inadequate to meet the therapeutic demands of the growing patient population. Conventional therapies, such as acetylcholinesterase inhibitors, face challenges like poor solubility, reduced absorption, and adverse side effects. Additionally, FDA-approved drugs for AD, such as rivastigmine, tacrine, galantamine, memantine, and donepezil, provide only symptomatic relief. The therapeutic efficacy of these drugs is further limited by issues like neurotoxicity, instability, poor bioavailability to neuronal membranes, and other unfavorable pharmacokinetic and pharmacodynamic properties (Song et al., 2023). As a result, there is an urgent need to explore alternative therapeutic strategies. Recently, natural herbal medicines have gained attention for their potential to target multiple pathways in AD, offering a promising new approach (Singh et al., 2021a). The BBB serves as a vital partition between the circulatory system and the central nervous system, not only blocking toxins but also impeding the entry of many therapeutic agents. Research shows that nearly 98% of small-molecule drugs struggle to cross BBB to reach the nervous system (Zhang et al., 2022a). Furthermore, the pharmacokinetic limitations of natural medicines, such as poor solubility in brain tissue, hinder their ability to traverse BBB effectively. As a result, patients often need to increase doses to achieve sufficient plasma concentrations, which can lead to toxicity. However, recent advances in nanotechnology have enabled the encapsulation of therapeutic agents in nanoparticles, facilitating their transport across BBB to the affected areas. This approach significantly enhances drug concentration in the nervous system, presenting a promising strategy for improving drug efficacy (Kaushal et al., 2024). This book chapter explores the latest advancements in the use of nanomaterials for AD treatment, with a focus on the pivotal role of various natural compounds. These innovations hold substantial potential for the future development of treatments for neurodegenerative disorders, including AD.

BBB and Alzheimer's Disease

The term "BBB" refers to the membrane that separates brain cells from the bloodstream via glial cells and capillary walls, as well as the membrane that divides plasma from cerebrospinal fluid through the choroid plexus. The BBB is a critical structure composed of vascular endothelial cells connected by adhesion and tight junction proteins (Alahmari, 2022). It plays a crucial role in regulating the passage of macromolecules into and out of the brain's neuronal system. The BBB restricts the entry of peripheral immune cells, macromolecular proteins, and harmful chemicals, thereby maintaining a stable environment within the central nervous system (CNS). However, this protective function also prevents many medications from entering the brain in sufficient amounts, posing a significant challenge in AD treatment (Pardridge, 2020). Additionally, drugs released prematurely from their carriers before reaching the brain may cause unwanted systemic side effects, complicating the therapy. To enhance drug delivery to the brain, a thorough understanding of the BBB's anatomy and physiology is essential. Various nanocarriers have been proposed in preliminary research as potential solutions for AD treatment, encapsulating therapeutic drugs to facilitate their passage through BBB.

Phytoherbals in Alzheimer's Disease

Currently approved drugs for AD, such as donepezil, tacrine, memantine, and galantamine, provide only symptomatic relief and are often accompanied by numerous side effects. As a result, multiple scientific studies have highlighted the potential of phytoconstituents, either used individually or in combination, as promising candidates for the development of novel, safer AD treatments that could offer advantages over existing drugs (Koul et al., 2023). Preclinical and clinical studies suggest that these phytochemicals have significant potential in treating AD by targeting multiple mechanisms, such as increasing α-secretase activity, reducing Aβ formation, decreasing tau hyperphosphorylation, and enhancing levels of antioxidant enzymes and anti-inflammatory markers. These actions collectively contribute to improvements in cognitive impairment, learning, and memory (Nagori et al., 2023). Moreover, a diet rich in fruits, vegetables, cereals, and nuts has been shown to promote healthy aging and lower the risk of age-related disorders, including AD (Sood et al., 2023b). However, the therapeutic application of herbal compounds for managing AD is often limited by their complex chemistry, large molecular weight, and poor solubility, which hinder absorption. Nanoparticle-mediated drug delivery offers a solution by enhancing the bioavailability of herbal compounds, thereby increasing their efficacy in AD treatment.

Nanotechnology in Alzheimer's Disease

Nanotechnology plays a crucial role in addressing both therapeutic and diagnostic challenges associated with AD. The primary obstacle in developing effective treatment strategies for AD lies in the limited permeability of drugs across BBB and CSF. Several nanotechnology-based approaches, including cubosomes, dendrimers, fullerenes, liposomes, nanoparticles, nanoemulsions, solid lipid nanoparticles, nanocapsules, and exosomes, enhance BBB/CSF permeability, facilitating the targeted delivery of drugs to affected brain regions in AD patients. These nanocarriers utilize multiple pathways, such as adsorption-mediated, carrier-mediated, cell-mediated, and receptor-mediated transport, to improve drug penetration (Afzal et al., 2022). Nanocarrier-based formulations offer several advantages, including improved adhesion, increased solubility, greater surface area for absorption, enhanced bioavailability, and controlled drug release. This leads to sustained therapeutic effects, better clinical outcomes, and reduced adverse drug reactions (Verma et al., 2024). Various nanoformulations have demonstrated the ability to inhibit Aβ accumulation, reduce NF-kB activity, and prevent tau hyperphosphorylation, making them promising candidates for AD treatment (Kanojia et al., 2023). The following section will explore the role of these nanomaterials in the development of herbal therapeutics aimed at combating the progression of AD.

Cubosomes

Cubosomes are nanostructured particles with a liquid crystalline composition, composed of biocompatible carriers. These particles are characterized by a 3D organized bi-continuous, curved lipid bilayer, which is divided into two aqueous channels. This unique structure facilitates interaction between proteins and bioactive components. One of the most significant characteristics of cubosomes is their ability to encapsulate hydrophobic, hydrophilic, and amphiphilic substances, allowing for controlled drug release and improved biological adhesion. Additionally, they exhibit thermodynamic stability, making them a promising method for drug delivery across various routes (Sivadasan et al., 2023).

Dendrimers

Dendrimers (DDs), often termed the "polymers of the 21st century," are recognized as promising nanocarriers for AD treatment due to their ability to cross BBB and enhance the absorption of conventional medications. Their unique structural properties have garnered significant research interest, offering advantages such as greater aqueous solubility, biocompatibility, low cytotoxicity, high stability, precise molecular weight, and polyvalence compared to conventional polymers. These attributes qualify dendrimers for targeted drug delivery to the brain. Moreover, DDs have shown potential in improving cellular absorption for specific cell types, acting as antioxidants, inhibiting amyloidogenic processes, and exhibiting anti-inflammatory properties. As a result, dendrimers may also serve as diagnostic tools for neurodegenerative disorders like AD (Arbez-Gindre et al., 2023).

Gold NPs

Gold nanoparticles (AuNPs) play a crucial role in facilitating drug distribution across BBB to treat NDs. Various formulations of AuNPs are utilized in diagnostic and therapeutic strategies for AD treatment (dos Santos et al., 2020). In a study involving an AD mouse model, intravenous administration of D-glutathione-stabilized gold nanoparticles demonstrated significant inhibitory effects against Aβ42 aggregation without inducing neurotoxic effects. Additionally, another study indicated that administering a gold nanoparticle formulation through intraperitoneal and intrahippocampal injections could enhance spatial learning, memory acquisition, and retention (Hou et al., 2020).

Liposomes

Nanosized liposomes (LPs) can exist as either unilamellar or multilamellar structures, characterized by their vesicular spherical shape and composed of lipid bilayer membranes. These LPs exhibit self-assembling and amphiphilic properties, presenting a promising approach for treating AD (Ross et al., 2018). LPs facilitate rapid distribution and enhanced effectiveness, allowing hydrophilic drugs to be incorporated into the aqueous core and lipophilic medicines to be integrated into the membrane. Functionalization and surface modulation of these drug delivery vehicles can be easily achieved using cell-penetrating peptides, functional proteins, and various polyethers. This customization offers several benefits, such as minimizing adverse effects on normal cells and enhancing targeted drug delivery across BBB, thereby improving drug efficacy and safety. Given the challenges faced by traditional small pharmaceuticals or biomolecules in advancing through clinical trials, tailored nano-LPs present a viable alternative for drug delivery in the context of AD (Naziris and Demetzos, 2021).

Nanoemulsions

Nanoemulsions (NEs) are extremely small colloidal dispersions consisting of dispersed droplets of an insoluble liquid phase. These nanovehicles are stabilized by adding surface-active agents, resulting in particle sizes ranging from 20 to 500 nm (Handa et al., 2021). Compared to traditional emulsions, the ultra-small size of NEs helps prevent particle aggregation, providing kinetic stability due to Brownian motion that overcomes gravitational forces. NE formulations enhance the effectiveness of medications targeting AD by allowing for more precise delivery to specific areas within CNS. For instance, a nanoemulsion was developed to encapsulate memantine for intranasal administration, which helps bypass the blood-brain barrier in the treatment of AD. Both *in vitro* and *in vivo* experiments have demonstrated promising results for nanoemulsions in combating AD (Vishwas et al., 2024).

Nanogels

Nanogels (NGs) are considered promising drug nanocarriers for targeted drug delivery. These materials are water-swollen three-dimensional hydrogels formed by crosslinking natural, synthetic, or hybrid polymeric nanoparticles, with sizes typically ranging from 10 to ~1000 nm, often within the 20-250 nm range. NGs can be dispersed in a high volume of aqueous medium, making them versatile for various applications. The characteristic features of NGs include size, amphiphilicity, porosity, network density, softness, surface electric charge, and chemical functional groups. These properties can be conveniently controlled and tailored to obtain NGs with desirable structural and functional characteristics (Duan et al., 2021). In a preclinical investigation, nanogels were utilized as carriers for intranasal insulin delivery, which is currently a leading medication for AD treatment, demonstrating high biocompatibility (Zhang et al., 2022b).

Niosomes

Niosomes are defined as nonimmunogenic, biodegradable, and biocompatible bilayer nanovesicles formed through the self-organization of non-ionized surfactants, specifically cholesterol and polyglycerol ether, which can be either di-alkyl or alkyl (Patil et al., 2022). Furthermore, niosomes demonstrate greater stability and cost-effectiveness compared to polymeric and lipid-based nanoparticles. They are capable of encapsulating both hydrophilic and hydrophobic medications, enhancing their solubility and penetration, regulating their release, and improving cellular absorption. Consequently, niosomal systems hold promise for a wide range of medication delivery applications.

Selenium Nanoparticles (SeNPs)

Selenium (Se) is a trace element renowned for its essential physiological and pharmacological effects. It plays a vital role in cellular function, detoxification, maintenance of redox homeostasis, and immune protection (Belenichev et al., 2021). As an essential micronutrient for the human body, Se has been extensively studied for its protective effects against neurodegenerative diseases, particularly AD. However, conventional selenium supplements are often limited by low absorption rates and notable toxic effects. This limitation has prompted the development of innovative nanocarrier systems aimed at improving bioavailability and facilitating controlled drug release. Various studies have demonstrated that selenium nano-formulations, such as selenite and SeNPs, exhibit enhanced bioavailability, improved antioxidant and anti-inflammatory effects, and reduced toxicity for AD treatment compared to conventional Se compounds (Malik et al., 2023).

Solid Lipid NPs

Solid lipid nanoparticles (SLNPs) have recently gained renewed attention as a potential drug delivery method for targeting the brain among various nanoparticulate formulations (Satapathy et al., 2021). SLNPs are considered one of the most cost-effective and safest drug carriers for addressing neurodegenerative diseases, thanks to their unique characteristics. These include a large surface area, high drug loading capacity, small particle size, enhanced drug stability, biocompatibility, and improved protection of pharmaceuticals from enzymatic metabolism. Moreover, SLNPs possess an inherent ability to penetrate the Blood-Brain Barrier, making them a promising option for administering medications to CNS (Scioli Montoto et al., 2020).

Carbon Dots

Carbon dots (CDs) are spherical or hemispherical nanomaterials composed of sp^2 hybridized carbon atoms, typically measuring less than 10 nm in size. Recognized as some of the most innovative and promising nanocarriers for use in nanomedicine, CDs exhibit several advantageous characteristics, including minimal cytotoxicity, adjustable photoluminescence, enhanced biocompatibility, excellent photostability, and remarkable chemical stability (Guo et al., 2022). Their unique properties, including favorable size distribution and low cytotoxicity, enable CDs to effectively penetrate the Blood-Brain Barrier, making them a viable option for AD treatment.

Nanophytoherbals in Alzheimer's Disease

With the advent of nanotechnology, it is now feasible to address various challenges and innovate new herbal formulations that offer numerous benefits, including increased plasma bioavailability, targeted delivery, and controlled drug release for treating AD (Table 1).

Table 1. List of nano-phytoherbal formulations used in Alzheimer's therapy

Drug	Chemical Structure	Type of nano formulation	Animal Model	Reference
Andrographolide	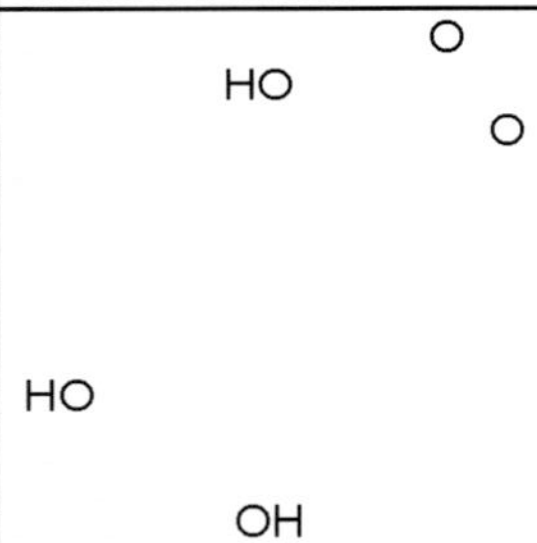	Human serum Nanoparticles	*In vitro* and *in-vivo* study using TgCRND8 mice	Bilia et al., 2019
Bacoposide	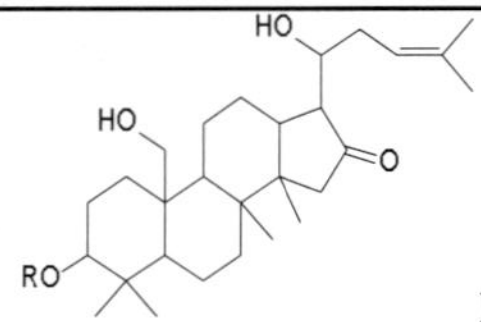	Polymersomes	5XFAD transgenic swiss albino mice	Abdul Manap et al., 2019
Berberin	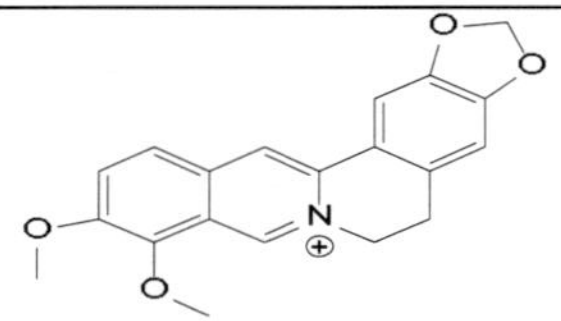	Nanoparticles	Aβ induced AD in mice	Singh et al., 2021b
Caffeic acid	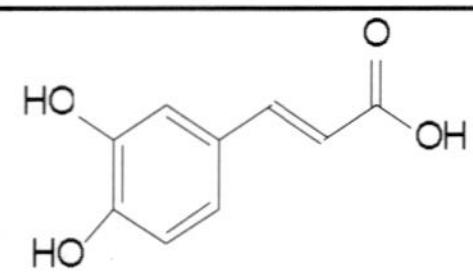	Liposomes	In-vitro study	Andrade et al., 2023
Curcumin	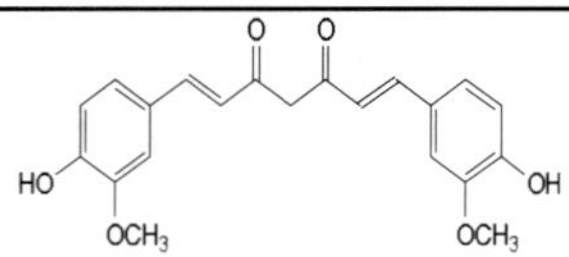	PLGA-NPs, Liposomes, nanosphere, nanocapsules	*In-vitro* study	Ege et al., 2021

Drug	Chemical Structure	Type of nano formulation	Animal Model	Reference

Epigallocatechin gallate	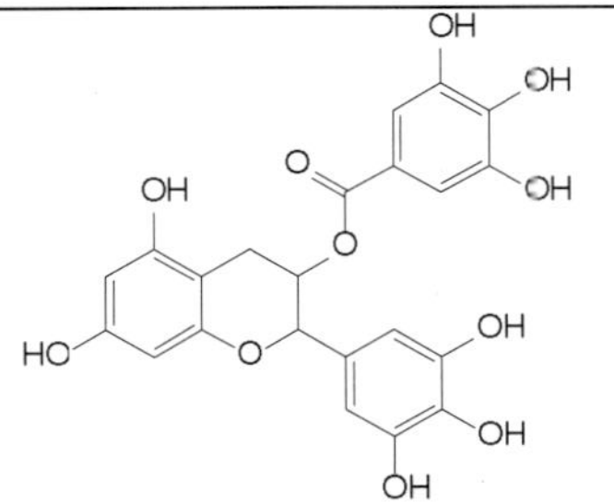	Selenium Nanoparticles	*In vitro* and *in-vivo* study	Zhang et al., 2020
Genistein	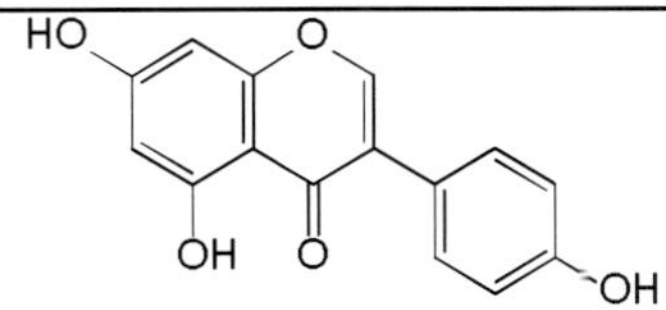	Fullerene and Multi-wall carbon nanotubes	*In-vivo* studies	Mehta and Shende, 2024
Naringenin	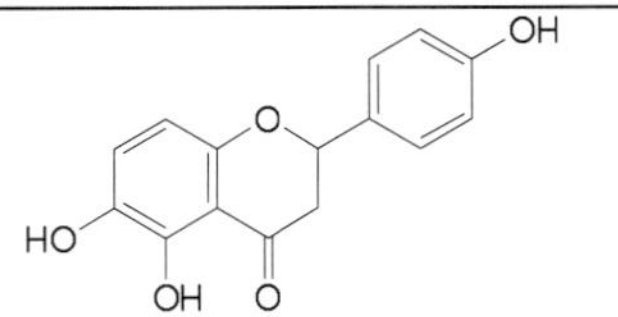	Nanoemulsion	Aβ25-35 induced PC12 cells and SH-SY5Y cells	Yan et al., 2024
Piperine	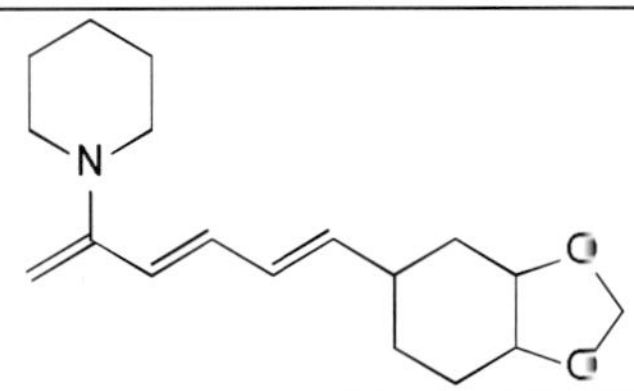	Nanoemulsion, Cubosomes, Nanoparticles	*In-vivo* study	Yusuf et al., 2018

Table 1. (Continued)

Drug	Chemical Structure	Type of nano formulation	Animal Model	Reference
Resveratrol	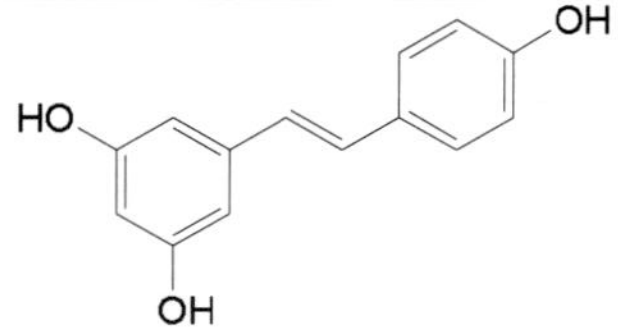	Lipid-core nanocapsules	Aβ-triggered oxidative stress in mice	Frozza et al., 2013b
		Mesoporous nano-selenium	Aβ1−42 induced neurotoxic	Sun et al., 2019
Quercetin	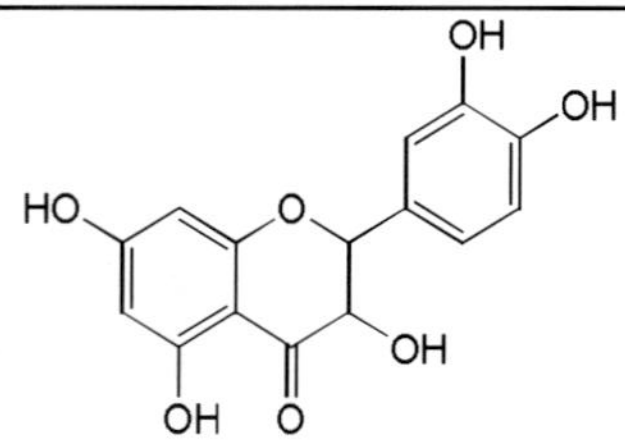	Liposomes, Nanocapsule	*In-vitro* and *in-vivo* study	Tomou et al., 2023
Withaferin	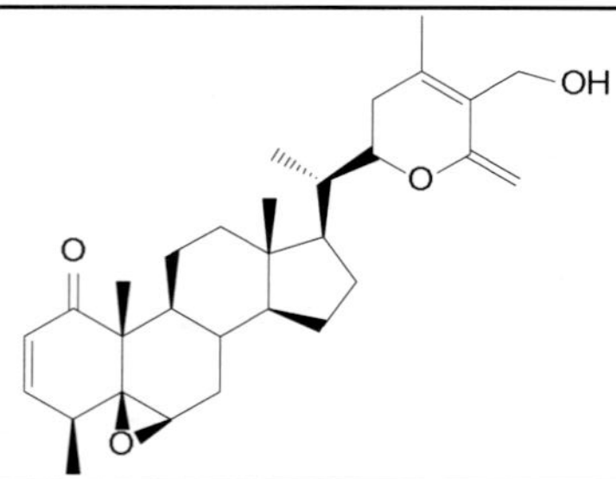	PLGA Nanoparticles	*In-Vitro*	Madhu et al., 2021

Andrographolides

Andrographolide (AG), a labdane diterpenoid derived from Andrographis paniculata, has been utilized as an alternative therapy for AD due to its anti-apoptotic, neuroprotective, antioxidant, and anti-inflammatory properties (Abedi et al., 2021). However, AG is reported to have a short biological half-life, low bioavailability, and difficulty crossing BBB, which limits its therapeutic benefits for neurological conditions. Recent research indicates that andrographolide-loaded human serum NPs (AGNPs) provide a promising avenue for AD treatment, demonstrating significant improvements in BBB penetration, non-toxicity, enhanced biocompatibility, high biodegradability, and better tolerability of AG in the affected brain regions of TgCRND8 AD mice (Bilia et al., 2019).

Bacoposide

The active ingredients of Bacopa monnieri, known as bacoposides, are well recognized for their neuroprotective properties. Polymersomes loaded with bacoposides have demonstrated significant neuroprotective benefits in treating AD, effectively removing amyloid plaques, restoring damaged neurons, stimulating the growth of new neurons, and attenuating AD-associated gene expression changes in the hippocampus of 5XFAD mice. Additionally, these polymersomes exhibited anti-inflammatory properties by inhibiting the activation of astrocytes and microglia. However, further investigation is necessary to explore the translational potential of this nanoformulation in human models of AD (Abdul Manap et al., 2019).

Berberine

Berberine (BRB) is an isoquinoline compound derived from traditional Chinese medicinal remedies such as *Coptis rhizoma*, *Cortex phellodendri*, and *Sanguinaria canadensis*. It has been studied for its antioxidant, antinociceptive, memory enhancement, and anti-inflammatory properties, particularly in improving spatial memory and learning in AD rat models. However, its selective penetration through BBB limits its clinical applicability. Research has shown that multi-walled carbon nanotubes coated with polysorbate and phospholipids, loaded with BRB, improve cognitive function and prevent AD-induced damage caused by β-amyloid in rats compared to the free form of berberine. Additionally, lipid-coated mesoporous silica nanoparticles loaded with BRB demonstrated an eightfold increase in BBB permeability compared to the oral intake of pure berberine (Singh et al., 2021b), suggesting their potential as a viable method for targeted drug delivery to the central nervous system.

Caffeic Acid

Caffeic acid (CA) shows promise for AD treatment due to its antioxidant, anti-inflammatory, and anti-amyloidogenic properties. However, its poor bioavailability and chemical instability limit its therapeutic potential in vivo. To address these challenges, transferrin was conjugated to the surfaces of liposomes, creating a potential approach for Alzheimer's treatment. This modification facilitates the transport of CA-loaded NPs across the blood-brain barrier, delaying the aggregation of Aβ1–42 monomers and reducing fibril formation, ultimately leading to the disaggregation of fully developed fibrils. These developed CA-loaded transferrin-functionalized NPs represent a promising method for treating AD, with future studies in animal models being essential to validate their therapeutic efficacy (Andrade et al., 2023).

Curcumin

Curcumin, a prominent natural polyphenol derived from *Curcuma longa* L., exhibits unique chemical properties that make it effective against Aβ and protein aggregation in neurodegenerative diseases like AD. Despite its therapeutic potential, curcumin faces challenges such as limited absorption and bioavailability. To overcome these limitations, various nanostructures, including nanoparticles, nanoliposomes, nanomicelles, and nanocapsules, have been developed to enhance curcumin's pharmacokinetics. *In vitro* studies have shown promising results, indicating that curcumin derivatives encapsulated in lipid-PEG liposomes significantly improved Aβ aggregation reduction and enhance BBB penetration. Similarly, functionalized nanoliposomes, such as TATCur-NL, demonstrated potential in preventing Aβ formation and reducing oxidative stress (Ege et al., 2021).

Epigallocatechin gallate

Epigallocatechin gallate (EGCG), an ester of gallic acid and epigallocatechin, is the main catechin found in tea and serves as the primary bioactive polyphenol in solid green tea extract. Numerous published *in vitro* and *in vivo* studies suggest the potential therapeutic use of EGCG in treating AD, indicating that this compound possesses neuroprotective properties. To mitigate the cytotoxicity of EGCG at elevated concentrations and inhibit Aβ fibrillation, EGCG was linked to the surface of selenium nanoparticles coated with the Tet-1 peptide (Zhang et al., 2020).

Genistein

A promising approach for treating AD involves utilizing natural substances such as genistein (GEN), a soybean-derived isoflavonoid known for its strong neuroprotective qualities that inhibit free radical production. Additionally, GEN combats AD by inhibiting Aβ aggregation, blocking the enzyme BACE1, and suppressing the expression of amyloid precursor protein (Fuloria et al., 2022). However, despite its potential, GEN faces challenges due to low solubility and limited penetration of BBB. Researchers are exploring carbon nanocarriers, such as multiwall carbon nanotubes and fullerene (C-60), to enhance its delivery, capitalizing on their biocompatibility, high loading capacity, and stability (Mehta and Shende, 2024). *In vivo* studies conducted on Wistar rats indicate regulated GEN release in CNS via intranasal delivery, suggesting its potential as an alternative treatment for AD.

Naringenin

Naringenin (NRG), a bioflavonoid found in various fruits, exhibits a range of beneficial properties, including antioxidant, free radical scavenging, anti-inflammatory, anticancer, immunomodulating, and memory-enhancing effects. Its antioxidant capabilities position it as a promising therapeutic agent for AD. However, challenges such as low aqueous solubility, gastrointestinal degradation, and poor transport across biological membranes hinder its clinical development and bioavailability. To address these limitations, a nanoemulsion formulation loaded with NRG has been explored. This formulation demonstrated a significant reduction in the neurotoxic effects of Aβ on PC12 and SH-SY5Y cells, potentially through the regulation of amyloidogenesis and tau hyperphosphorylation. Therefore, it presents a promising therapeutic option for AD (Yan et al., 2024).

Piperine

Piperine (PIP), a potent alkaloid found in the fruits of piper species, has been extensively studied for its effects on CNS, particularly its influence on acetylcholine levels. However, PIP faces challenges in oral bioavailability due to its high lipophilicity and low aqueous solubility. To address these issues, researchers have explored various formulations, including Tween-added monoolein cubosomes (T-cubs) and microemulsions loaded with piperine. In AD models, PIP-encapsulated T-cubs demonstrated superior efficacy in restoring cognitive function. Furthermore, intranasal delivery of PIP-filled chitosan NPs proved to be an effective treatment for AD, requiring a lower dosage of PIP compared to PIP alone. Similarly, a PIP microemulsion showed enhanced clinical outcomes and improved brain distribution compared to untreated AD subjects (Etman et al., 2018). Piperine solid lipid nanoparticles (PIP-SLNs) coated with polysorbate 80 (PS80) reduced SOD1 enzyme immobility while increasing acetylcholinesterase levels. Histopathological evaluations also revealed decreased plaque and tangle formations (Yusuf et al., 2018).

Resveratrol

Resveratrol (RSV), chemically known as 3, 5, 4-trihydroxy stilbene, is a dietary polyphenolic compound found naturally in various fruits, including berries, grapes, pomegranates, and peanuts. It exhibits a wide range of biological effects, such as anti-inflammatory, anti-aging, cardioprotective, chemopreventive, anticarcinogenic, and antioxidant properties. *In vitro* studies have demonstrated the antioxidant and anti-apoptotic potential of RSV-loaded polymeric micelles in PC12 cells. Additionally, an improved formulation of RSV-loaded lipid core nanoparticles (RSVLNC) presents a promising therapeutic approach for AD by modulating Aβ-triggered neuroinflammation and oxidative stress *in vitro*. RSVLNC also restored Aβ1−42-induced neurotoxic effects in rats (Frozza et al., 2013b). Furthermore, RSV-loaded mesoporous nanoselenium administration systems prevented the aggregation of Aβ, suppressed tau hyperphosphorylation, mitigated oxidative stress, and improved memory deficits in PS1/PSS mice (Sun et al., 2019).

Quercetin

Quercetin (QC) is a well-known bioflavonoid recognized for its neuroprotective, antioxidant, and anti-inflammatory properties, found in various vegetables, fruits, and certain herbal oils. However, challenges such as inadequate dissolution and low absorption have impeded its initial therapeutic uses. To address these limitations, alternative nanoformulations of QC, including microspheres, nanocapsules, nanosuspensions, nanogels, and liposomes, have been proposed. In a specific study, QC-loaded nanolipid carriers (NLCs) demonstrated improved bioavailability and targeted delivery to the brain, along with enhanced antioxidant activity (Tomou et al., 2023).

Withaferin

Withaferin-A, derived from the plant Ashwagandha (*Withania somnifera*, family Solanaceae), commonly known as Indian winter cherry or Indian ginseng, plays a significant role in the Ayurvedic medicinal system of India. This herb aids in removing amyloid-beta (Aβ) plaques in the brains of AD patients and possesses a unique ability to heal injured neurons and rebuild neuronal synapses and networks, thereby improving cognition and memory. To address the challenge of drug transport to the brain due to BBB, Withaferin-A was encapsulated in polymeric nanoparticles made of poly(lactic-co-glycolic acid) (PLGA) to specifically target CNS for AD. The results suggested that it may serve as a useful alternative for AD treatment, exhibiting significant antioxidant effects (Madhu et al., 2021).

Future Prospects

AD, a refractory neurological illness, is characterized by tau hyperphosphorylation and amyloid-β deposition in CNS tissue. The development of effective drugs primarily targets these two pathological features. However, challenges such as BBB penetration, peripheral adverse effects, and absorption hinder the efficacy of anti-AD medications. Currently, these treatments only address symptoms without slowing disease progression. Since 2003, FDA-approved AD medications have been scarce. Recent research suggests that artificial intelligence (AI)-enabled nanodrugs may identify optimal combinations of nanomedicine for neurodegenerative diseases like AD. Nanoparticles enhance targeting, improve bioavailability, and facilitate BBB penetration while minimizing peripheral side effects and reducing clearance by endothelial cells and enzymatic degradation. To effectively encapsulate herbal drugs with significant anti-apoptotic and anti-inflammatory properties, it is crucial to develop nanoparticles with high BBB penetrability. The characteristics of nanoparticles can influence drug binding, delivery, BBB crossing, localization, and release. Future research should focus on designing multifunctional and multicomponent nanoparticles by integrating diverse functions, shapes, and sizes while maximizing their distinct features. However, the clinical translation of nanomedicine remains challenging. Safety is paramount; while some studies suggest that natural drug-loaded nanoparticles are less hazardous, these findings are primarily preclinical. Drug-loaded NPs may also induce neuroinflammation, excitotoxicity, DNA damage, and allergic reactions, necessitating further investigation. A deeper understanding of these systems will aid in optimizing formulations, reducing or replacing harmful components, and minimizing adverse events. Although functionalized NPs can target drugs effectively, their large surface area and nanoscale dimensions may limit particle accumulation and drug loading. Consequently, more advanced nanostructures are needed for improved therapeutic efficacy.

Conclusion

The prevalence of NDs is rising alongside global life expectancy, highlighting the need for innovative treatment strategies to enhance symptoms and improve the quality of life for patients. The CNS is protected by several barriers, necessitating that suitable drugs successfully cross BBB to reach their target. While various drug delivery technologies exist, phytochemical-based nanocarriers are particularly promising due to their reliability, environmental friendliness, low toxicity, affordability, and ease of scalability, along with the ability to provide controlled particle size and shape. Plant-mediated nanosystems can enhance brain penetration, prevent the formation of aggregates in the brain, and improve the pharmacokinetic properties and absorption of phytotherapeutic compounds within the CNS. Numerous studies have demonstrated that NPs can restore neurological abnormalities in preclinical models; however, further research is essential to address safety concerns. In the realm of neurological medicine, the efficacy of NPs requires long-term evaluation. It is crucial to consider nanoformulations tailored for specific brain cells and types of neurological disorders, ensuring targeted and effective therapeutic outcomes.

References

Abdul Manap, A. S., Vijayabalan, S., Madhavan, P., Chia, Y. Y., Arya, A., Wong, E. H., Rizwan, F., Bindal, U., & Koshy, S. (2019). *Bacopa monnieri*, a neuroprotective lead in Alzheimer disease: a review on its properties, mechanisms of action, and preclinical and clinical studies. *Drug Target Insights*, 13, 1177392819866412.

Abedi, Z., Basri, H., Hassan, Z., Mat, L. N. I., Khaza'ai, H., & Mohamad, N. A. (2021). A review of the neuroprotective effects of andrographolide in Alzheimer's disease. *Advances in Traditional Medicine*, 21, 253-266.

Afzal O, Altamimi ASA, Nadeem MS, Alzarea SI, Almalki WH, Tariq A, Mubeen B, Murtaza BN, Iftikhar S, Riaz N, Kazmi I. Nanoparticles in Drug Delivery: From History to Therapeutic Applications. *Nanomaterials*, 12(24), 4494.

Alahmari, A. (2021). Blood-brain barrier overview: Structural and functional correlation. *Neural Plasticity*, 2021, 1-10.

Andrade, S., Pereira, M. C., & Loureiro, J. A. (2023). Caffeic acid loaded into engineered lipid nanoparticles for Alzheimer's disease therapy. *Colloids and Surfaces B: Biointerfaces*, *225*, 113270.

Arbez-Gindre, C., Steele, B. R., & Micha-Screttas, M. (2023). Dendrimers in Alzheimer's Disease: Recent Approaches in Multi-Targeting Strategies. *Pharmaceutics*, 15(3), 898.

Belenichev, I. F., Gorchakova, N. O., Bukhtiyarova, N. V., Samura, I. B., Savchenko, N. V., & Popazova, O. O. (2021). Pharmacological properties of selenium and its preparations: from antioxidant to neuroprotector. *Research Results in Pharmacology*, 7(4), 29-40.

Bilia, A. R., Nardiello, P., Piazzini, V., Leri, M., Bergonzi, M. C., Bucciantini, M., & Casamenti, F. (2019). Successful brain delivery of andrographolide loaded in human albumin nanoparticles to TgCRND8 mice, an Alzheimer's disease mouse model. *Frontiers in pharmacology*, 10, 910.

Dos Santos Tramontin, N., da Silva, S., Arruda, R., Ugioni, K. S., Canteiro, P. B., de Bem Silveira, G., Mendes, C., Silveira, P. C. L., & Muller, A. P. (2020). Gold Nanoparticles Treatment Reverses Brain Damage in Alzheimer's Disease Model. *Molecular neurobiology*, 57(2), 926–936.

Duan, Q. Y., Zhu, Y. X., Jia, H. R., Wang, S. H., & Wu, F. G. (2023). Nanogels: Synthesis, properties, and recent biomedical applications. *Progress in Materials Science*, 101167.

Ege, D. (2021). Action mechanisms of curcumin in Alzheimer's disease and its brain targeted delivery. *Materials*, 14(12), 3332.

Etman, S. M., Elnaggar, Y. S., Abdelmonsif, D. A., & Abdallah, O. Y. (2018). Oral brain-targeted microemulsion for enhanced piperine delivery in Alzheimer's disease therapy: *In vitro* appraisal, *in vivo* activity, and nanotoxicity. *AAPS pharmscitech*, 19, 3698-3711.

Frozza, R. L., Bernardi, A., Hoppe, J. B., Meneghetti, A. B., Battastini, A. M., Pohlmann, A. R., Guterres, S. S., & Salbego, C. (2013). Lipid-core nanocapsules improve the effects of resveratrol against Abeta-induced neuroinflammation. *Journal of biomedical nanotechnology*, 9(12), 2086-2104.

Frozza, R. L., Bernardi, A., Hoppe, J. B., Meneghetti, A. B., Matté, A., Battastini, A. M., Pohlmann, A. R., Guterres, S. S., & Salbego, C. (2013b). Neuroprotective effects of resveratrol against Aβ administration in rats are improved by lipid-core nanocapsules. *Molecular neurobiology*, 47(3), 1066–1080.

Fuloria, S., Yusri, M. A. A., Sekar, M., Gan, S. H., Rani, N. N. I. M., Lum, P. T., Ravi, S., Subramaniyan, V., Azad, A. K., Jeyabalan, S., Wu, Y. S., Meenakshi, D. U., Sathasivam, K. V., & Fuloria, N. K. (2022). Genistein: A Potential Natural Lead Molecule for New Drug Design and Development for Treating Memory Impairment. *Molecules*, 27(1), 265.

Guo, F., Li, Q., Zhang, X., Liu, Y., Jiang, J., Cheng, S., Yu, S., Zhang, X., Liu, F., Li, Y., Rose, G., & Zhang, H. (2022). Applications of Carbon Dots for the Treatment of Alzheimer's Disease. *International Journal of Nanomedicine*, 6621-6638.

Handa, M., Tiwari, S., Yadav, A. K., Almalki, W. H., Alghamdi, S., Alharbi, K. S., Shukla, R., & Beg, S. (2021). Therapeutic potential of nanoemulsions as feasible wagons for targeting Alzheimer's disease. *Drug Discovery Today*, 26(12), 2881-2888.

Hou, K., Zhao, J., Wang, H., Li, B., Li, K., Shi, X., Wan, K., Ai, J., Lv, J., Wang, D., Huang, Q., Wang, H., Cao, Q., Liu, S., & Tang, Z. (2020). Chiral gold nanoparticles enantioselectively rescue memory deficits in a mouse model of Alzheimer's disease. *Nature communications*, 11(1), 4790.

Kanojia, N., Thapa, K., Kaur, G., Sharma, A., Puri, V., & Verma, N. (2023). Update on Therapeutic potential of emerging nanoformulations of phytocompounds in Alzheimer's and Parkinson's disease. *Journal of Drug Delivery Science and Technology*, 79, 104074.

Kaushal, M. A., Patel, N. A., Xavier, G., & Prajapati, B. G. (2024). Roles of nano medicine in diagnosis of Alzheimer's disease. In *Alzheimer's Disease and Advanced Drug Delivery Strategies* (pp. 115-138). Academic Press.

Koul, B., Farooq, U., Yadav, D., & Song, M. (2023). Phytochemicals: A Promising Alternative for the Prevention of Alzheimer's Disease. *Life*, 13(4), 999.

Madhu, S., Komala, M., & Pandian, P. (2021). Formulation development and characterization of withaferin-A loaded polymeric nanoparticles for Alzheimer's disease. *BioNanoScience*, 11, 559-566.

Malik, J. A., AjgarAnsari, J., Ahmed, S., Rani, A., Ansari, S. Y., & Anwar, S. (2023). Emerging Selenium Nanoparticles for CNS Intervention. In *Biotechnology-Biosensors, Biomaterials and Tissue Engineering Annual Volume 2023*. IntechOpen.

Mehta, P., & Shende, P. (2024). Collation of fullerenes and carbon nanotubes with genistein for synergistic anti-Alzheimer's activity by amyloid-β deaggregation. *Journal of Drug Delivery Science and Technology*, 91, 105205.

Nagori, K., Nakhate, K. T., Yadav, K., Ajazuddin, & Pradhan, M. (2023). Unlocking the Therapeutic Potential of Medicinal Plants for Alzheimer's Disease: Preclinical to Clinical Trial Insights. *Future Pharmacology*, 3(4), 877-907.

Naziris, N., & Demetzos, C. (2021). Liposomes: Production methods and application in Alzheimer's Disease. In *GeNeDis 2020: Genetics and Neurodegenerative Diseases* (pp. 385-394). Springer International Publishing.

Pardridge, W. M. (2020). Treatment of Alzheimer's disease and blood–brain barrier drug delivery. *Pharmaceuticals*, *13*(11), 394.

Patil, A. C., Patil, A. S., Desai, S. P., Phalke, T. M., & Saralaya, M. G. (2022). Niosomes: A Future Of Targeted Drug Delivery Systems As Promising Nanocarrier Through Blood-Brain Barrier For Natural Drug Delivery. *NeuroQuantology,* 20(17), 1547.

Pugazhenthi, S., Qin, L., & Reddy, P. H. (2017). Common neurodegenerative pathways in obesity, diabetes, and Alzheimer's disease. *Biochimica et biophysica acta (BBA)-molecular basis of disease*, 1863(5), 1037-1045.

Ross, C., Taylor, M., Fullwood, N., & Allsop, D. (2018). Liposome delivery systems for the treatment of Alzheimer's disease. *International journal of nanomedicine*, 8507-8522.

Satapathy, M. K., Yen, T. L., Jan, J. S., Tang, R. D., Wang, J. Y., Taliyan, R., & Yang, C. H. (2021). Solid lipid nanoparticles (SLNs): an advanced drug delivery system targeting brain through BBB. *Pharmaceutics*, 13(8), 1183.

Scioli Montoto, S., Muraca, G., & Ruiz, M. E. (2020). Solid lipid nanoparticles for drug delivery: pharmacological and biopharmaceutical aspects. *Frontiers in molecular biosciences*, 7, 319.

Singh, A. K., Rai, S. N., Maurya, A., Mishra, G., Awasthi, R., Shakya, A., Chellappan, D. K., Dua, K., Vamanu, E., Chaudhary, S. K., & Singh, M. P. (2021a). Therapeutic potential of phytoconstituents in management of Alzheimer's disease. *Evidence-based complementary and alternative medicine*, 2021, 1-19.

Singh, A. K., Singh, S. S., Rathore, A. S., Singh, S. P., Mishra, G., Awasthi, R., Mishra, S. K., Gautam, V., & Singh, S. K. (2021b). Lipid-coated MCM-41 mesoporous silica nanoparticles loaded with berberine improved inhibition of acetylcholine esterase and amyloid formation. *ACS Biomaterials Science & Engineering*, 7(8), 3737-3753.

Sivadasan, D., Sultan, M. H., Alqahtani, S. S., & Javed, S. (2023). Cubosomes in Drug Delivery—A Comprehensive Review on Its Structural Components, Preparation Techniques and Therapeutic Applications. *Biomedicines*, 11(4), 1114.

Song, N., Sun, S., Chen, K., Wang, Y., Wang, H., Meng, J., Guo, M., Zhang, X. D., & Zhang, R. (2023). Emerging nanotechnology for Alzheimer's disease: From detection to treatment. *Journal of Controlled Release*, 360, 392-417.

Sood, P., Singh, V., & Shri, R. (2023a). Morus Alba Fruit Extract and its Fractions Ameliorate Streptozotocin Induced Cognitive Deficit in Mice via Modulating Oxidative and Cholinergic Systems. *Neurochemical Research*, 1-14.

Sood, P., Singh, V., & Shri, R. (2023b). Morus alba fruit diet ameliorates cognitive deficit in mouse model of streptozotocin-induced memory impairment. *Metabolic Brain Disease*, 38(5), 1657-1669.

Sun, J., Wei, C., Liu, Y., Xie, W., Xu, M., Zhou, H., & Liu, J. (2019). Progressive release of mesoporous nano-selenium delivery system for the multi-channel synergistic treatment of Alzheimer's disease. *Biomaterials*, 197, 417-431.

Tomou, E. M., Papakyriakopoulou, P., Saitani, E. M., Valsami, G., Pippa, N., & Skaltsa, H. (2023). Recent Advances in Nanoformulations for Quercetin Delivery. *Pharmaceutics*, 15(6), 1656.

Vaiserman, A., Koliada, A., & Lushchak, O. (2020). Neuroinflammation in pathogenesis of Alzheimer's disease: Phytochemicals as potential therapeutics. *Mechanisms of Ageing and Development*, 189, 111259.

Verma, N., Sharma, S., Thakur, N., Kaur, N., & Dua, K. (2024). Nanotherapeutics for Alzheimer's disease using metal nanocomposites. *Metal Nanocomposites in Nanotherapeutics for Oxidative Stress-Induced Metabolic Disorders*, 372-391.

Vishwas, S., Bashir, B., Birla, D., Khandale, N., Chaitanya, M. V. N. L., Chellappan, D. K., Gupta, G., Negi, P., Dua, K., & Singh, S. K. (2024). Neuroprotective Role of Phytoconstituents-based Nanoemulsion for the Treatment of Alzheimer's Disease. *Current Topics in Medicinal Chemistry.*

Xu, X., Ray, R., Gu, Y., Ploehn, H. J., Gearheart, L., Raker, K., & Scrivens, W. A. (2004). Electrophoretic analysis and purification of fluorescent single-walled carbon nanotube fragments. *Journal of the American Chemical Society*, 126(40), 12736-12737.

Yan, C., Gu, J., Yin, S., Wu, H., Lei, X., Geng, F., Zhang, N., & Wu, X. (2024). Design and preparation of naringenin loaded functional biomimetic nano-drug delivery system for Alzheimer's disease. *Journal of Drug Targeting*, *32*(1), 80-92.

Yarns, B. C., Holiday, K. A., Carlson, D. M., Cosgrove, C. K., & Melrose, R. J. (2022). Pathophysiology of Alzheimer's Disease. *Psychiatric Clinics*, 45(4), 663-676.

Yusuf, M., Khan, M., Khan, R. A., & Ahmed, B. (2013). Preparation, characterization, *in vivo* and biochemical evaluation of brain targeted Piperine solid lipid nanoparticles in an experimentally induced Alzheimer's disease model. *Journal of drug targeting*, 21(3), 300-311.

Zhang, S., Gan, L., Cao, F., Wang, H., Gong, P., Ma, C., Ren, L., Lin, Y., & Lin, X. (2022). The barrier and interface mechanisms of the brain barrier, and brain drug delivery. *Brain Research Bulletin*, *190*, 69-83.

Zhang, S., Zhu, Q., Chen, J. Y., OuYang, D., & Lu, J. H. (2020). The pharmacological activity of epigallocatechin-3-gallate (EGCG) on Alzheimer's disease animal model: A systematic review. *Phytomedicine*, 79, 153316.

Zhang, Y., Zou, Z., Liu, S., Miao, S., & Liu, H. (2022b). Nanogels as novel nanocarrier systems for efficient delivery of CNS therapeutics. *Frontiers in Bioengineering and Biotechnology*, 10, 954470.

Chapter 5

Applications of Nanophytoherbals in Parkinson's Therapy

Navidha Aggarwal[1]
Sumnit Wadhwa[1]
Simran[1]
and Prinsy Rana[1,*]
M.M. College of Pharmacy, Maharishi Markandeshwar (Deemed to be University), Mullana, Haryana, India

Abstract

Parkinson's disease (PD) is a neurological condition that primarily affects the elderly, characterized by the degeneration of dopaminergic neurons in the ventrolateral midbrain. Numerous studies have been conducted to evaluate the disease's clinical features and diagnostic accuracy. The advent of nanotechnology presents promising opportunities to address the challenges associated with PD. This advanced technique offers personalized and targeted treatments for neurodegenerative diseases by specifically targeting damaged neurons to reduce oxidative stress and inflammation, which are significant contributors to PD. The field of nano-phytoherbs is emerging as a promising area of study that could enhance treatment efficacy for neurological conditions, including PD and other neurodegenerative disorders. Recently, phytoherbs have gained attention in managing PD, with certain Ayurvedic medicines, such as *Bacopa monnieri* and *Mucuna pruriens*, showing potential as neuroprotective agents. Moreover, the effectiveness of various phytoherbs in treating PD has been supported by clinical trials. This chapter explores the findings regarding the use of nano-phytoherbs for PD treatment, discussing the approaches of nano-phyto formulations to facilitate the delivery of phytoconstituents across the blood-brain barrier and enhance their pharmacological effects. In conclusion, preclinical studies highlight the therapeutic potential of natural products and herbal medicines in offering protective benefits against the key attributes of PD.

Keywords: Parkinson's disease, blood brain barrier, nano-phytoherbs, nano formulations, neurological disorders, nanotechnology

---

* Corresponding Author's Email: princy.rana65@gmail.com.

In: Phyto-Nanomedicine
Editors: Hitesh Chopra, Vinod Kumar Gauttam, Ajmer Singh Grewal et al.
ISBN: 979-8-89530-317-7

Introduction

Neurological diseases have increasingly dominated the landscape of human health concerns, with Parkinson's disease ranking as the second most common neurodegenerative disorder after Alzheimer's. Recent estimates indicate that our city reported 120.5 cases of Parkinson's disease per 100,000 people within a year. The incidence of new cases surged significantly after the age of 60, reaching 854.7 cases per 100,000 person-years in the 85-89 age group, before declining in individuals aged 90-99 (Driver et al., 2009). Over the past 25 years, the prevalence of Parkinson's disease has doubled, with approximately 8.5 million people affected globally in 2019. The disease contributed to 5.8 million disability-adjusted life years and 329,000 deaths that same year, representing an increase of over 100% since 2000 (Parkinson Disease, n.d.). The national economic burden of Parkinson's disease in developed nations, such as the United States, is estimated to exceed $52 billion (New Study Shows the Economic Burden of Parkinson's Disease Double Previous Estimates | Parkinson's Foundation, n.d.). In underdeveloped countries like India, patients' average gross national income was found to cover only 16.7% to 41.7% of their treatment costs (Bovolenta et al., 2017). Characterized by the accumulation of misfolded α-synuclein in intracytoplasmic structures known as Lewy bodies, the disease leads to the degeneration of dopaminergic neurons in the substantia nigra pars compacta. By the time patients are diagnosed, a substantial number of dopaminergic neurons have already been lost, and neurodegeneration has typically spread to other regions of the central nervous system (Figure 1).

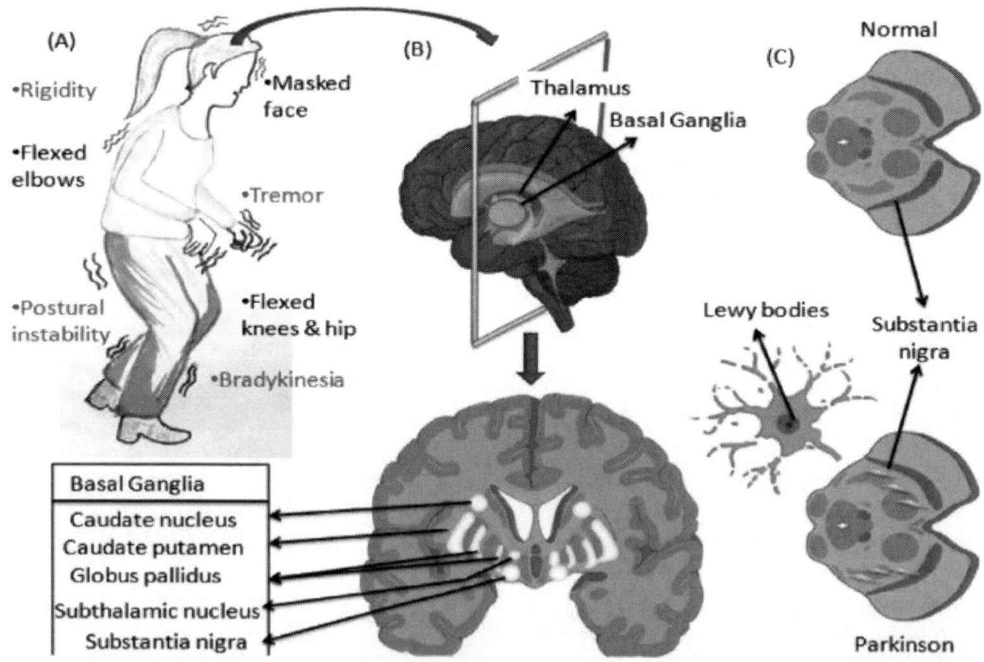

Figure 1. Sign and symptoms of Parkinson's disease.

While the etiology of Parkinson's disease remains unclear for the majority of cases, hereditary factors account for 5%–10% of instances. Deep brain stimulation is an elective treatment option for patients in later stages of the disease. Current medications for Parkinson's disease effectively manage motor symptoms but do not halt disease progression or the increasing disability of patients. However, nanotechnology holds promise for enhancing treatment efficacy through innovative carrier-based platforms that ensure customized and controlled drug release while improving delivery by modulating or bypassing the blood-brain barrier (Singh et al., 2024). The challenge of delivering neurotherapeutics to the brain arises from the highly effective and dense blood-brain barrier, which, in concert with enzymes, limits the entry of drugs and many neurotherapeutics to maintain the brain's internal environment (Abbott & Romero, 1996). Previous studies have demonstrated that nearly all low molecular weight medications and all macromolecular drugs cannot cross the blood-brain barrier (Abbott & Romero, 1996). It has been demonstrated in previous outbreaks that almost all low molecular weight medications and all macromolecular drugs are unable to cross the blood-brain barrier (Roney et al., 2005). Research has investigated the advantages of the nasal route for delivering phytoconstituents, highlighting its ability to bypass the blood-brain barrier, avoid first-pass metabolism in the liver, and provide practical, safe, and user-friendly options (Chopra et al., 2023; Pardeshi et al., 2012).

Conventional Therapies in Parkinson's Disease

The primary strategy for managing Parkinson's disease has focused on addressing the deficiency of dopaminergic neurotransmission to alleviate core motor symptoms. Since the discovery of dopamine cell loss in the substantia nigra of patients with Parkinson's disease, Levodopa therapy has transformed treatment, serving as the cornerstone for alleviating motor symptoms. However, its long-term use has introduced new clinical challenges, particularly the emergence of motor complications such as dyskinesias. As a response, dopamine receptor agonists are often prescribed earlier in the disease progression due to their ability to reduce Parkinsonian symptoms while posing a lower risk of troublesome dyskinesias compared to Levodopa. This shift in treatment strategy has occurred as the complications associated with Levodopa have become increasingly apparent. Extensive randomized controlled trials of second-generation medications such as pramipexole and ropinirole have confirmed their effectiveness. However, it is now recognized that dopamine receptor agonists can also lead to motor complications, sometimes more severe than those associated with Levodopa. This emergence of both motor and non-motor side effects from all forms of dopamine replacement therapy underscores that treatments aimed at "normalizing" dopaminergic transmission may offer only limited benefits over the course of the disease. The development of a model of basal ganglia circuitry has significantly influenced treatment approaches for Parkinson's disease patients. Deep brain stimulation (DBS), which targets specific brain regions, has become the standard surgical intervention for certain patients with advanced Parkinson's disease. Initially, surgeons favored ablative techniques that targeted the internal pallidal segment or the subthalamic nucleus. While subthalamic nucleus DBS has shown clear benefits for alleviating motor symptoms of Parkinson's disease, recent findings indicating significant non-motor side effects have raised concerns about selecting appropriate candidates for this treatment (Benabid et al., 2009).

Herbs Used in Parkinson's Disease

Herbs have been shown to contain various bioactive compounds and exhibit numerous medicinal properties (Figure 2) (Sharma et al., 2022). The use of herbs aims to alleviate the symptoms of Parkinson's disease and slow its progression through natural products. Notable plants such as Ashwagandha, Brahmi, and Mucuna pruriens are rich in antioxidants and offer neuroprotective effects. These herbs have demonstrated significant potential in reducing oxidative stress and enhancing motor abilities, among other benefits, thanks to their antioxidant properties. Incorporating these herbs into nanoparticle formulations can improve their absorption into the bloodstream, facilitating their therapeutic effects. Below, we discuss the research studies on several herbs in the context of Parkinson's disease:

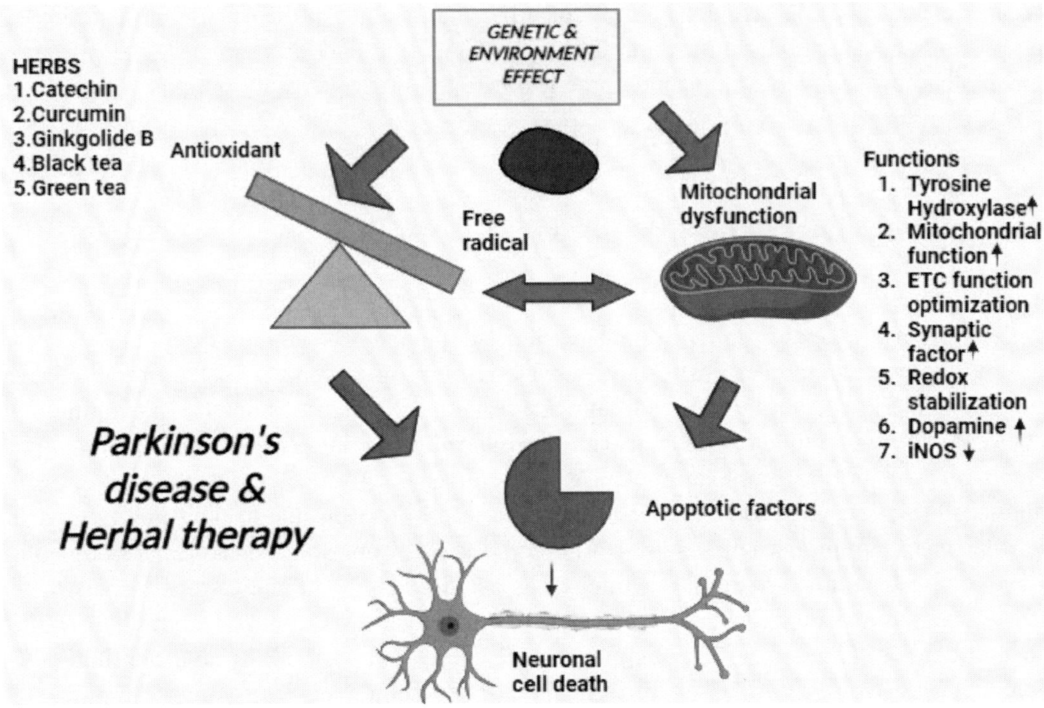

Figure 2. Various herbs and their functions in Parkinson's disease.

Bacopa monnieri or Brahmi

Brahmi, also known as *Bacopa monnieri*, possesses various pharmacological activities, including antioxidative (Kumar & Mondal, 2016) anti-inflammatory (Srivastav et al., 2017), antimicrobial, neuroprotective (Uabundit et al., 2010), and memory-enhancing (Morgan & Stevens, 2010) properties. Additionally, *Bacopa monnieri* extracts have demonstrated cognitive-enhancing abilities (Hazra et al., 2017; Kumar et al., 2016a). Research indicates that *Bacopa monnieri* extracts exhibit anti-parkinsonism effects in both transgenic and toxin-induced animal models, suggesting potential utility for Parkinson's disease treatment. In these models, *Bacopa monnieri* has shown protective effects against paraquat toxin by mitigating oxidative stress in both Drosophila and mice. Similar protective effects have been observed in Parkinson's disease models, where Drosophila treated with rotenone exhibited benefits from *Bacopa monnieri* extract supplementation, leading to reduced oxidative stress and apoptosis. In transgenic Parkinson's disease models, *Bacopa monnieri* extract supplementation decreased α-synuclein aggregation and minimized dopaminergic neuron degeneration. The extract has been shown to counteract the cytotoxic effects of rotenone on dopaminergic neurons by increasing antioxidant enzyme activity and restoring redox balance, thereby normalizing oxidative stress. Studies demonstrate that *Bacopa monnieri* supplementation decreases oxidative markers such as H_2O_2, protein carbonyl content, and malondialdehyde (Hosamani & Muralidhara, 2009). Furthermore, it enhances mitochondrial function by restoring the activity of electron transport chain complexes (Singh et al., 2012) and maintaining mitochondrial membrane potential (Ψm) and the activity of complex I in dopaminergic cell lines treated with paraquat and 1-methyl-4-phenyl-pyridinium iodide. *Bacopa monnieri* extract also elevates neurogenic gene expression in the substantia nigra region and enhances tyrosine hydroxylase activity. Studies on animal models of Parkinson's disease have shown that *Bacopa monnieri* extract can improve motor and locomotor activity, as well as cognitive function. Consequently, *Bacopa monnieri* exhibits promising properties as a potential monotherapy for Parkinson's disease. However, further studies are necessary to elucidate the mechanisms underlying its neuroprotective effects, indicating that *Bacopa monnieri* could be a valuable medicinal product for targeting Parkinson's disease.

Mucuna pruriens (Mp)

Mucuna pruriens, commonly known as velvet bean, is primarily utilized in the traditional Ayurvedic system of medicine. Recent findings have suggested its neuroprotective effects, making it a potential treatment for Parkinson's disease due to its levodopa content. However, current evidence indicates that its significance may extend beyond merely serving as an adjunct to levodopa therapy, highlighting the need to explore other bioactive compounds present in the seeds. Historically, *Mucuna pruriens* has been used for centuries in Ayurvedic medicine to alleviate symptoms of Parkinson's disease, underscoring its longstanding importance in managing this condition (Ovallath & Deepa, 2013a). Levodopa (Damodaran & Ramaswamy, 1937), the active compound found in *Mucuna pruriens* seeds, is a standard treatment for Parkinson's disease, yet its role might encompass more than just levodopa supplementation. Consequently, further studies are warranted to investigate the potential effects of other constituents within Mucuna pruriens seeds for treating Parkinson's disease. Therefore, more studies are required to examine the roles of other ingredients in *Mucuna pruriens* seed for Parkinson's disease. Research involving both human subjects (Singhal et al., 2003) and has demonstrated that incorporating *Mucuna pruriens* seeds into the diet enhances locomotor behavior. The plant's antioxidative and metal-chelating properties contribute to reducing oxidative stress and improving redox status. Additionally, the seed extract of *Mucuna pruriens* has been shown to enhance synaptic and mitochondrial functions essential for neuronal survival, as well as increase the expression of tyrosine hydroxylase in Parkinson's disease-affected mice and Drosophila. Studies indicate that *Mucuna pruriens* seed powder acts quickly and remains effective for an extended period without side effects. Notably, *Mucuna pruriens* seed extract has been reported to be a more effective treatment for Parkinson's disease than synthetic levodopa. This advantage may stem from other compounds present in the seeds that could help combat the disease. Thus, further research is essential to deepen our understanding of *Mucuna pruriens*. Comparisons between *Bacopa monnieri* extract and *Mucuna pruriens* seed extract have shown that *Bacopa monnieri* extract exhibits superior efficacy in mouse models.

Withania somnifera **or Ashwagandha**

Withania somnifera, commonly known as ashwagandha in Ayurveda, has been used as a restorative herb in India (Rai et al., 2016a). It is considered a potential nerve tonic that enhances memory and learning. *Withania somnifera* possesses significant therapeutic potential, with its roots containing antioxidant, anti-inflammatory, anti-carcinogenic (Rai et al., 2016b), anxiolytic-antidepressant (Bhattacharya et al., 2000), and memory-enhancing (Shivamurthy et al., 2016) properties. These characteristics underline its efficacy in managing Parkinson's disease. Research indicates that *Withania somnifera* root extract increases levels of glutathione and glutathione peroxidase, thereby normalizing oxidative stress in 1-methyl-4-phenyl-1,2,3,6-tetrahydropyridine (MPTP)-induced mouse models. *In vivo* studies have shown that *Withania somnifera* treatment leads to increased dopamine levels within the striatum. Additionally, a separate study utilizing a Maneb-parquat mouse model of Parkinson's disease demonstrated that ethanolic extract of *Withania somnifera* reduces inducible NO synthase expression and improves locomotor function in mice. Consequently, research using various Parkinson's disease models in mice illustrates the potential of *Withania somnifera* in preventing the progression of Parkinson's disease (De Rose et al., 2016).

Curcuma longa **or Tumeric**

Curcuma longa, commonly known as turmeric, has been used in traditional medicine for a long time to treat sprains and swelling resulting from injuries (Ammon & Wahl, 1991). Extensive research has demonstrated that *Curcuma longa* possesses significant therapeutic potential, evidenced by its antioxidative (Motterlini et al., 2000; Srivastava et al., 2016), anti-inflammatory (Surh et al., 2001), anti-microbial (Gunes et al., 2016), anti-carcinogenic (Allegra et al., 2017; Chaurasia et al., 2016a), and antidepressant (Chaurasia et al., 2016b) properties. Additionally, *Curcuma longa* exhibits neuroprotective effects against brain aging, neuronal death, behavioral abnormalities (Wang et al., 2005), and blood-brain barrier damage (Jiang et al., 2007). Moreover, studies have investigated its efficacy in neurodegenerative diseases such as Parkinson's and Alzheimer's. Research in rat models of Parkinson's disease has shown that curcumin, the active component of *Curcuma longa*, provides antioxidant benefits and increases striatal dopamine levels. Curcumin treatment protects against protein oxidation by mitigating the effects of glutathione depletion in dopaminergic neuronal cells and mice. It also maintains the activity of mitochondrial complex I (Jagatha et al., 2008), protects against nitrosamine stress, and prevents *in vitro* brain mitochondrial damage. Another study demonstrated that curcumin protects against neuronal abnormalities in the substantia nigra region of the brain in rat models of Parkinson's disease induced by 6-hydroxydopamine, reducing malondialdehyde levels while increasing superoxide dismutase and glutathione peroxidase levels. Furthermore, elevated levels of dopamine and acetylcholine were observed (Song et al., 2016). Recent studies have shown that pre-treatment with curcumin followed by exposure to paraquat in PINK1 siRNA cells resulted in enhanced mitochondrial respiration, ATP production, restoration of mitochondrial membrane potential, and decreased apoptosis (Van der Merwe et al., 2016). All the literature supports the potential effects of curcumin against Parkinson's disease. Additionally, curcumin-glucoside, a synthetic derivative of curcumin, can bind to α-synuclein in its oligomeric form, thereby preventing the further fibrillization of α-synuclein (Shrikanth Gadad et al., 2012). Based on these studies, *Curcuma longa* appears to be a promising candidate for managing Parkinson's disease, warranting further clinical studies for greater clarity.

Camellia sinensis

Teas made from *Camellia sinensis* are widely recognized for their diverse range, including green, black, oolong, and white teas. Black tea is the most popular variety, accounting for over 70% of all tea produced (Sharangi, 2009a). The beneficial value of tea is attributed to the various flavonoids and other antioxidants it contains, which contribute to its health-promoting properties. Dried and steamed *Camellia sinensis* leaves are used to prepare green tea (Cabrera et al., 2006), which demonstrates various beneficial properties. The polyphenols in *Camellia sinensis* exhibit antioxidative (Chan et al., 2007; Chen et al., 2008), anti-microbial (Chan et al., 2011), anti-inflammatory (Chen et al., 2012), anti-carcinogenic (Ravindranath et al., 2006), anti-arthritic (Kim et al., 2008), and neuroprotective (Boadas-Vaello & Verdú, 2015) effects. Studies suggest that *Camellia sinensis* supplementation may reduce the risk of Parkinson's disease (Tanaka et al., 2011). The active component, catechin, possesses antioxidative and iron-chelating capabilities, particularly epigallocatechin-3-gallate, which demonstrates neuroprotection in MPTP-induced animal models of Parkinson's disease. These effects are achieved by scavenging free radicals, which typically damage dopaminergic neurons in the striatum and midbrain (Guo et al., 2007). A notable study confirmed that the polyphenols found in *Camellia sinensis* protect mice's dopaminergic neurons from 1-methyl-4-phenylpyridinium (MPP+) toxicity by inhibiting the dopamine transporter, thereby preventing MPP+ uptake (Pan et al., 2003). Further research demonstrated that epigallocatechin gallate from *Camellia sinensis* suppresses inducible NO synthase in MPTP-induced models of Parkinson's disease (Kim et al., 2010). Recent studies in mouse models showed that epigallocatechin gallate protects dopaminergic neurons from MPTP toxicity by reducing oxidative stress and decreasing iron levels in the nigral area of the brain (Xu et al., 2016).

Black tea, the commonly consumed oxidized form of tea produced through fermentation, is recognized for its medicinal compound theaflavin (Sharangi, 2009b). The flavonoid content in theaflavin is comparable to the catechins found in green tea, and research has highlighted its anti-oxidative (Leung et al., 2001a), and neuroprotective properties (Joghataie et al., 2004). Studies show that black tea can protect dopaminergic neurons in a 6-hydroxydopamine-induced rat model, as evidenced by enhanced tyrosine hydroxylase expression in the substantia nigra region of the brain. Pre-treatment with black tea before 6-hydroxydopamine administration further enhances its neuroprotective effects (Chaturvedi et al., 2006). The mechanism behind theaflavin's neuroprotective properties remains unclear, although its potent antioxidant effect is recognized. Theaflavin has also been shown to increase the expression of tyrosine hydroxylase and dopamine transporter in the nigral region of the brain in C57BL/6 mice treated with MPTP. Additionally, it has demonstrated anti-apoptotic effects in the MPTP-induced mouse model of Parkinson's disease, indicated by a reduction in Caspase expression (Leung et al., 2001b). In a transgenic Drosophila model of Parkinson's disease expressing human α-synuclein, black tea consumption reduced oxidative stress and increased dopaminergic levels (Anandhan et al., 2012). Furthermore, black tea contains chlorogenic acid, which has been shown to elevate human total plasma homocysteine levels (Olthof et al., 2001). Elevated homocysteine levels have been associated with Parkinson's disease patients (Blandini et al., 2001), and may influence mitochondria-mediated neuronal cell death (Mattson & Shea, 2003).

Innovations of Phyto-Nanotechnology for the Treatment of Parkinson's Disease

Innovations in plant-based drug formulations for Parkinson's disease represent a significant advancement in precision drug delivery, with phytochemicals being better absorbed and utilized. This improvement is primarily due to the rise of nanofunctionalization in nanoparticles, which enhances the effectiveness and stability of phytomedicines, ensuring highly specific and potent treatment. Nanoscience, particularly in the field of plant-based nanoformulations, plays a crucial role in this process. Nanophyto therapeutics offer the potential to overcome the brain barriers, allowing for direct delivery of active agents to the brain, thereby optimizing treatment outcomes for neurodegenerative conditions like Parkinson's disease (Goldsmith et al., 2014). Furthermore, drug delivery methods based on nanotechnology employ various strategies to enhance cellular absorption. Liposomes, solid lipid nanoparticles, and polymeric nanoparticles, for instance, increase a drug's surface area and improve its ability to bind and penetrate cell membranes. These techniques also enhance the drug's stability in biological fluids, prolonging its residence time (Bhattacharya et al., 2022a). Nano phyto-technologies offer a key advantage in their ability to enhance a drug's permeability across the blood-brain barrier, increasing the likelihood of the drug reaching the brain directly. Due to the unique properties of nano formulations, such as optimal size, physico-chemical characteristics, and functional potential, they show significant promise in transporting drugs across the blood-brain barrier. Another critical factor is the metabolism of phytochemicals, which are plant-derived organic compounds believed to have therapeutic effects on Parkinson's disease. However, the pharmacokinetic properties of these phytochemicals limit their efficacy in treating Parkinson's. By encapsulating them in nanoparticles, their pharmacokinetic characteristics—such as prolonged circulation time, increased potency, and improved central nervous system penetration—can be enhanced. This may boost the therapeutic effectiveness of phytoherbs for Parkinson's disease through nanotechnology-based delivery methods (Burns et al., 2023a). In this context, numerous research studies have been conducted. A recent study on *Withania somnifera* demonstrated its ability to reduce stress, enhance motor function, and improve the quality of life in patients with Parkinson's disease (Jin et al., 2022a). Its potent antioxidant, anti-peroxidant, and free radical-quenching activities may help reduce oxidative stress associated with neurological disorders like Parkinson's disease. *Withania somnifera* has also shown strong protective effects against mitochondrial damage, a key factor linked to the etiology of Parkinson's disease (Wongtrakul et al., 2021). The neuroprotective effects of *Withania somnifera* in models of Parkinson's disease are attributed to the inhibition of apoptotic pathways, leading to improved motor function and a reduction in parkinsonian symptoms. Studies using an extract of *Withania somnifera* root have demonstrated significant behavioral and biochemical improvements in animal models of Parkinson's disease, highlighting the potency of this compound against the disease through multiple pathways (Lerose et al., 2024). Furthermore, *Bacopa monnieri* has been reported to be neuroprotective against the effects of oxidative stress and neurotoxicity in models of Parkinson's disease. The extract demonstrated an increase in lifespan, improved locomotor function, and protection of mitochondria from damage caused by oxidative stress in Parkinson's disease models. Through its anti-inflammatory properties, the extract may also reduce the neuroinflammation associated with Parkinson's disease (Siddique et al., 2014). It may help enhance memory and cognitive abilities in individuals with Parkinson's disease (Jin et al., 2022b). Moreover, the seeds of *Mucuna pruriens* have a high concentration of levodopa, which has been utilized since ancient times in Ayurvedic medicine to treat symptoms associated with Parkinson's disease. Extracts of *Mucuna pruriens*, with their favorable pharmacokinetic profile, may help alleviate motor symptoms of Parkinson's disease and reduce the risk and severity of dyskinesias (Ovallath & Deepa, 2013b). Its anti-inflammatory activity contributes to decreasing astrocyte reactivity related to Parkinson's disease. It also protects against nephrotoxicity and enhances neurological activity (Rai et al., 2017). Ultimately, all the innovations demonstrate that nanoparticle-based herbal formulations hold the potential to maximize the efficacy of phytochemical deliveries, such as *Withania somnifera*, *Bacopa monnieri*, and *Mucuna pruriens*, in the treatment of Parkinson's disease. These phytochemicals exhibit neuroprotective, antioxidant, and anti-inflammatory properties and can be used in managing and reducing the progression of Parkinson's disease.

Clinical Translation

According to prior studies, the symptoms of Parkinson's disease are primarily caused by neurodegeneration in the nigrostriatal pathway, which connects the substantia nigra pars compacta in the midbrain to the dorsal striatum. Several theories explain this neurological deterioration. Neurodegeneration in Parkinson's disease may result from a combination of various factors, including apoptosis, immune response mechanisms, abnormalities in proteolysis, oxidative stress, disrupted mitochondria, disorders related to iron metabolism, and misfolded proteins (Pan et al., 2008). Currently, there are no conclusive studies available for a verified diagnostic method for Parkinson's disease. Nonetheless, the initial diagnostic parameters are clinical characteristics, which include the cardinal motor features previously mentioned. Clinical symptoms of Parkinson's disease can overlap with those of other syndromes, making early diagnosis difficult (Tolosa et al., 2006). Studies have shown that certain herbs are more reliable and effective than conventional medications. In Ayurveda, velvet bean is a popular herb used to treat Parkinson's disease (Katzenschlager, 2004). The Mucuna plant possesses therapeutic qualities in all its parts, and studies on M. pruriens extracts have demonstrated a wide range of pharmacological effects, including neuroprotective, anti-inflammatory, anti-diabetic, and antioxidant properties (Lampariello et al., 2012). At four distinct dosages, *Mucuna pruriens* has shown no observable toxic effects, either acute or chronic, in mice or rodents. Furthermore, its effectiveness has been validated in the intrastriatal 6-hydroxydopamine Parkinsonian animal model, which is used to induce symptoms resembling Parkinson's disease by killing dopaminergic neurons in the striatum. This research into the nasal drug delivery system, which bypasses the blood-brain barrier and hepatic first-pass effect, is intensively pursued due to its convenience and non-intrusive nature. It has become essential to assess *Mucuna pruriens* bioavailability, safety, and effectiveness as an antiparkinsonian agent (Hussian & Manyam, 1997). Clinical trials comparing *Mucuna pruriens* to levodopa in terms of safety and efficacy have been conducted. These studies demonstrate that *Mucuna pruriens* is not inferior to levodopa based on all safety and efficacy outcome measures, and it is more tolerable. Specifically, compared to an equivalent dosage of levodopa prepared pharmaceutically alone, high-dose *Mucuna pruriens* powder produced noticeably fewer adverse effects (Cilia et al., 2017). The potential of using *Withania somnifera* (Ashwagandha) in the treatment of Parkinson's disease has also been examined, and several preclinical investigations have been conducted. According to these studies, ashwagandha can help improve impaired dopaminergic activity and dopamine depletion, restore antioxidant capacity, and enhance motor movements in mice. It can also counteract Parkinson-like symptoms. By enhancing motor function and lowering catalase peaks while raising nitrite and lipid oxidation levels, ashwagandha has been shown to have a neuro-ameliorative effect on Parkinsonian mouse models (Zahiruddin et al., 2020). However, there are currently not enough human-based clinical trials to evaluate the well-being status of ashwagandha. Although some studies have been conducted on humans with Parkinson's disease, it remains challenging to conclude whether the herbal remedy ashwagandha can effectively treat the disease. Many studies tend to incorporate ashwagandha into broader formulas that include other herbs (i.e., polyherbal formulations). In a trial involving patients with Parkinson's disease, ashwagandha root extract was administered, resulting in various observed pharmacological effects. The study group received 300 mg of ashwagandha root extract twice daily for eight weeks, while the control group received placebo capsules. Outcome measures in subjects included memory, visual perception, brain control, and focus abilities. The findings showed that ashwagandha root extract significantly enhanced several cognitive functioning domains (Choudhary et al., 2017). Consequently, more investigation is required to confirm the therapeutic efficacy and clinical translation of ashwagandha for the management of Parkinson's disease (Dar & MuzamilAhmad, 2020). The current issues with ashwagandha in Parkinson's disease highlight the need for further research to evaluate its therapeutic efficacy. Moreover, the neuroprotective properties, anti-aging effects, and potential to enhance cognitive function of *Bacopa monnieri* extract are drawing the attention of researchers. Studies on *Bacopa monnieri* extract have revealed its anti-inflammatory, antioxidative, and mitochondrial properties through preclinical research. The ongoing issues with ashwagandha in Parkinson's disease necessitate more studies to evaluate its therapeutic efficacy. *Bacopa monnieri* has demonstrated promising potential to preserve the body's basic vitality while providing neuroprotection. The extract comprises various phytoconstituents, including flavonoids, alkaloids, bacosides, and saponins. These phytoconstituents have been shown to enhance *Bacopa monnieri* extract's antioxidative, behavioral, and cognitive abilities (Abdul Manap et al., 2019). *Bacopa monnieri* has been included in several clinical trials involving human participants to enhance cognitive function. In one study, serum calcium levels and memory tests significantly improved in 60 medical students from Government Medical College, Nagpur, India, after taking a standardized 150 mg extract of Bacopa monnieri for 15 days (Kumar et al., 2016b). *Furthermore, Bacopa monnieri* not only improves cognition but also enhances learning capacity. At the University of Wollongong in Australia, 76 participants aged 40 to 65 experienced significant improvements in their ability to retain new information after consuming Bacopa monnieri for three months (Roodenrys, 2002). Numerous *in vitro* studies have been conducted, showing good therapeutic efficacy and synergistic effects as illustrated in Table 1. However, clinical trials still need to be conducted to ensure the safety profile of nanophytoherbs.

Table 1. Effects of nano-phytomedicines on *in vitro* Parkinson's disease models

Nano-Phytomedicine	PD Model	Effects observed	Reference
Curcumin nanoparticles	PC12 cells	Reduced α-synuclein aggregation	(Zhao et al., 2018)
Resveratrol-loaded nanoparticles	SH-SY5Y cells	Enhanced neuroprotection in MPP+-induced	(Niblett et al., 2017)
Quercetin-loaded nanoemulsion	SH-SY5Y cells	Improved antioxidant activity in 6-OHDA-treated SH-SY5Y cells	(Ferreira et al., 2020)
Naringenin-loaded chitosan nanoparticles	SH-SY5Y cells	Decreased oxidative stress in rotenone-induced SH-SY5Y cells	(Marcuello et al., 2020)
Berberine-loaded liposomes	PC12 cells	Reduced α-synuclein aggregation	(Ambardekar et al., 2018)

Future Perspectives and Biosafety

Research on Parkinson's disease is anticipated to focus on several key areas to improve diagnosis, therapies, and management. Various studies have been conducted to develop techniques targeting neuroinflammation and mitochondrial dysfunction to prevent the progression of this medical condition. Future investigations into nano-phytomedicines and nanoparticle delivery systems could yield more precise and potent treatments for Parkinson's disease, enhancing drug delivery across the blood-brain barrier and improving treatment outcomes (Burns et al., 2023b). Nanotechnology holds the potential to revolutionize the treatment of Parkinson's disease by facilitating the delivery of more clinically effective agents to the brain (Bhattacharya et al., 2022b). A meta-analysis study has shown a complementary effect in Parkinson's disease patients using phytomedicines alongside synthetic medications. Despite their promising in vitro efficacy, the pharmacokinetic properties of phytomedicines require further development. Challenges include stability, lipophilicity, and molecular size, which may limit their effectiveness *in vivo* (Shan et al., 2018; Gunasekaran et al., 2014). For phytoherbs to be integrated into clinical practice, more research is needed to evaluate their effectiveness, safety, and mechanisms of action in Parkinson's disease. Addressing clinical application, production, biocompatibility, and pricing will be essential for advancing nano-phytomedicine as a potential treatment for Parkinson's disease (Sainz et al., 2015; Hua et al., 2018). Current research is concentrating on developing safe and efficient methods for clinical applications of nanotechnology-based phytochemical delivery systems in Parkinson's disease. Further investigation and clinical trials are necessary to confirm the effectiveness, safety, and therapeutic potential of these natural substances and innovative delivery methods for treating Parkinson's disease (Balakrishnan et al., 2021).

Conclusion

Combining phytoherbs with nanotechnology presents a promising strategy for treating Parkinson's disease. Nanotechnology offers innovative methods to enhance phytochemical delivery to the brain, significantly improving the bioavailability and therapeutic effectiveness of these compounds. Literature surveys on current studies involving nano-phytoconstituents indicate that these technologies have shown neuroprotective effects in animal models of Parkinson's disease, effectively reducing motor symptoms and protecting against key characteristics of the disease, such as α-synuclein aggregation, mitochondrial dysfunction, and dopaminergic neuronal death. Nanoparticles have demonstrated the ability to enhance the transport of phytochemicals across the blood-brain barrier, enabling targeted delivery to the brain and potentially improving treatment outcomes for Parkinson's disease. Encapsulating herbal extracts in nanoparticle form is an effective approach to maximizing the therapeutic efficacy of treatments aimed at this condition. Various phyto-constituents have been identified as beneficial in treating neurological disorders. For example, studies on the extract of Mucuna pruriens have revealed antioxidant properties that exhibit synergistic effects in managing Parkinson's patients. Similarly, Ashwagandha roots have shown a range of benefits, including antioxidant, anti-inflammatory, anxiolytic, antidepressant, anti-carcinogenic, and memory-enhancing qualities. The application of nanoparticles for delivering phytochemicals derived from plants is known as nano-phytomedicine, which has shown promise in enhancing therapeutic effectiveness. Numerous nano phytoconstituents, such as quercetin and epigallocatechin, have been utilized without significant side effects. Ongoing research indicates the potential for developing more targeted and effective therapeutic strategies through the application of nanotechnology in the treatment of Parkinson's disease. By leveraging the unique properties of nanoparticles, researchers can optimize drug delivery, enhance drug efficacy, and minimize off-target effects. To fully realize the potential of nano-phytomedicines in improving the management and outcomes of Parkinson's disease, further research and development in this area are essential.

References

Abbott, N. J., & Romero, I. A. (1996). Transporting therapeutics across the blood-brain barrier. *Molecular Medicine Today*, *2*(3), 106–113. https://doi.org/10.1016/1357-4310(96)88720-X.

Abdul Manap, A. S., Vijayabalan, S., Madhavan, P., Chia, Y. Y., Arya, A., Wong, E. H., Rizwan, F., Bindal, U., & Koshy, S. (2019). *Bacopa monnieri*, a Neuroprotective Lead in Alzheimer Disease: A Review on Its Properties, Mechanisms of Action, and Preclinical and Clinical Studies. *Drug Target Insights*, *13*, 117739281986641. https://doi.org/10.1177/1177392819866412.

Allegra, A., Innao, V., Russo, S., Gerace, D., Alonci, A., & Musolino, C. (2017). Anticancer Activity of Curcumin and Its Analogues: Preclinical and Clinical Studies. *Cancer Investigation*, *35*(1), 1–22. https://doi.org/10.1080/07357907.2016.1247166.

Ambardekar, V. V., Wakaskar, R. R., Ye, Z., Curran, S. M., McGuire, T. R., Coulter, D. W., Singh, R. K., & Vetro, J. A. (2018). Complexation of Chol-DsiRNA in place of Chol-siRNA greatly increases the duration of mRNA suppression by polyplexes of PLL(30)-PEG(5K) in primary murine syngeneic breast tumors after i.v. administration. *International Journal of Pharmaceutics*, *543*(1–2), 130–138. https://doi.org/10.1016/j.ijpharm.2018.03.045.

Ammon, H., & Wahl, M. (1991). Pharmacology of *Curcuma longa*. *Planta Medica*, *57*(01), 1–7. https://doi.org/10.1055/s-2006-960004.

Anandhan, A., Tamilselvam, K., Radhiga, T., Rao, S., Essa, M. M., & Manivasagam, T. (2012). Theaflavin, a black tea polyphenol, protects nigral dopaminergic neurons against chronic MPTP/probenecid induced Parkinson's disease. *Brain Research*, *1433*, 104–113. https://doi.org/10.1016/j.brainres.2011.11.021.

Balakrishnan, R., Azam, S., Cho, D. Y., Su-Kim, I., & Choi, D. K. (2021). Natural Phytochemicals as Novel Therapeutic Strategies to Prevent and Treat Parkinson's Disease: Current Knowledge and Future Perspectives. *Oxidative Medicine and Cellular Longevity*, *2021*, 1–32. https://doi.org/10.1155/2021/6680935.

Benabid, A. L., Chabardes, S., Mitrofanis, J., & Pollak, P. (2009). Deep brain stimulation of the subthalamic nucleus for the treatment of Parkinson's disease. *The Lancet Neurology*, *8*(1), 67–81. https://doi.org/10.1016/S1474-4422(08)70291-6.

Bhattacharya, S. K., Bhattacharya, A., Sairam, K., & Ghosal, S. (2000). Anxiolytic-antidepressant activity of Withania somnifera glycowithanolides: an experimental study. *Phytomedicine*, *7*(6), 463–469. https://doi.org/10.1016/S0944-7113(00)80030-6.

Bhattacharya, T., Soares, G. A. B. e, Chopra, H., Rahman, Md. M., Hasan, Z., Swain, S. S., & Cavalu, S. (2022a). Applications of Phyto-Nanotechnology for the Treatment of Neurodegenerative Disorders. *Materials*, *15*(3), 804. https://doi.org/10.3390/ma15030804.

Bhattacharya, T., Soares, G. A. B. e, Chopra, H., Rahman, Md. M., Hasan, Z., Swain, S. S., & Cavalu, S. (2022b). Applications of Phyto-Nanotechnology for the Treatment of Neurodegenerative Disorders. *Materials*, *15*(3), 804. https://doi.org/10.3390/ma15030804

Blandini, F., Fancellu, R., Martignoni, E., Mangiagalli, A., Pacchetti, C., Samuele, A., & Nappi, G. (2001). Plasma Homocysteine and l-DOPA Metabolism in Patients with Parkinson Disease. *Clinical Chemistry*, *47*(6), 1102–1104. https://doi.org/10.1093/clinchem/47.6.1102.

Boadas-Vaello, P., & Verdú, E. (2015). Epigallocatechin-3-gallate treatment to promote neuroprotection and functional recovery after nervous system injury. *Neural Regeneration Research*, *10*(9), 1390. https://doi.org/10.4103/1673-5374.165502.

Bovolenta, T. M., de Azevedo Silva, S. M. C., Arb Saba, R., Borges, V., Ferraz, H. B., & Felicio, A. C. (2017). Systematic Review and Critical Analysis of Cost Studies Associated with Parkinson's Disease. *Parkinson's Disease*, *2017*, 1–11. https://doi.org/10.1155/2017/3410946.

Burns, J., Buck, A. C., D' Souza, S., Dube, A., & Bardien, S. (2023a). Nanophytomedicines as Therapeutic Agents for Parkinson's Disease. *ACS Omega*, *8*(45), 42045–42061. https://doi.org/10.1021/acsomega.3c04862.

Burns, J., Buck, A. C., D' Souza, S., Dube, A., & Bardien, S. (2023b). Nanophytomedicines as Therapeutic Agents for Parkinson's Disease. *ACS Omega*, *8*(45), 42045–42061. https://doi.org/10.1021/acsomega.3c04862.

Cabrera, C., Artacho, R., & Giménez, R. (2006). Beneficial Effects of Green Tea—A Review. *Journal of the American College of Nutrition*, *25*(2), 79–99. https://doi.org/10.1080/07315724.2006.10719518.

Chan, E. W. C., Lim, Y. Y., & Chew, Y. L. (2007). Antioxidant activity of Camellia sinensis leaves and tea from a lowland plantation in Malaysia. *Food Chemistry*, *102*(4), 1214–1222. https://doi.org/10.1016/j.foodchem.2006.07.009.

Chan, EricW. C., Tie, P., Soh, E., & Law, Y. (2011). Antioxidant and antibacterial properties of green, black, and herbal teas of Camellia sinensis. *Pharmacognosy Research*, *3*(4), 266. https://doi.org/10.4103/0974-8490.89748.

Chaturvedi, R. K., Shukla, S., Seth, K., Chauhan, S., Sinha, C., Shukla, Y., & Agrawal, A. K. (2006). Neuroprotective and neurorescue effect of black tea extract in 6-hydroxydopamine-lesioned rat model of Parkinson's disease. *Neurobiology of Disease*, *22*(2), 421–434. https://doi.org/10.1016/j.nbd.2005.12.008.

Chaurasia, S., Chaubey, P., Patel, R. R., Kumar, N., & Mishra, B. (2016a). Curcumin-polymeric nanoparticles against colon-26 tumor-bearing mice: cytotoxicity, pharmacokinetic and anticancer efficacy studies. *Drug Development and Industrial Pharmacy*, *42*(5), 694–700. https://doi.org/10.3109/03639045.2015.1064941.

Chaurasia, S., Chaubey, P., Patel, R. R., Kumar, N., & Mishra, B. (2016b). Curcumin-polymeric nanoparticles against colon-26 tumor-bearing mice: cytotoxicity, pharmacokinetic and anticancer efficacy studies. *Drug*

Development and Industrial Pharmacy, *42*(5), 694–700. https://doi.org/10.3109/03639045.2015.1064941.

Chen, B.-T., Li, W.-X., He, R.-R., Li, Y.-F., Tsoi, B., Zhai, Y.-J., & Kurihara, H. (2012). Anti-Inflammatory Effects of a Polyphenols-Rich Extract from Tea (*Camellia sinensis*) Flowers in Acute and Chronic Mice Models. *Oxidative Medicine and Cellular Longevity*, *2012*, 1–7. https://doi.org/10.1155/2012/537923.

Chen, H., Zhang, M., Qu, Z., & Xie, B. (2008). Antioxidant activities of different fractions of polysaccharide conjugates from green tea (Camellia Sinensis). *Food Chemistry*, *106*(2), 559–563. https://doi.org/10.1016/j.foodchem.2007.06.040.

Chopra, H., Goyal, R., Agarwal, N., Mishra, D., & Gautam, R. K. (2023). Edible Mushroom assisted synthesis and applications of metal nanoparticles: A comprehensive review. Journal of Integrated Science and Technology, 11(1), 427-427. https://pubs.thesciencein.org/journal/index.php/jist/article/view/427.

Choudhary, D., Bhattacharyya, S., & Bose, S. (2017). Efficacy and Safety of Ashwagandha (*Withania somnifera* (L.) *Dunal*) Root Extract in Improving Memory and Cognitive Functions. *Journal of Dietary Supplements*, *14*(6), 599–612. https://doi.org/10.1080/19390211.2017.1284970.

Cilia, R., Laguna, J., Cassani, E., Cereda, E., Pozzi, N. G., Isaias, I. U., Contin, M., Barichella, M., & Pezzoli, G. (2017). *Mucuna pruriens* in Parkinson disease. *Neurology*, *89*(5), 432–438. https://doi.org/10.1212/WNL.0000000000004175.

Damodaran, M., & Ramaswamy, R. (1937). Isolation of *l* -3:4-dihydroxyphenylalanine from the seeds of *Mucuna pruriens*. *Biochemical Journal*, *31*(12), 2149–2152. https://doi.org/10.1042/bj0312149.

Dar, N. J., & MuzamilAhmad. (2020). Neurodegenerative diseases and Withania somnifera (L.): An update. *Journal of Ethnopharmacology*, *256*, 112769. https://doi.org/10.1016/j.jep.2020.112769.

De Rose, F., Marotta, R., Poddighe, S., Talani, G., Catelani, T., Setzu, M. D., Solla, P., Marrosu, F., Sanna, E., Kasture, S., Acquas, E., & Liscia, A. (2016). Functional and Morphological Correlates in the Drosophila LRRK2 loss-of-function Model of Parkinson's Disease: Drug Effects of Withania somnifera (Dunal) Administration. *PLOS ONE*, *11*(1), e0146140. https://doi.org/10.1371/journal.pone.0146140.

Driver, J. A., Logroscino, G., Gaziano, J. M., & Kurth, T. (2009). Incidence and remaining lifetime risk of Parkinson disease in advanced age. *Neurology*, *72*(5), 432–438. https://doi.org/10.1212/01.wnl.0000341769.50075.bb.

Ferreira, L. A. B., dos Reis, S. B., do Nascimento da Silva, E., Cadore, S., Bernardes, J. da S., Durán, N., & de Jesus, M. B. (2020). Thiol-antioxidants interfere with assessing silver nanoparticle cytotoxicity. *Nanomedicine: Nanotechnology, Biology and Medicine*, *24*, 102130. https://doi.org/10.1016/j.nano.2019.102130.

Goldsmith, M., Abramovitz, L., & Peer, D. (2014). Precision Nanomedicine in Neurodegenerative Diseases. *ACS Nano*, *8*(3), 1958–1965. https://doi.org/10.1021/nn501292z.

Gunasekaran, T., Haile, T., Nigusse, T., & Dhanaraju, M. D. (2014). Nanotechnology: an effective tool for enhancing bioavailability and bioactivity of phytomedicine. *Asian Pacific Journal of Tropical Biomedicine*, *4*, S1–S7. https://doi.org/10.12980/APJTB.4.2014C980.

Gunes, H., Gulen, D., Mutlu, R., Gumus, A., Tas, T., & Topkaya, A. E. (2016). Antibacterial effects of curcumin. *Toxicology and Industrial Health*, *32*(2), 246–250. https://doi.org/10.1177/0748233713498458.

Guo, S., Yan, J., Yang, T., Yang, X., Bezard, E., & Zhao, B. (2007). Protective Effects of Green Tea Polyphenols in the 6-OHDA Rat Model of Parkinson's Disease Through Inhibition of ROS-NO Pathway. *Biological Psychiatry*, *62*(12), 1353–1362. https://doi.org/10.1016/j.biopsych.2007.04.020.

Hazra, S., Kumar, S., Saha, G. K., & Mondal, A. C. (2017). Reversion of BDNF, Akt and CREB in Hippocampus of Chronic Unpredictable Stress Induced Rats: Effects of Phytochemical, *Bacopa Monnieri*. *Psychiatry Investigation*, *14*(1), 74. https://doi.org/10.4306/pi.2017.14.1.74.

Hosamani, R., & Muralidhara. (2009). Neuroprotective efficacy of Bacopa monnieri against rotenone induced oxidative stress and neurotoxicity in Drosophila melanogaster. *NeuroToxicology*, *30*(6), 977–985. https://doi.org/10.1016/j.neuro.2009.08.012.

Hua, S., de Matos, M. B. C., Metselaar, J. M., & Storm, G. (2018). Current Trends and Challenges in the Clinical Translation of Nanoparticulate Nanomedicines: Pathways for Translational Development and Commercialization. *Frontiers in Pharmacology*, *9*. https://doi.org/10.3389/fphar.2018.00790.

Hussian, G., & Manyam, B. V. (1997). Mucuna pruriens proves more effective thanl-DOPA in Parkinson's disease animal model. *Phytotherapy Research*, *11*(6), 419–423. https://doi.org/10.1002/(SICI)1099-1573(199709)11:6<419::AID-PTR120>3.0.CO;2-Q.

Jagatha, B., Mythri, R. B., Vali, S., & Bharath, M. M. S. (2008). Curcumin treatment alleviates the effects of glutathione depletion *in vitro* and *in vivo*: Therapeutic implications for Parkinson's disease explained via in silico studies. *Free Radical Biology and Medicine*, *44*(5), 907–917. https://doi.org/10.1016/j.freeradbiomed.2007.11.011.

Jiang, J., Wang, W., Sun, Y. J., Hu, M., Li, F., & Zhu, D. Y. (2007). Neuroprotective effect of curcumin on focal cerebral ischemic rats by preventing blood–brain barrier damage. *European Journal of Pharmacology*, *561*(1–3), 54–62. https://doi.org/10.1016/j.ejphar.2006.12.028.

Jin, C., Cho, K.-H., Kwon, S., Lee, H.-G., Kim, T.-H., Jung, W.-S., Moon, S.-K., Cho, S.-Y., Kang, B.-K., Park, J.-M., Park, H.-J., & Ko, C.-N. (2022a). Effectiveness and safety of herbal medicine Ukgansan for clinical symptoms in Parkinson's disease: A pilot, randomized, assessor-blinded clinical trial. *Frontiers in Neurology*, *13*. https://doi.org/10.3389/fneur.2022.1025269.

Jin, C., Cho, K. H., Kwon, S., Lee, H. G., Kim, T. H., Jung, W. S., Moon, S. K., Cho, S. Y., Kang, B. K., Park, J. M., Park, H. J., & Ko, C.-N. (2022b). Effectiveness and safety of herbal medicine Ukgansan for clinical symptoms in Parkinson's disease: A pilot, randomized, assessor-blinded clinical trial. *Frontiers in Neurology*, *13*. https://doi.org/10.3389/fneur.2022.1025269.

Joghataie, M. T., Roghani, M., Negahdar, F., & Hashemi, L. (2004). Protective effect of caffeine against neurodegeneration in a model of Parkinson's disease in rat: behavioral and histochemical evidence. *Parkinsonism & Related Disorders*, *10*(8), 465–468. https://doi.org/10.1016/j.parkreldis.2004.06.004.

Katzenschlager, R. (2004). Mucuna pruriens in Parkinson's disease: a double blind clinical and pharmacological study. *Journal of Neurology, Neurosurgery & Psychiatry*, *75*(12), 1672–1677. https://doi.org/10.1136/jnnp.2003.028761.

Kim, H. R., Rajaiah, R., Wu, Q. L., Satpute, S. R., Tan, M. T., Simon, J. E., Berman, B. M., & Moudgil, K. D. (2008). Green Tea Protects Rats against Autoimmune Arthritis by Modulating Disease-Related Immune Events. *The Journal of Nutrition*, *138*(11), 2111–2116. https://doi.org/10.3945/jn.108.089912.

Kim, J. S., Kim, J. M., O, J. J., & Jeon, B. S. (2010). Inhibition of inducible nitric oxide synthase expression and cell death by (−)-epigallocatechin-3-gallate, a green tea catechin, in the 1-methyl-4-phenyl-1,2,3,6-tetrahydropyridine mouse model of Parkinson's disease. *Journal of Clinical Neuroscience*, *17*(9), 1165–1168. https://doi.org/10.1016/j.jocn.2010.01.042.

Kumar, N., Abichandani, L. G., Thawani, V., Gharpure, K. J., Naidu, M. U. R., & Venkat Ramana, G. (2016a). Efficacy of Standardized Extract of *Bacopa monnieri* (Bacognize®) on Cognitive Functions of Medical Students: A Six-Week, Randomized Placebo-Controlled Trial. *Evidence-Based Complementary and Alternative Medicine*, *2016*, 1–8. https://doi.org/10.1155/2016/4103423.

Kumar, N., Abichandani, L. G., Thawani, V., Gharpure, K. J., Naidu, M. U. R., & Venkat Ramana, G. (2016b). Efficacy of Standardized Extract of *Bacopa monnieri* (Bacognize®) on Cognitive Functions of Medical Students: A Six-Week, Randomized Placebo-Controlled Trial. *Evidence-Based Complementary and Alternative Medicine*, *2016*, 1–8. https://doi.org/10.1155/2016/4103423.

Kumar, S., & Mondal, A. C. (2016). Neuroprotective, Neurotrophic and Anti-oxidative Role of Bacopa monnieri on CUS Induced Model of Depression in Rat. *Neurochemical Research*, *41*(11), 3083–3094. https://doi.org/10.1007/s11064-016-2029-3.

Lampariello, L. R., Cortelazzo, A., Guerranti, R., Sticozzi, C., & Valacchi, G. (2012). The Magic Velvet Bean of Mucuna pruriens. *Journal of Traditional and Complementary Medicine*, *2*(4), 331–339. https://doi.org/10.1016/S2225-4110(16)30119-5.

Lerose, V., Ponticelli, M., Benedetto, N., Carlucci, V., Lela, L., Tzvetkov, N. T., & Milella, L. (2024). Withania somnifera (L.) Dunal, a Potential Source of Phytochemicals for Treating Neurodegenerative Diseases: A Systematic Review. *Plants*, *13*(6), 771. https://doi.org/10.3390/plants13060771.

Leung, L. K., Su, Y., Zhang, Z., Chen, Z.-Y., Huang, Y., & Chen, R. (2001a). Theaflavins in Black Tea and Catechins in Green Tea Are Equally Effective Antioxidants. *The Journal of Nutrition*, *131*(9), 2248–2251. https://doi.org/10.1093/jn/131.9.2248.

Leung, L. K., Su, Y., Zhang, Z., Chen, Z.-Y., Huang, Y., & Chen, R. (2001b). Theaflavins in Black Tea and Catechins in Green Tea Are Equally Effective Antioxidants. *The Journal of Nutrition*, *131*(9), 2248–2251. https://doi.org/10.1093/jn/131.9.2248.

Marcuello, C., Foulon, L., Chabbert, B., Aguié-Béghin, V., & Molinari, M. (2020). Atomic force microscopy reveals how relative humidity impacts the Young's modulus of lignocellulosic polymers and their adhesion with cellulose nanocrystals at the nanoscale. *International Journal of Biological Macromolecules*, *147*, 1064–1075. https://doi.org/10.1016/j.ijbiomac.2019.10.074.

Mattson, M. P., & Shea, T. B. (2003). Folate and homocysteine metabolism in neural plasticity and neurodegenerative disorders. *Trends in Neurosciences*, *26*(3), 137–146. https://doi.org/10.1016/S0166-2236(03)00032-8.

Morgan, A., & Stevens, J. (2010). Does *Bacopa monnieri* Improve Memory Performance in Older Persons? Results of a Randomized, Placebo-Controlled, Double-Blind Trial. *The Journal of Alternative and Complementary Medicine*, *16*(7), 753–759. https://doi.org/10.1089/acm.2009.0342.

Motterlini, R., Foresti, R., Bassi, R., & Green, C. J. (2000). Curcumin, an antioxidant and anti-inflammatory agent, induces heme oxygenase-1 and protects endothelial cells against oxidative stress. *Free Radical Biology and Medicine*, *28*(8), 1303–1312. https://doi.org/10.1016/S0891-5849(00)00294-X.

New Study Shows the Economic Burden of Parkinson's Disease Double Previous Estimates | Parkinson's Foundation. (n.d.). Retrieved April 25, 2024, from https://www.parkinson.org/about-us/news/economic-burden-of-parkinsons-disease-study.

Niblett, D., Porter, S., Reynolds, G., Morgan, T., Greenamoyer, J., Hach, R., Sido, S., Karan, K., & Gabbott, I. (2017). Development and evaluation of a dimensionless mechanistic pan coating model for the prediction of coated tablet appearance. *International Journal of Pharmaceutics*, *528*(1–2), 180–201. https://doi.org/10.1016/j.ijpharm.2017.05.060.

Olthof, M. R., Hollman, P. C., Zock, P. L., & Katan, M. B. (2001). Consumption of high doses of chlorogenic acid, present in coffee, or of black tea increases plasma total homocysteine concentrations in humans. *The American Journal of Clinical Nutrition*, *73*(3), 532–538. https://doi.org/10.1093/ajcn/73.3.532.

Ovallath, S., & Deepa, P. (2013a). The history of parkinsonism: Descriptions in ancient Indian medical literature. *Movement Disorders*, *28*(5), 566–568. https://doi.org/10.1002/mds.25420.

Ovallath, S., & Deepa, P. (2013b). The history of parkinsonism: Descriptions in ancient Indian medical literature. *Movement Disorders*, *28*(5), 566–568. https://doi.org/10.1002/mds.25420.

Pan, T., Fei, J., Zhou, X., Jankovic, J., & Le, W. (2003). Effects of green tea polyphenols on dopamine uptake and on MPP+-induced dopamine neuron injury. *Life Sciences*, *72*(9), 1073–1083. https://doi.org/10.1016/S0024-3205(02)02347-0.

Pan, T., Kondo, S., Le, W., & Jankovic, J. (2008). The role of autophagy-lysosome pathway in neurodegeneration associated with Parkinson's disease. *Brain*, *131*(8), 1969–1978. https://doi.org/10.1093/brain/awm318.

Pardeshi, C. V., Rajput, P. V., Belgamwar, V. S., & Tekade, A. R. (2012). Formulation, optimization and evaluation of spray-dried mucoadhesive microspheres as intranasal carriers for Valsartan. *Journal of Microencapsulation*, *29*(2), 103–114. https://doi.org/10.3109/02652048.2011.630106.

Parkinson disease. (n.d.). Retrieved April 25, 2024, from https://www.who.int/news-room/fact-sheets/detail/parkinson-disease.

Rai, M., Jogee, P. S., Agarkar, G., & Santos, C. A. dos. (2016a). Anticancer activities of *Withania somnifera*: Current research, formulations, and future perspectives. *Pharmaceutical Biology*, *54*(2), 189–197. https://doi.org/10.3109/13880209.2015.1027778.

Rai, M., Jogee, P. S., Agarkar, G., & Santos, C. A. dos. (2016b). Anticancer activities of *Withania somnifera*: Current research, formulations, and future perspectives. *Pharmaceutical Biology*, *54*(2), 189–197. https://doi.org/10.3109/13880209.2015.1027778.

Rai, S. N., Birla, H., Singh, S. S., Zahra, W., Patil, R. R., Jadhav, J. P., Gedda, M. R., & Singh, S. P. (2017). Mucuna pruriens Protects against MPTP Intoxicated Neuroinflammation in Parkinson's Disease through NF-κB/pAKT Signaling Pathways. *Frontiers in Aging Neuroscience*, *9*. https://doi.org/10.3389/fnagi.2017.00421.

Ravindranath, M. H., Saravanan, T. S., Monteclaro, C. C., Presser, N., Ye, X., Selvan, S. R., & Brosman, S. (2006). Epicatechins Purified from Green Tea (Camellia sinensis) Differentially Suppress Growth of

Gender-Dependent Human Cancer Cell Lines. *Evidence-Based Complementary and Alternative Medicine*, *3*(2), 237–247. https://doi.org/10.1093/ecam/nel003.

Roney, C., Kulkarni, P., Arora, V., Antich, P., Bonte, F., Wu, A., Mallikarjuana, N. N., Manohar, S., Liang, H.-F., Kulkarni, A. R., Sung, H.-W., Sairam, M., & Aminabhavi, T. M. (2005). Targeted nanoparticles for drug delivery through the blood–brain barrier for Alzheimer's disease. *Journal of Controlled Release*, *108*(2–3), 193–214. https://doi.org/10.1016/j.jconrel.2005.07.024.

Roodenrys, S. (2002). Chronic Effects of Brahmi (Bacopa monnieri) on Human Memory. *Neuropsychopharmacology*, *27*(2), 279–281. https://doi.org/10.1016/S0893-133X(01)00419-5.

Sainz, V., Conniot, J., Matos, A. I., Peres, C., Zupanðið, E., Moura, L., Silva, L. C., Florindo, H. F., & Gaspar, R. S. (2015). Regulatory aspects on nanomedicines. *Biochemical and Biophysical Research Communications*, *468*(3), 504–510. https://doi.org/10.1016/j.bbrc.2015.08.023.

Shan, C. S., Xu, Q. Q., Shi, Y. H., Wang, Y., He, Z. X., & Zheng, G. Q. (2018). Chuanxiong Formulae for Migraine: A Systematic Review and Meta-Analysis of High-Quality Randomized Controlled Trials. *Frontiers in Pharmacology*, *9*. https://doi.org/10.3389/fphar.2018.00589.

Sharangi, A. B. (2009a). Medicinal and therapeutic potentialities of tea (Camellia sinensis L.) – A review. *Food Research International*, *42*(5–6), 529–535. https://doi.org/10.1016/j.foodres.2009.01.007.

Sharangi, A. B. (2009b). Medicinal and therapeutic potentialities of tea (Camellia sinensis L.) – A review. *Food Research International*, *42*(5–6), 529–535. https://doi.org/10.1016/j.foodres.2009.01.007.

Sharma, R. K., Bibi, S., Chopra, H., Khan, M. S., Aggarwal, N., Singh, I., ... & Kabra, A. (2022). In Silico and *In Vitro* Screening Constituents of Eclipta alba Leaf Extract to Reveal Antimicrobial Potential. *Evidence-Based Complementary and Alternative Medicine*, *2022*(1), 3290790. https://doi.org/10.1155/2022/3290790.

Shivamurthy, S., Manchukonda, R., & Ramadas, D. (2016). Evaluation of learning and memory enhancing activities of protein extract of Withania somnifera (Ashwagandha) in Wistar albino rats. *International Journal of Basic and Clinical Pharmacology*, 453–457. https://doi.org/10.18203/2319-2003.ijbcp20160761.

Shrikanth Gadad, B., K. Subramanya, P., Pullabhatla, S., S. Shantharam, I., & K.S., R. (2012). Curcumin-glucoside, A Novel Synthetic Derivative of Curcumin, Inhibits α-Synuclein Oligomer Formation: Relevance to Parkinson's Disease. *Current Pharmaceutical Design*, *18*(1), 76–84. https://doi.org/10.2174/138161212798919093.

Siddique, Y. H., Mujtaba, S. F., Faisal, M., Jyoti, S., & Naz, F. (2014). The effect of Bacopa monnieri leaf extract on dietary supplementation in transgenic Drosophila model of Parkinson's disease. *European Journal of Integrative Medicine*, *6*(5), 571–580. https://doi.org/10.1016/j.eujim.2014.05.007.

Singh, R., Kumar, P., Kuma, N., Chopra, H., & Kumar, V. (2024). Alopecia areata: review of epidemiology, pathophysiology, current treatments and nanoparticulate delivery system. *Therapeutic Delivery*, *15*(3), 193-210. https://doi.org/10.4155/tde-2023-0071.

Singh, M., Murthy, V., & Ramassamy, C. (2012). Standardized Extracts of Bacopa monniera Protect Against MPP+- and Paraquat-Induced Toxicity by Modulating Mitochondrial Activities, Proteasomal Functions, and Redox Pathways. *Toxicological Sciences*, *125*(1), 219–232. https://doi.org/10.1093/toxsci/kfr255.

Singhal, B., Lalkaka, J., & Sankhla, C. (2003). Epidemiology and treatment of Parkinson's disease in India. *Parkinsonism & Related Disorders*, *9*, 105–109. https://doi.org/10.1016/S1353-8020(03)00024-5.

Song, S., Nie, Q., Li, Z., & Du, G. (2016). Curcumin improves neurofunctions of 6-OHDA-induced parkinsonian rats. *Pathology - Research and Practice*, *212*(4), 247–251. https://doi.org/10.1016/j.prp.2015.11.012.

Srivastav, S., Fatima, M., & Mondal, A. C. (2017). Important medicinal herbs in Parkinson's disease pharmacotherapy. *Biomedicine & Pharmacotherapy*, *92*, 856–863. https://doi.org/10.1016/j.biopha.2017.05.137.

Srivastava, S., Saksena, A. K., Khattri, S., Kumar, S., & Dagur, R. S. (2016). Curcuma longa extract reduces inflammatory and oxidative stress biomarkers in osteoarthritis of knee: a four-month, double-blind, randomized, placebo-controlled trial. *Inflammopharmacology*, *24*(6), 377–388. https://doi.org/10.1007/s10787-016-0289-9.

Surh, Y. J., Chun, K. S., Cha, H. H., Han, S. S., Keum, Y. S., Park, K. K., & Lee, S. S. (2001). Molecular mechanisms underlying chemopreventive activities of anti-inflammatory phytochemicals: down-regulation of COX-2 and iNOS through suppression of NF-κB activation. *Mutation Research/Fundamental and Molecular Mechanisms of Mutagenesis*, *480–481*, 243–268. https://doi.org/10.1016/S0027-5107(01)00183-X.

Tanaka, K., Miyake, Y., Fukushima, W., Sasaki, S., Kiyohara, C., Tsuboi, Y., Yamada, T., Oeda, T., Miki, T., Kawamura, N., Sakae, N., Fukuyama, H., Hirota, Y., & Nagai, M. (2011). Intake of Japanese and Chinese teas reduces risk of Parkinson's disease. *Parkinsonism & Related Disorders*, *17*(6), 446–450. https://doi.org/10.1016/j.parkreldis.2011.02.016.

Tolosa, E., Wenning, G., & Poewe, W. (2006). The diagnosis of Parkinson's disease. *The Lancet Neurology*, *5*(1), 75–86. https://doi.org/10.1016/S1474-4422(05)70285-4.

Uabundit, N., Wattanathorn, J., Mucimapura, S., & Ingkaninan, K. (2010). Cognitive enhancement and neuroprotective effects of Bacopa monnieri in Alzheimer's disease model. *Journal of Ethnopharmacology*, *127*(1), 26–31. https://doi.org/10.1016/j.jep.2009.09.056.

Van der Merwe, J. W., Rugunanan, M., Ras, J., Röscher, E.-M., Henderson, B. D., & Joubert, G. (2016). Patient preferences regarding the dress code, conduct and resources used by doctors during consultations in the public healthcare sector in Bloemfontein, Free State. *South African Family Practice*, *58*(3), 1. https://doi.org/10.4102/safp.v58i3.5666.

Wang, Q., Sun, A. Y., Simonyi, A., Jensen, M. D., Shelat, P. B., Rottinghaus, G. E., MacDonald, R. S., Miller, D. K., Lubahn, D. E., Weisman, G. A., & Sun, G. Y. (2005). Neuroprotective mechanisms of curcumin against cerebral ischemia-induced neuronal apoptosis and behavioral deficits. *Journal of Neuroscience Research*, *82*(1), 138–148. https://doi.org/10.1002/jnr.20610.

Wongtrakul, J., Thongtan, T., Kumrapich, B., Saisawang, C., & Ketterman, A. J. (2021). Neuroprotective effects of Withania somnifera in the SH-SY5Y Parkinson cell model. *Heliyon*, *7*(10), e08172. https://doi.org/10.1016/j.heliyon.2021.e08172.

Xu, Q., Langley, M., Kanthasamy, A., & Reddy, M. (2016). Neurorescue Effect of EGCG in an Animal Model of Parkinson's Disease. *The FASEB Journal*, *30*(S1). https://doi.org/10.1096/fasebj.30.1_supplement.1174.11.

Zahiruddin, S., Basist, P., Parveen, A., Parveen, R., Khan, W., Gaurav, & Ahmad, S. (2020). Ashwagandha in brain disorders: A review of recent developments. *Journal of Ethnopharmacology*, *257*, 112876. https://doi.org/10.1016/j.jep.2020.112876.

Zhao, X., Tang, D., Yang, T., & Wang, C. (2018). Facile preparation of biocompatible nanostructured lipid carrier with ultra-small size as a tumor-penetration delivery system. *Colloids and Surfaces B: Biointerfaces*, *170*, 355–363. https://doi.org/10.1016/j.colsurfb.2018.06.017.

Chapter 6

Nanophytoherbals for Enhanced Parkinson's Treatment: Harnessing Nanotechnology

Arushi[1,*]
Vinod Kumar Gauttam[1]
Kavita Munjal[2]
Vaibhav Jaiswal[3]
and Jyotiram Arjun Sawale[4]

[1]Department of Pharmacy, Shiva Institute of Pharmacy, Bilaspur, Himachal Pradesh, India
[2]Amity Institute of Pharmacy, Amity University, Noida, Uttar Pradesh, India
[3]I.E.S. Institute of Pharmacy, I.E.S. University, Bhopal, Madhya Pradesh, India
[4]Krishna Institute of Pharmacy, Krishna Vishwa Vidyapeeth (Deemed to be University), Karad, Maharashtra, India

Abstract

Neurodegenerative disorders (NDs) are primarily characterized by the loss of neurons, with Parkinsonism being one of the more prevalent NDs. Parkinson's disease is a complex neurodegenerative condition that worsens over time. Its characteristic features include bradykinesia (slowness of movement), tremor, and stiffness. Some individuals may also develop postural instability as the disease progresses. Developing treatments for neurodegenerative diseases is particularly challenging due to the presence of the blood-brain barrier (BBB). The BBB, consisting of closely spaced epithelial cells and blood vessels, creates obstacles for drug penetration into the brain. However, nanotechnology offers a promising solution by using small molecules ranging from 1 to 100 nm in size. Among various nanotechnology-based treatments, products derived from medicinal herbs, known as nanophytoherbals, have gained prominence in the development of innovative neurotherapeutics. Their natural abundance, ability to be designed for targeted brain delivery, and reduced potential for undesirable side effects make them highly appealing. Previous studies have demonstrated that phytoconstituents such as curcumin and resveratrol, when administered as nanoformulations, significantly improve the condition of patients suffering from NDs. These nanoformulations enhance bioavailability, improve the compounds' ability to cross the BBB, and offer more potent neuroprotective, anti-

* Corresponding Author's Email: arushi75086@gmail.com.

In: Phyto-Nanomedicine
Editors: Hitesh Chopra, Vinod Kumar Gauttam, Ajmer Singh Grewal et al.
ISBN: 979-8-89530-317-7

inflammatory, and antioxidant effects compared to conventional herbal formulations. This chapter will discuss the effects and applications of additional phytoherbals and their nanoformulations in the treatment of Parkinsonism, as well as a comparative analysis with traditional herbal formulations.

Keywords: BBB, nanoformulations, nanoparticles, Parkinsonism, phytoherbals

Abbreviations

AChE	Acetylcholine E
AD	Alzheimer's disease
ALS	Amyotrophic Lateral Sclerosis
BBB	Blood Brain Barrier
CNS	Central Nervous System
HD	Huntington disease
PD	Parkinson Disease
ND	Neurodegenerative disease
WHO	World Health Organization

Introduction

Neurodegeneration has been identified as a primary pathophysiological change in most brain-related diseases. Despite relentless efforts by modern science to provide surgical or pharmaceutical treatments, the outcomes have not been promising. Neurodegenerative disorders (NDs) such as dementia and Alzheimer's continue to be major clinical concerns, particularly for older adults (Gadhave et al., 2024; Malik et al., 2015). One of the most significant obstacles to the effective management of NDs is the highly selective blood-brain barrier (BBB). While several successful procedures and minimally invasive approaches have been developed, their clinical adoption has been limited due to concerns about long-term safety and potential BBB damage (Verma et al., 2024; Satyavert et al., 2021). Nanotherapeutics, which possess the ability to cross the BBB without causing damage, have emerged as a promising alternative to halt or reverse neurodegeneration in several instances (Cooper et al., 2024). The growing popularity of nanotherapeutics is attributed to their numerous advantages over traditional dosing forms. Neurons, fundamental to the brain's healthy functioning, play an essential role in communication (Butt et al., 2024). While neurons are present throughout the body, most originate in the brain. Neural stem cells produce the bulk of neurons during childhood, but in adulthood, the number of new neurons is significantly lower (Kunoh et al., 2024). Recent research suggests that a single neurodegenerative illness may result from multiple underlying disorders (Ricci, 2024). Depending on the type and stage of the disease, neurodegenerative disorders can be extremely dangerous or even fatal. While some treatments focus on symptom relief, pain management, and restoring movement or balance, many NDs progress without remission (Wang, 2024). Neurodegenerative disorders are now among the most prevalent and disabling health issues, surpassing cancer, myocardial infarction, and stroke, and have become the fourth leading cause of death. These disorders severely disrupt cognitive functions, skilled movements, emotions, and memory, causing both short- and long-term disabilities (Upadhyay et al., 2024). As the global population ages, the prevalence of neurodegenerative diseases is expected to rise, emphasizing the need for comprehensive solutions. Regulatory efforts to develop disease-modifying treatments have increased in recent years, driven by a deeper understanding of the pathogenesis of these debilitating conditions (Arora and Baldi, 2024). Nanoengineered particles offer a less invasive approach by crossing the BBB. Given the lack of proven clinical treatments for neurodegenerative diseases, this chapter explores nanotechnological approaches as a potential solution for these conditions.

The Real Problem of Neurodegenerative Diseases

Age-related illnesses, such as NDs, are on the rise globally due to an increase in the elderly population. However, the main issue is not merely the rising incidence, but the lack of effective therapies (Mitra, 2024). Although NDs were first identified in the early 1900s according to historical records, there are still no proven therapies for these conditions in modern medicine. In some cases, integrative medicine can both prevent certain diseases and slow their progression (Karalis, 2024). Synthetic medications have shown encouraging results in the treatment of common NDs. However, their long-term use is often linked to several negative side effects, rendering them unsuitable for prolonged medical care. Given these unfavorable consequences, scientists are gradually shifting their focus to phytochemicals, which tend to have fewer side effects, as a potential alternative to synthetic medications (Yates et al., 2024). Neurodegenerative disorders exhibit a variety of clinical symptoms, leading to severe behavioral and cognitive abnormalities. For instance, prion diseases impact many individuals worldwide. As a result, NDs have a profound effect on society, healthcare systems, and the economy. One of the major challenges in managing NDs is the BBB, which acts as a defensive mechanism, obstructing the entry of many medications. This barrier limits therapies to addressing only the symptoms of the disease, rather than the underlying causes. In addition, the diagnostic markers commonly used for NDs are often invalidated, meaning that only tentative or approximate diagnoses can be made (Zhang et al., 2024). NDs such as Alzheimer's, Parkinson's, Huntington's, and amyotrophic lateral sclerosis (ALS) are closely associated with aging. As the global population continues to age, these conditions present significant challenges for many societies. A hallmark feature of these illnesses is the accumulation of misfolded and aggregated proteins in the brain. In light of these developments, it is crucial for societies to adopt a holistic approach that includes not only medical interventions but also social support systems (Hossain et al., 2024). Table 1 provides a list of various plants used in the management of neurodegenerative disorders.

The Role of Nanotechnology in Neurodegenerative Disorders

Although there isn't a cure for NDs, researchers are continually working to develop new treatment approaches. NDs are primarily influenced by genetic factors and environmental conditions.

Table 1. Plants used in neuron disease management

Plants used	Disease	Mechanism	Reference
Ginkgo biloba	Huntington disease	Increased striatal MDA, increased SDH activity, and increased locomotor activity.	Liu et al., 2024).
Bacopa monnieri	Alzheimer's disease	Decrease neuron density in all hippocampus area.	Jain et al., 2024
Camellia sinensis	Alzheimer's disease	Inhibit amyloidic plaque formation.	AnhPhan et al., 2024
Allium Sativum	Alzheimer's disease	Increase GAD 65 and 67 in Hippocampal region, increase VGLUT 1.	Shukla et al., 2024
Withania somnifera	Huntington disease	Decrease MDA and NO, increase catalase and decrease LDH activity in cortex and straitum region.	Lerose et al., 2024
Centella asiatica	NDs	Reduces the amount of Aβ deposited in the brain and also lowers ferric ion levels and restores GSH levels by upregulating GST activity.	Ling et al., 2024
Panax ginseng	Anxiety	Suppress AchE activity in cells and improve cholinergic metabolism.	Rosanti et al., 2024
Acorus calamus	Sedative	Down regulation of Bcl-w and Bcl-2, leads to the activation of caspase-3 and phosphorylation of c-Jun N-terminal kinase.	Banerjee et al., 2024
Curcuma longa	Synaptic dysfunction	Aβ oligomerization and fibril production are inhibited.	Zhang et al., 2024
Glycyrrhiza glabra	Improved learning and memory on scopolamine induced disorders	lowers the glutathione levels, raises the superoxide dismutase level, and lowers the MDA level.	Murck et al., 2024

A significant focus has been placed on neuroimmune interactions, as studies have identified several risks associated with genes that are critical to the immune system. The immune response markers in disease states play a crucial role in identifying cellular indicators and signaling pathways, which can enhance the diagnosis and treatment of NDs. Extensive research has shown that NDs are associated with heightened pro-inflammatory immune responses (Garmendia et al., 2024). It's important to note that two primary cell types are responsible for phagocytosis and cytokine release: microglia and astrocytes. Astrocytes are also involved in the formation of glial scars and the maintenance of the BBB. Treatments targeting microglial pathways have shown potential. Across the globe, researchers are developing new drugs aimed at addressing neuroinflammation and overcoming the challenge of BBB transmigration (Jacob et al., 2024). The effectiveness of current treatments for central nervous system (CNS) disorders has been limited by poor drug delivery methods. Compounding the challenge are factors such as the adverse effects of prolonged medication use, aging, and comorbidities associated with aging. The BBB is a major obstacle, making drug administration difficult. Despite recent advancements in understanding the pathophysiology of CNS disorders, early diagnosis and treatment remain challenging, with most current therapies focusing on symptomatic relief. The development of new drugs, especially proteins and peptides, faces obstacles including poor pharmacokinetics and nonspecific targeting, leading to potential side effects (Khatua et al., 2024). Given the limited response of NDs to conventional therapies, researchers are now exploring plant-based drugs using nanotechnological approaches. One such promising area of research is nanotheranostics, which integrates diagnosis and treatment through the use of nanoparticles. This approach has gained attention due to its ability to directly target damaged areas and its aggressive therapeutic potential. Additionally, nanotheranostics can be personalized to meet the specific needs of patients, adapting the treatment based on the type of disorder (He et al., 2024). Recent advances in nanotechnology indicate that it could be a valuable tool in both the diagnosis and treatment of CNS disorders. Nanotechnology involves the manipulation of materials at the nanoscale (one billionth of a meter), which gives nanomaterials unique properties compared to their larger counterparts. These materials exhibit altered surface atom spacing and molecular organization, offering numerous applications in biomarker detection, therapy, and theranostics. Nanomaterials can be engineered to target and repair damaged tissues and cells at the molecular level. Moreover, they can improve drug delivery by increasing bioavailability, protecting compounds from degradation, and enabling controlled drug release. Functionalized nanomaterials can also be designed to cross the BBB and extend their presence in the bloodstream (Nag et al., 2024).

Recent Trends of Neuro-Phytoherbals

Recent advances in nanotechnology and green chemistry offer promising avenues for the theranostic development of treatments for NDs such as Alzheimer's disease (AD) and Parkinson's disease (PD). The use of chemically synthesized compounds, though effective, is often limited by their high cost and potential toxicity. Recent research has explored the neuroprotective properties of biogenic gold nanoparticles (NPs) derived from Terminalia arjuna (Naseem et al., 2024). The results demonstrated significant neuroprotection and biocompatibility of these biogenic gold NPs. These particles effectively reduced Aβ fibrillation, inhibited acetylcholinesterase (AChE), and destabilized mature fibrils at low doses (Al et al., 2024). The inclusion of trehalose in the synthesis of gold nanoparticles further enhanced their ability to prevent protein aggregation and disintegrate mature fibrils, which holds promise for applications in photothermal therapy (Roy et al., 2024). Functionalizing gold nanoparticles with anti-amyloidogenic compounds is another promising approach to boost their neuroprotective capabilities. Additionally, biosynthesizing biogenic platinum NPs using Bacopa monnieri as a neuroprotective agent has yielded notable results, particularly when functionalized with phytochemicals (Lala, 2021; Munjal et al., 2023). Another development involves selenium nanoparticles functionalized with polyphenols, specifically EGCG (epigallocatechin gallate) from tea, which has demonstrated neuroprotective activity and inhibition of amyloid-forming proteins, including amyloid beta, transthyretin, α-synuclein, and huntingtin, all of which are associated with AD (Illes et al., 2024; Munjal et al., 2020). Further enhancement of the therapeutic potential of these nanoparticles has been achieved by coating them with Tet-1, a protein with a high affinity for neurons. Similarly, curcumin and its derivatives have shown promise in treating AD. The combination of benzothiazolinone and curcumin, both of which bind strongly to amyloid plaques, has been effective in targeting curcumin or similar natural compounds in AD treatment (Francisco et al., 2024).

Table 2. Nanoparticles used in neurodegeneration disease (Kaur et al., 2024)

Sr. No.	Nanoparticles used	Disease Treatment
1.	Polymeric nanoparticles Liposomes Solid lipid nanoparticles Lipoprotein based nanoparticles	Alzheimer's disease
2.	Carbon nanotube Polymer bases Nano-capsules Polymeric micelles Dendrimers Nano-emulsions Exosomes	Parkinson disease
3.	Magnetic nanoparticles Solid-lipid nanoparticles Polymeric nanoparticles	Huntington disease

In another approach, methoxypolyethylene glycol nanoparticles coated with tween 80 were produced using the nanoprecipitation method to enhance the pharmacological activity and specificity toward rotundine (RIN), a neuroprotective compound. The encapsulation of RIN within PLGA nanoparticles did not affect its neuroprotective properties, showing potential for targeted neurodegenerative treatments. Phyto-nanomedicines, which combine phytochemicals with nanotechnology, appear to offer a promising alternative to existing ND treatments. These compounds exhibit anti-inflammatory, antioxidative, and anticholinesterase properties, making them well-suited for ND management. However, further research is required to fully explore the neuroprotective mechanisms of these compounds and to investigate the potential for combination therapies that may act synergistically as neuroprotectants (Qneibi et al., 2024). Despite their potential, phyto-nanomedicines face several limitations. Kumar (2020) pointed out that differences in neuro functioning, individual traits, and DNA prevent the development of a universal treatment strategy. Additionally, there are challenges related to the monitoring and efficacy of the treatment, which complicates tracking its progress and effects. The high cost of these methods further adds to the challenge of their widespread clinical application (Kaur et al., 2024). Applications of nanoparticles in various neurodegenerative diseases are illustrated in the following Table 2.

Nanoparticles Based on Proteins

Biopolymers like proteins are increasingly used in nanoparticle formulations for functional and therapeutic purposes due to their safety profile and biodegradability (Kumar et al., 2024). Proteins play specialized roles in both biology and industry, making them useful building blocks for nanoparticles. The small size of protein nanoparticles allows for endocytic trafficking. Protein nanoparticles are an effective drug delivery system due to their biodegradability, stability, surface modifiability, ease of particle size control, and lack of toxicity-related issues like immunogenicity. Specifically, protein nanoparticles can enhance a drug's stability, activity, and half-life by protecting it from enzymatic breakdown and renal clearance. Moreover, due to their non-antigenic properties, protein nanoparticles are used for targeted therapies, including cancer, tumor treatments, and vaccinations. When incorporated into biodegradable polymers, protein nanoparticles can release drugs over an extended period. The primary goal of nanoparticle design is to control surface area and particle size, ensuring the desired amount of drug can be encapsulated within nanoparticles that release active ingredients for site-specific action (Arora et al., 2024). Fibroin protein, which is found in silk fibers, makes up about 65–85% of the total protein composition. The outer sericin from the silk, obtained from Bombyx mori silkworms, is removed through degumming with Na_2CO_3, a common method to extract fibroin. Fibroin is a popular choice for nanoparticle synthesis due to its strength, flexibility, minimal environmental impact, biodegradability, and biocompatibility. Fibroin nanoparticles exhibit a negative zeta potential, but a positively charged polymer, such as chitosan, can act as a crosslinking agent to modify the surface charge. Various factors, such as molecular weight, crystallinity, drug encapsulation, fibroin characteristics, and manufacturing conditions, can influence the physical properties of the nanoparticles. Because fibroin nanoparticles can address challenges associated with loading low-molecular-weight drugs, they have been extensively studied for pharmaceutical delivery. All fibroin nanoparticles loaded with nano-sized/low-molecular-weight drugs have demonstrated improvements in drug solubility and stability, inhibiting drug degradation and reducing toxicity, which leads to enhanced therapeutic outcomes (Bashir et al., 2024). HSA is a protein with a molecular weight of 66 kDa and consists of approximately 585 amino acids. The bloodstream contains the majority of HSA. HSA's three primary components each contain subunits A and B, with primary binding sites located at Sudlow's sites I and II in subunits IIA and IIIA. When hydrophobic molecules are used as carriers for other substances, HSA increases their solubility in the blood, facilitating the delivery of various substances to specific tissues (Liu et al., 2024). HSA is stable at a pH range of 4–9 and a temperature of 60°C for up to 10 hours. Additionally, it offers the advantage of being derived from natural (biological) sources due to its high solubility, biodegradability, non-toxicity, and non-immunogenicity. Due to these characteristics, both bovine and human HSAs are commonly used in evaluating the efficacy of protein binding and targeted drug delivery. Owing to HSA's high affinity for a wide range of drugs, these compounds can be effectively incorporated into an HSA nanoparticle matrix (Alam et al., 2024).

Polymeric Nanomaterials

Polymeric nanoparticles are colloidal particles ranging from 1 to 1000 nm in size, containing a drug encapsulated within a biodegradable and biocompatible polymeric carrier system. One of the most extensively studied polymers is lactide-glycolide copolymer. In an animal study on AD, curcumin-loaded nanoparticles demonstrated the ability to reduce tau phosphorylation and amyloid-beta deposition (Eissa et al., 2024). Additionally, these nanoparticles promote hippocampal neurogenesis and the proliferation of neural stem cells. Due to curcumin's poor water solubility, its ability to reach neuronal levels in AD is believed to be enhanced by nanoparticle formulation. PLGA-coated curcumin nanoparticles have shown inhibition of amyloid formation and free radicals while also targeting the Tet-1 gene in an experimental animal model of AD (Gao et al., 2024). Importantly, research on cell survival capacity has indicated that these nanoparticles do not damage cells (Pandya et al., 2024).

Conclusion

Nanotechnology holds significant potential in revolutionizing the development of nanotechnology-enabled medicines for treating NDs. It may also reshape our understanding of neuronal disorders and therapeutic interventions, paving the way for innovative approaches and methods. As research in neuropathology and neurophysiology advances, it will simultaneously contribute to the development of nanotechnology that offers neuroprotection and promotes CNS healing. Nanotechnology could serve as an alternative to conventional therapeutics in diagnosing, managing, and treating NDs, addressing challenges associated with current therapies, such as non-targeted drug delivery, low efficacy, and limited drug penetration due to size and BBB. To fully explore the potential of nanotechnology in drug design and delivery, a collaborative research approach is crucial. Stakeholders, including neurosurgeons, neurologists, neuroscientists, novel drug researchers, and formulation development scientists, must work together to expand the capabilities of nanotechnology. Given the deeply multidisciplinary nature of therapeutic and medical sciences, it is essential to consider the impact of advances in basic and clinical neuroscience, as well as other novel approaches like nano-informatics and nanotechnology, in building robust therapeutic strategies against NDs.

References

Al-Radadi, N. S., Al-Bishri, W. M., Salem, N. A., & El Shebiney, S. A. (2024). Plant-mediated green synthesis of gold nanoparticles using an aqueous extract of Passifloraligularis, optimization, characterizations, and their neuroprotective effect on propionic acid-induced autism in Wistar rats. *Saudi Pharmaceutical Journal*, *32*(2), 101921.

Alam, M. J., Rahman, M. H., Hossain, M. A., Hoque, M. R., & Aktaruzzaman, M. (2024). Bioinformatics and Systems Biology Approaches to Identify the Synergistic Effects of Alcohol Use Disorder on the Progression of Neurological Diseases. *Neuroscience*, *543*, 65-82.

AnhPhan, D. T., Tran, H. T., Le, H. P., Khuong, T. H., Ha, H. T., Nguyen, D. T., Nguyen, G. T., Le, M. V., & Ly, T. H. (2024). Exploring the Therapeutic Potential of Camellia longii Orel & Luu Leaf Extracts for Memory Loss in Alzheimer's disease: Novel Findings and Functional Food Applications. *ACS Omega*, 29651-29665.

Arora, R., & Baldi, A. (2024). Revolutionizing Neurological Disorder Treatment: Integrating Innovations in Pharmaceutical Interventions and Advanced Therapeutic Technologies. *Current Pharmaceutical Design*, *30*(19), 1459-1471.

Arora, S., Bajaj, T., Kumar, J., Goyal, M., Singh, A., & Singh, C. (2024). Recent advances in delivery of peptide and protein therapeutics to the brain. *Journal of Pharmacology and Experimental Therapeutics*, *388*(1), 54-66.

Banerjee, S., Das, K. K., Pal, G., & Bose, S. (2024). Acoruscalamus L. (Sweet Flag): Bioactive Compounds, Medicinal Properties, and Biological Activity. In *Advances in Medicinal and Aromatic Plants* (pp. 1-21). Apple Academic Press.

Bashir, M., Un-Nisa, A., Bashir, D. J., Ganie, N. A., Dar, K. A., Qadri, S. F. I., Sofi T. A., & Mohi-ud-Din, M. (2024). Fibroin Nanoparticles: Use in Drug Delivery. *Advances in Research*, *25*(3), 77-84.

Butt, A. M., Abdullah, N., Sattar, A., Hussain, T., Pandey, M., Garg, U., Rathee, T. K., Jain, N., & Abeer, M. M. (2024). Advantages of Nanomedicine Over Conventional Therapeutics. In *Nanomedicine in Treatment of Diseases* (pp. 45-85). Singapore: Springer Nature Singapore.

Cooper, C. G., Kafetzis, K. N., Patabendige, A., & Tagalakis, A. D. (2024). Blood–brain barrier disruption in dementia: Nano-solutions as new treatment options. *European Journal of Neuroscience*, *59*(6), 1359-1385.

Eissa, M. A., Hashim, Y. Z., & Badawi, N. M. (2024). Unlocking the potential of chitosan-based polymeric nanoparticles for the treatment of neurological disorders. *Nanomedicine Journal*, *11*(2), 107-118.

Francisco, T. N., Malafaia, D., Melo, L., Silva, A. M., & Albuquerque, H. M. (2024). Recent Advances in Fluorescent Theranostics for Alzheimer's Disease: A Comprehensive Survey on Design, Synthesis, and Properties. *ACS Omega*, *9*(12), 13556-13591.

Gadhave, D. G., Sugandhi, V. V., Jha, S. K., Nangare, S. N., Gupta, G., Singh, S. K., Dua, K., Cho, H., Hansbro, P. M., & Paudel, K. R. (2024). Neurodegenerative Disorders: Mechanisms of Degeneration and Therapeutic Approaches with Their Clinical Relevance. *Ageing Research Reviews*, 99, 102357.

Gao, J., Xia, Z., Gunasekar, S., Jiang, C., Karp, J. M., & Joshi, N. (2024). Precision drug delivery to the central nervous system using engineered nanoparticles. *Nature Reviews Materials*, 9, 567-588.

Garmendia, J. V., De Sanctis, C. V., Das, V., Annadurai, N., Hajduch, M., & De Sanctis, J. B. (2024). Inflammation, autoimmunity and neurodegenerative diseases, therapeutics and beyond. *Current Neuropharmacology*, *22*(6), 1080

Giri, P. M., Banerjee, A., Ghosal, A., & Layek, B. (2024). Neuroinflammation in Neurodegenerative Disorders: Current Knowledge and Therapeutic Implications. *International Journal of Molecular Sciences*, *25*(7), 3995.

He, S., Abarrategi, J. S., Bediaga, H., Arrasate, S., & González-Díaz, H. (2024). On the additive artificial intelligence-based discovery of nanoparticle neurodegenerative disease drug delivery systems. *Beilstein Journal of Nanotechnology*, *15*(1), 535-555.

Hossain, M. U., Arefin, M. S., & Yukongdi, V. (2024). Personality traits, social self-efficacy, social support, and social entrepreneurial intention: The moderating role of gender. *Journal of Social Entrepreneurship*, *15*(1), 119-139.

Illes-Toth, E., Rempel, D. L., & Gross, M. L. (2024). Exploration of Resveratrol as a Potent Modulator of α-Synuclein Fibril Formation. *ACS Chemical Neuroscience*, *15*(3), 503-516.

Jacob, S., Kaushik, P., & Parvez, S. (2024). Organ-on-a-chip for blood–brain barrier studies. In *Human Organs-on-a-Chip Technology* (pp. 309-325). Academic Press.

Jain, N., Tambekar, O., Goel, T., Bodhankar, S. L., & Bansode, D. A. (2024). A Comprehensive Mini Review on the Natural Product Bacopamonnieri for the Management of Alzheimer's Disease. *The Natural Products Journal*, *14*(2), 2-13.

Karalis, V. D. (2024). The integration of artificial intelligence into clinical practice. *Applied Biosciences*, *3*(1), 14-44.

Kaur, G., Chirayimmel, A. J., Rana, P., Sharma, S., Bose, J. C., Rath, S. K., & Dwibedi, V. (2024). Nanomaterials for Diagnosis and Treatment of Common Neurological Disorders. In *Nanomaterials for Drug Delivery and Neurological Diseases Management* (pp. 171-199). Singapore: Springer Nature Singapore.

Khatua, R., Bhar, B., Dey, S., Jaiswal, C., Victoria, J., & Mandal, B. B. (2024). Advances in engineered nanosystems: immunomodulatory interactions for therapeutic applications. *Nanoscale*, 16, 12820-12856.

Kumar, M., Mahmood, S., Chopra, S., & Bhatia, A. (2024). Biopolymer based nanoparticles and their therapeutic potential in wound healing–A review. *International Journal of Biological Macromolecules*, 267, 131335.

Kunoh, S., Nakashima, H., & Nakashima, K. (2024). Epigenetic Regulation of Neural Stem Cells in Developmental and Adult Stages. *Epigenomes*, *8*(2), 22.

Lala, S. (2021). Nanoparticles as Elicitors and Harvesters of Economically Important Secondary Metabolites in Plants. *IET Nanobiotechnology*, 15(1), 28-57.

Lerose, V., Ponticelli, M., Benedetto, N., Carlucci, V., Lela, L., Tzvetkov, N. T., & Milella, L. (2024). Withania somnifera (L.) Dunal, a Potential Source of Phytochemicals for Treating Neurodegenerative Diseases: A Systematic Review. *Plants*, *13*(6), 771.

Ling, Z., Zhou, S., Zhou, Y., Zhong, W., Su, Z., & Qin, Z. (2024). Protective role of made cassoside from Centella asiatica against protein L-isoaspartyl methyl transferase deficiency-induced neurodegeneration. *Neuropharmacology*, *246*, 109834.

Liu, Q., Wang, J., Gu, Z., Ouyang, T., Gao, H., Kan, H., & Yang, Y. (2024). Comprehensive Exploration of the Neuroprotective Mechanisms of Ginkgo biloba Leaves in Treating Neurological Disorders. *American Journal of Chinese Medicine*, 52(4), 1053-1086.

Liu, Y., Li, Y., Wei, X., Ullah, I., Uddin, S., Wang, J., Xia R. & Li, H. (2024). A comparative study on the effects of human serum albumin and α-melanocyte-stimulating hormone fusion proteins on the anti-neuroinflammatory in the central nervous system of adult mice. *Neuropeptides*, *104*, 102410.

Malik, J., Munjal, K., & Deshmukh, R. (2015). Attenuating effect of standardized lyophilized *Cinnamomum zeylanicum* bark extract against streptozotocin-induced experimental dementia of Alzheimer's type. *Journal of Basic and Clinical Physiology and Pharmacology*, 26(3), 275-285.

Mitra, S. (2024). Special Issue 'Advances in Neurodegenerative Diseases Research and Therapy 2.0'. *International Journal of Molecular Sciences*, 25(9), 4709.

Murck, H., Karailiev, P., Karailievova, L., Puhova, A., & Jezova, D. (2024). Treatment with Glycyrrhiza glabra Extract Induces Anxiolytic Effects Associated with Reduced Salt Preference and Changes in Barrier Protein Gene Expression. *Nutrients*, *16*(4), 515.

Munjal, K., Ahmad, S., Gupta, A., Haye, A., Amin, S., Mir, S. R. (2020). Polyphenol-enriched fraction and the compounds isolated from *Garcinia indica* fruits ameliorate obesity through suppression of digestive enzymes and oxidative stress. *Pharmacognosy Magazine*, 16(70), S236-S245.

Munjal K., Gautam, V. K., Goel, Y., Ahamad, J., & Mir, S. R. (2023). Qualitative Diagnostic Features of Alkaloidal Spices. In *Analysis of Food Spices* (pp. 135-150). CRC Press.

Nag, S., Bhatt, M., Ghosh, S., Dey, A., Paul, S., Dutta, S., J. Gowda, & Ahmed, M. G. (2024). Drug Delivery for Neurological Disorders Using Nanotechnology. In *Theranostic Applications of Nanotechnology in Neurological Disorders* (pp. 135-165). Singapore: Springer Nature Singapore.

Naseem, K., Aziz, A., Khan, M. E., Ali, S., & Khalid, A. (2024). Bioinorganic metal nanoparticles and their potential applications as antimicrobial, antioxidant and catalytic agents: a review. *Reviews in Inorganic Chemistry*, https://doi.org/10.1515/revic-2023-0040.

Pandya, T., Kulkarni, M., Acharya, S., & Prajapati, B. G. (2024). PLGA mediated drug delivery for Alzheimer's disease. In *Alzheimer's Disease and Advanced Drug Delivery Strategies* (pp. 181-196). Academic Press.

Perluigi, M., Di Domenico, F., & Butterfield, D. A. (2024). Oxidative damage in neurodegeneration: roles in the pathogenesis and progression of Alzheimer disease. *Physiological Reviews*, *104*(1), 103-197.

Qneibi, M., Bdir, S., Maayeh, C., Bdair, M., Sandouka, D., Basit, D., & Hallak, M. (2024). A Comprehensive Review of Essential Oils and Their Pharmacological Activities in Neurological Disorders: Exploring Neuroprotective Potential. *Neurochemical Research*, *49*(2), 258-289.

Rahm, C. (2024). White Paper on Neurodegenerative Disease and Related Disorders and Associated Case Study. *Practice*, *4*, 31-42.

Ricci, C. (2024). Neurodegenerative Disease: From Molecular Basis to Therapy. *International Journal of Molecular Sciences*, *25*(2), 967.

Rosanti, A. (2024). The Effect of Giving Ginseng Tea on Anxiety During Premenopause in the Mekarjaya Village Area, Purwakarta Regency, Indonesia. *Eureka Herba Indonesia*, *5*(1), 423-425.

Roy, S., Srinivasan, V. R., Arunagiri, S., Mishra, N., Bhatia, A., Shejale, K. P., Prajapati, K. P., Kar, K., & Anand, B. G. (2024). Molecular insights into the phase transition of lysozyme into amyloid nanostructures: Implications of therapeutic strategies in diverse pathological conditions. *Advances in Colloid and Interface Science*, 331, 103205.

Sahu, S., Gantayat, D., Sahu, S. K., Kaur, G., Dwibedi, V., & Rath, S. K. (2024). Nanomaterials and Neurological Disorders Management. In *Nanomaterials for Drug Delivery and Neurological Diseases Management* (pp. 81-107). Singapore: Springer Nature Singapore.

Satyavert, Gupta, S., Choudhury, H., Jacob, S., Nair, A. B., Dhanawat, M., & Munjal, K. (2021). Pharmacokinetics and tissue distribution of hydrazinocurcumin in rats. *Pharmacological Reports, 73*(6), 1734-1743.

Shukla, D., Jaiswal, A. K., Suryavanshi, A., Asati, V., Mahapatra, D. K., Kumar, V., & Bharti, S. K. (2024). Role of garlic and onion for better cognition and maintenance of neurodegenerative diseases. In *Nutraceutical Fruits and Foods for Neurodegenerative Disorders* (pp. 333-352). Academic Press.

Upadhyay, S. K., Dan, S., & Ali, S. A. (2024). *Evidence-Based Neurological Disorders: Symptoms, Causes, and Therapy*. CRC Press.

Verma, K., Kapoor, D., Jain, S., Singh, R., & Sharma, S. (2024). Transporter Systems and Metabolism at the Blood–Brain Barrier and Blood–CSF Barrier. In *Drug Delivery Strategies in Neurological Disorders: Challenges and Opportunities* (pp. 47-73). Singapore: Springer Nature Singapore.

Vinutha, B., & Borse, B. B. (2024). Prevention, Diagnosis, and Understanding Mechanisms of Metabolic Diseases Using Systems Biology. In *Systems Biology Approaches: Prevention, Diagnosis, and Understanding Mechanisms of Complex Diseases* (pp. 561-588). Springer, Singapore.

Wang, W., Pan, D., Liu, Q., Chen, X., & Wang, S. (2024). L-Carnitine in the Treatment of Psychiatric and Neurological Manifestations: A Systematic Review. *Nutrients*, *16*(8), 1232.

Yates, P., Janiol, J., Li, C., & Song, B. H. (2024). Nematocidal Potential of Phenolic Acids: A Phytochemical Seed-Coating Approach to Soybean Cyst Nematode Management. *Plants*, *13*(2), 319.

Zhang, Y., Yang, J., Gong, Y., He, S., Wen, P., Jiang, Y., He, J., Zhu, B., & Li, L. (2024). *In Vitro* and *In Vivo* Supplementation with Curcumin Promotes Hippocampal Neuronal Synapses Development in Rats by Inhibiting GSK-3β and activating β-catenin. *Molecular Neurobiology*, *61*(4), 2390-2410.

Zhang, Z. F., Fan, Y. Y., Lu, X. M., Min, X. Z., Ma, W. L., Liu, L. Y., Li, Y. F., & Li, W. L. (2024). Seasonal patterns, fate and ecological risk assessment of pharmaceutical compounds in a wastewater treatment plant with Bacillus bio-reactor treatment. *Journal of Environmental Management*, *357*, 120732.

Chapter 7

Applications of Nanophytoherbals in Cardiovascular Therapy

Karan Goel[1]
Manisha Bhatia[1,*]
Isha Chawla[1]
Kavita Munjal[2]
Jyoti Uikey[3]
and Hitesh Chopra[4]

[1]M. M. College of Pharmacy, Maharishi Markandeshwar (Deemed to be University), Mullana, Ambala, Haryana, India
[2]Department of Pharmacy, Amity Institute of Pharmacy, Amity University, Noida, Uttar Pradesh, India
[3]I.E.S. Institute of Pharmacy, I.E.S. University, Bhopal, Madhya Pradesh, India
[4]Department of Biosciences, Saveetha School of Engineering, Saveetha Institute of Medical and Technical Sciences, Chennai, Tamil Nadu, India

Abstract

The unique characteristics of nanoscale materials provide promising opportunities for medical nanotechnology, with the potential to fundamentally transform the fields of illness detection, treatment, and prevention. This discussion will focus on nanoparticles and nanophytoherbals, which are distinct but interconnected phenomena. Nanoparticles possess unique physical and chemical characteristics that enable more accurate delivery of medicine and enhance therapeutic outcomes, despite their small size. Phytochemicals have garnered significant attention as prospective therapeutic agents for cardiovascular diseases, which are the leading cause of mortality globally. Encapsulating phytochemicals in nanoparticles enhances their efficacy in decreasing inflammation and oxidative stress, which are significant contributors to cardiovascular disorders. Nanophytoherbals show promise in the treatment of cardiovascular conditions, with evidence of both beneficial and adverse effects. However, it is necessary to address concerns such as the expenses associated with research and the potential long-term harmful effects. One possible future approach in personalized medicine is to enhance treatment outcomes by combining nanophytoherbals with conventional drugs. Further study is required to comprehensively

* Corresponding Author's Email: manisha181979@mmumullana.org.

In: Phyto-Nanomedicine
Editors: Hitesh Chopra, Vinod Kumar Gauttam, Ajmer Singh Grewal et al.
ISBN: 979-8-89530-317-7

understand the potential advantages and disadvantages of using nanophytoherbals in cardiovascular treatment, encompassing their regulated release and targeted distribution, as well as any synergistic impacts they may exhibit alongside conventional treatments.

Keywords: nanoparticles, nanophytoherbals, cardiovascular diseases, phytochemicals, targeted delivery

Abbreviations

CT	Computed tomography
MRI	Magnetic resonance imaging
CAD	Coronary artery disease
HHD	hypertensive heart disease
ABI	Ankle-brachial index
CVDs	Cardiovascular diseases
ABI	Ankle-brachial index
ROS	Reactive oxygen species
LDL	Low density lipoprotein
ACE	Angiotensin-converting enzyme
ENOS	Endothelial nitric oxide synthase

Introduction

Nanophytoherbals, a unique nexus of nanotechnology and phytotherapy, offer a promising future for the improvement of cardiovascular treatment. This rapidly expanding field enhances the transport, bioavailability, and therapeutic efficacy of plant-based phytochemicals by utilizing the unique properties of nanoparticles. The potential health benefits of phytochemicals have been recognized for quite some time (Pebam et al., 2023) The anti-inflammatory, antioxidant, and lipid-lowering characteristics of these compounds are particularly useful in treating cardiovascular diseases (CVDs). However, there are some challenges associated with these molecules that limit their therapeutic use, including low solubility, rapid breakdown in the body, and restricted bioavailability. One potential solution that nanotechnology offers is the capacity to encapsulate phytochemicals in nanocarriers. This process enhances their stability, allows for targeted distribution to specific tissues or cells, and preserves the active components. The therapeutic advantages of phytochemicals are enhanced, and the possibility of unwanted effects is reduced with this personalized strategy. Consequently, nanophytoherbals provide a safer and more effective option for patients (Akhileshwar Jha et al., 2024; Pebam et al., 2023). Treatments that are both effective and convenient for patients are in high demand due to the rising global prevalence of CVDs. Research and clinical studies are currently underway to explore the full potential of nanophytoherbals and integrate them into evidence-based medicine. This exploration delves into the various functions that nanophytoherbals fulfill in managing cardiovascular ailments. Topics presented include research on the action mechanisms of these natural compounds, clinical trials, and their significance for evidence-based medicine (Akhileshwar Jha et al., 2024; Amjad & Mahdi, 2023). The objective of our study is to provide a thorough examination of this innovative therapeutic strategy, which has the potential to greatly transform the management and treatment of cardiovascular illnesses. To achieve this, we will conduct a comprehensive analysis of these individual elements.

Nanotechnology in Medicine

Innovative medical applications are made possible by the unique qualities of nanoscale materials through nanotechnology in medicine. This technology enhances illness prevention, treatment, and diagnostics (Karahmet Sher et al., 2024). The size of nanoparticles can be measured in nanometers, ranging from one to one hundred. Despite their small size, their large surface area gives them distinctive physical and chemical characteristics. One of the many medicinal applications of nanoparticles is the encapsulation of medications, which allows for regulated release and protection against degradation (Aschner, 2009). Because they can be tailored to target specific cells or organs, nanoparticles have the potential to increase therapy effectiveness while reducing the risk of adverse effects. For instance, chemotherapy drugs can be delivered directly to tumor cells using liposomes and polymeric nanoparticles. Additionally, nanoparticles may serve as potential contrast agents for diagnostic and imaging procedures such as computed tomography (CT), magnetic resonance imaging (MRI), and fluorescence imaging. Their incorporation enhances the sensitivity and resolution of these procedures, making it easier to diagnose illnesses in their early stages (Dufort et al., 2012; Sharma et al., 2024). Optical imaging may also benefit from the use of gold nanoparticles to increase contrast. There is speculation that nanoparticles could have therapeutic applications in medicine. Target therapy involves using an external magnetic field to direct magnetic nanoparticles to specific regions of the body. Nanoparticle biosensors can detect trace amounts of biomarkers, pathogens, or other substances in a process known as biosensing. These sensors appear to be particularly useful for early illness detection and monitoring (Aschner, 2009; Singh, 2016).

Nanophytoherbals

Nanophytoherbals is an area that combines conventional herbal treatment with nanotechnology. Nanoparticle encapsulation is one potential strategy for increasing the bioavailability, stability, and efficacy of plant-based active compounds or herbal extracts. Nanophytoherbals aim to circumvent some of the limitations of conventional herbal remedies while leveraging the medicinal benefits of naturally occurring chemicals (Jose et al., 2022; Babazadeh et al., 2018). Many natural compounds exhibit low water solubility and bioavailability, making this strategy particularly effective. Encapsulating these substances in nanoparticles may enhance their solubility and absorption within the body. Additionally, nanoparticles can protect sensitive herbal components from environmental stresses such as heat, light, and oxygen. Thus, nanoparticles serve dual purposes: protection and stability (Jalili et al., 2023; Jose et al., 2022). This enhances the stability and shelf life of herbal compositions. To ensure that herbal components reach the relevant cells or tissues, nanophytoherbals can be designed for targeted distribution. This targeted approach holds promise for increasing therapeutic efficacy while decreasing side effects. Furthermore, herbal compounds can be administered through controlled release using nanoparticle compositions, allowing for longer-lasting medicinal effects. Phytochemicals such as curcumin, resveratrol, and quercetin have benefited from nanotechnology, which has improved their delivery. For instance, curcumin has poor bioavailability on its own but is significantly more effective when encapsulated in nanoparticles (Jalili et al., 2023; Jose et al., 2022).

Cardiovascular Diseases

The heart and blood vessels are the primary targets of CVDs. They account for over 17.9 million fatalities each year, or almost a third of all deaths globally, making them the leading cause of mortality according to the World Health Organization. Examples of cardiovascular illnesses include coronary artery disease (CAD), hypertensive heart disease (HHD), arrhythmias, and various congenital anomalies affecting the arteries or blood vessels in children (Farley et al., 2012; "Global, Regional, and National Age–Sex Specific All-Cause and Cause-Specific Mortality for 240 Causes of Death, 1990–2013: A Systematic Analysis for the Global Burden of Disease Study 2013," 2015). CVDs have surpassed all other causes of death in both industrialized and developing countries, causing intricate damage to the delicate and fragile arteries. The negative effects of CVDs profoundly impact patients' physiology and psyche, affecting their daily lives. Two of the most serious CVDs requiring immediate medical intervention are ischemic heart disease and stroke (Petersen & Kris-Etherton, 2021). Epidemiological research has linked habit-forming behavioral risk factors, such as smoking, alcohol use, inadequate fruit and vegetable consumption, lack of physical exercise, and hypertension, to CVDs. Essential components of prevention include maintaining a healthy weight, engaging in regular physical activity, and avoiding tobacco products. With appropriate therapy and lifestyle adjustments, many individuals with CVD can lead long, active lives, and early detection is possible through screenings, which allows for better management (Farley et al., 2012; "Global, Regional, and National Age–Sex Specific All-Cause and Cause-Specific Mortality for 240 Causes of Death, 1990–2013: A Systematic Analysis for the Global Burden of Disease Study 2013," 2015; Petersen & Kris-Etherton, 2021).

Type of Cardiovascular Diseases

CVDs encompass a variety of conditions affecting the heart and blood vessels. They are a leading cause of global mortality and morbidity (Farley et al., 2012). CVDs can be classified into various types (Table 1).

Prevalence

Every year, cardiovascular illnesses claim the lives of around 17.8 million individuals worldwide. Heart attacks and strokes kill more than 80% of people with CVDs. CVD-related mortality rates have increased significantly. Nearly 23% of all fatalities in India are attributed to CVDs, and these diseases account for around 53% of all deaths in the country. India has a far higher mortality rate from CVD than the world average, with 272 deaths per 100,000 people, according to a 2010 study by the Global Burden of Disease. Heart disease accounts for 20.3% of male fatalities and 16.9% of female fatalities in India each year, out of an estimated 10.5 million total deaths. When it comes to CVDs, diabetes plays a significant role, particularly among the elderly. The accumulation of glucose in the blood while fasting is the primary cause of diabetic cardiomyopathy, a condition that connects the two diseases and causes heart damage (Zhang et al., 2024).

Phytochemicals in Cardiovascular Health

Protective effects against CVDs are only one of the many health advantages associated with phytochemicals, which are naturally occurring substances found in plants. They work in various ways, including enhancing endothelial function, modulating lipid metabolism, reducing inflammation, and acting as antioxidants (Farley et al., 2012; Pai et al., 2023; Thijssen et al., 2023). Some important phytochemicals and their roles in heart health are presented in Table 2.

The Role of Nanophytoherbals in Cardiovascular Therapy

When utilized in herbal remedies, nanophytoherbals significantly enhance therapeutic potential, particularly in cardiovascular treatment, by integrating the benefits of nanotechnology with phytochemicals. This novel approach offers several advantages, including reduced side effects, targeted distribution, controlled release, and improved bioavailability. For example, curcumin is known for its limited bioavailability and poor water solubility. Encapsulation in nanoparticles markedly improves the absorption and efficacy of such compounds, thereby effectively reducing oxidative stress and inflammation—two critical risk factors for CVDs (Babazadeh et al., 2018; He et al., 2024; Jalili et al., 2023). Nanocarriers can be constructed to transport phytochemicals to specific cells or tissues with pinpoint accuracy. To avoid endothelial dysfunction and atherosclerosis, for example, nanoparticles laden with polyphenols from green tea may target endothelial cells and exhibit anti-inflammatory and antioxidant actions. Furthermore, nanocarriers can release phytochemicals in a regulated and sustained manner, ensuring that their therapeutic benefits remain constant over time. One example is the use of resveratrol-loaded nanoparticles, which help manage chronic cardiovascular problems by maintaining therapeutic amounts in the body for long durations. Additionally, nanophytoherbals lessen the likelihood of adverse effects by limiting phytochemical exposure to non-target tissues and preventing the premature release of phytochemicals. The risk of gastrointestinal irritation or toxicity may be reduced by encasing phytochemicals within nanoparticles, which limits direct interaction with the gastrointestinal system. Nanoparticles also increase the stability and longevity of herbal preparations by shielding delicate phytochemicals from breakdown caused by light, heat, and oxygen. Nanoparticle formulations stabilize flavonoids, which are susceptible to degradation, allowing them to retain their potency until they reach the target location (Abdi Syahputra et al., 2024; He et al., 2024; Jalili et al., 2023; Pebam et al., 2023). Another benefit of nanophytoherbals is their multifunctional therapeutic potential. Cardiovascular treatment may take a multipronged approach using nanocarriers that co-deliver phytochemicals or combine them with conventional medications. The anti-inflammatory and blood-clot-preventing properties of aspirin and quercetin, for instance, may work in tandem if delivered via a nanoparticle system. Nanophytoherbals are essential for the prevention and management of CVDs because they enhance the antioxidant and anti-inflammatory effects of phytochemicals. Atherosclerosis may be slowed or halted by using nanoparticles containing polyphenols from grape seeds, which lower inflammation and oxidative stress (Babazadeh et al., 2018; He et al., 2024). Nanotechnology enhances the lipid metabolism regulation capabilities of phytochemicals. For better management of hyperlipidemia, garlic extracts can be nano-encapsulated to improve their efficacy in lowering cholesterol levels. Nanophytoherbals may also augment the anticoagulant and antiplatelet effects of certain phytochemicals, increasing their effectiveness in combating blood clots. For instance, nanoparticles containing gingerol have been shown to reduce platelet aggregation, thereby lowering the risk of thrombosis in cardiovascular patients (Jalili et al., 2023; Jose et al., 2022; Abid et al., 2024).

Research Studies on Nanophytoherbals in Cardiovascular Therapy

Several *in vitro* and *in vivo* investigations have explored the effectiveness, action mechanisms, and potential therapeutic advantages of nanophytoherbals in cardiovascular treatment (Table 3). Research of this nature illuminates how nanophytoherbals may contribute to cardiovascular health.

Clinical Trials and Evidence-Based Practice

Several clinical studies are currently investigating the use of nanophytoherbals in cardiovascular treatment to determine their safety, effectiveness, and potential advantages. These trials consist of various stages, each with its own specific goals. For example, phase I studies are being conducted in healthy volunteers to assess the best methods for dosing and evaluating the safety of nano-encapsulated curcumin (He et al., 2024; Jalili et al., 2023). In phase II studies, researchers are examining the effects of nano-encapsulated garlic extract on blood pressure in hypertensive patients and the efficacy of nano-encapsulated resveratrol in reducing LDL cholesterol levels in individuals with hyperlipidemia. Expanded studies are evaluating the long-term cardioprotective advantages of nano-encapsulated green tea polyphenols in patients with coronary artery disease and comparing the effects of nano-encapsulated flavonoids on endothelial function with traditional antihypertensive drugs in phase III. After the commercial release of nano-encapsulated phytosterols for cholesterol management, phase IV studies will track their efficacy and safety over the long term (du Toit et al., 2022; Firdous et al., 2021).

Table 1. Overview of CVDs: descriptions, risk factors, signs and symptoms, diagnosis, and treatment strategies

Type of CVD	Description	Common Risk Factors	Signs and Symptoms	Diagnosis	Treatment	Reference
Coronary Artery Disease (CAD)	Narrowing/blockage of coronary arteries, leading to chest pain and heart attacks	High cholesterol, smoking, high blood pressure, diabetes, obesity	Chest pain (angina), shortness of breath, heart attack	ECG, stress tests, coronary angiography, blood tests	Lifestyle changes, medications (e.g., statins, beta-blockers), angioplasty, stent placement, bypass surgery	(Khan et al., 2023)
Hypertension (High Blood Pressure)	Consistently elevated blood pressure	Obesity, high salt intake, lack of physical activity, excessive alcohol intake, genetics	Often asymptomatic; severe cases may cause headaches, shortness of breath, or nosebleeds	Blood pressure measurement, ambulatory blood pressure monitoring	Lifestyle changes, antihypertensive medications (e.g., ACE inhibitors, diuretics)	(Binka et al., 2023)
Heart Failure	The inability of the heart to pump blood effectively	CAD, hypertension, diabetes, obesity, heart valve diseases	Shortness of breath, fatigue, swollen legs, rapid heartbeat	Echocardiogram, chest X-ray, blood tests, ECG, stress tests	Lifestyle changes, medications (e.g., ACE inhibitors, beta-blockers), devices (pacemakers), surgery	(Blumer et al., 2024)
Cardiomyopathy	Diseases of the heart muscle leading to weakened heart function	Genetic factors, infections, alcohol abuse, drug abuse, hypertension	Breathlessness, swelling of the legs, fatigue, irregular heartbeat	Echocardiogram, MRI, genetic testing, blood tests, ECG	Medications, lifestyle changes, implanted devices, surgery, heart transplant	(Ezzeddine et al., 2024)
Arrhythmias	Abnormal heart rhythms, including tachycardia, bradycardia, and irregular rhythms	CAD, high blood pressure, smoking, alcohol abuse, stress	Palpitations, dizziness, fainting, chest discomfort	ECG, Holter monitoring, electrophysiological study, tilt table test	Medications, lifestyle changes, catheter ablation, pacemaker or defibrillator implantation	(Pai et al., 2023)
Valvular Heart Disease	Disorders of the heart valves, affecting blood flow	Rheumatic fever, infections, aging, congenital defects	Fatigue, shortness of breath, irregular heartbeat, swelling of ankles	Echocardiogram, chest X-ray, MRI, cardiac catheterization	Medications, valve repair or replacement surgery, lifestyle changes	(Feng et al., 2023)
Peripheral Artery Disease (PAD)	Narrowing/blockage of arteries in the limbs	Smoking, diabetes, high cholesterol, hypertension	Leg pain/cramps while walking, numbness or weakness in legs, cold feet	Ankle-brachial index (ABI), Doppler ultrasound, angiography, blood tests	Lifestyle changes, medications (antiplatelets), angioplasty, bypass surgery	(Matsushita et al., 2022)

Table 1. (Continued)

Type of CVD	Description	Common Risk Factors	Signs and Symptoms	Diagnosis	Treatment	Reference
Stroke	Interruption of blood flow to the brain can be ischemic or hemorrhagic	High blood pressure, smoking, atrial fibrillation, high cholesterol	Sudden numbness, confusion, trouble speaking, vision problems, dizziness	CT scan, MRI, carotid ultrasound, blood tests	Emergency treatment (thrombolytics, surgery), rehabilitation, medications (antiplatelets, anticoagulants)	(Sun & Lynch, 2023)
Congenital Heart Defects	Structural heart abnormalities present at birth	Genetic factors, maternal health issues during pregnancy	Cyanosis, rapid breathing, fatigue, poor weight gain	Echocardiogram, chest X-ray, MRI, cardiac catheterization	Medications, surgical repair, catheter-based procedures, monitoring	(Liu et al., 2023)
Aortic Disease	Conditions affecting the aorta, including aneurysms and dissections	Hypertension, atherosclerosis, genetic factors, connective tissue disorders	Sudden severe chest or back pain, difficulty breathing, fainting	CT scan, MRI, echocardiogram, angiography	Medications (blood pressure management), surgery (aneurysm repair, stenting), lifestyle changes	(Thijssen et al., 2023)

Table 2. Phytochemicals, their mechanisms, cardiovascular benefits, and dietary sources

Phytochemical	Phytochemical	Mechanisms	Cardiovascular Benefits	Reference
Flavonoids	Berries, apples, onions, dark chocolate, green tea, red wine	• Scavenge free radicals • Inhibit enzymes involved in ROS production • Modulate nitric oxide levels	• Reduce oxidative stress • Lower blood pressure • Reduce LDL oxidation • Prevent platelet aggregation	(Abdi Syahputra et al., 2024)
Phenolic Acids	Coffee, fruits, whole grains, vegetables	• Antioxidant effects through radical scavenging • Inhibit inflammatory cytokines	• Protect blood vessel integrity • Reduce arterial stiffness • Lower risk of atherosclerosis	(Queiroz et al., 2024)
Carotenoids	Carrots, sweet potatoes, spinach, tomatoes	• Quench singlet oxygen • Reduce lipid peroxidation • Lower risk of LDL oxidation • Improve overall antioxidant status	• Lower risk of LDL oxidation • Improve overall antioxidant status	(Moissl et al., 2023)
Omega-3 Fatty Acids	Flaxseeds, chia seeds, walnuts	• Inhibit synthesis of pro-inflammatory eicosanoids • Enhance membrane fluidity	• Lower triglycerides • Reduce inflammation • Improve endothelial function	(Huang et al., 2023)
Sterols and Stanols	Vegetable oils, nuts, seeds, legumes	• Block absorption of cholesterol in the intestines • Increase cholesterol excretion	• Lower total and LDL cholesterol levels • Reduce the risk of coronary heart disease	(Plat et al., 2019)
Lignans	Flaxseeds, sesame seeds, whole grains	• Act as phytoestrogens • Modulate estrogen receptors • Inhibit oxidative enzymes	• Lower blood pressure • Improve lipid profiles • Reduce oxidative stress	(Jenkins et al., 2021)
Sulfur-Containing Compounds	Garlic, onions, leeks	• Increase nitric oxide production • Inhibit angiotensin-converting enzyme (ACE) • Reduce platelet aggregation	• Lower blood pressure • Reduce total cholesterol and LDL levels • Inhibit clot formation	(Jikah & Edo, 2023)
Resveratrol	Grapes, red wine, peanuts	• Activate sirtuin proteins • Inhibit NF-kB pathway • Enhance endothelial nitric oxide synthase (eNOS)	• Improve vascular function • Lower blood pressure • Reduce inflammation	(Zordoky et al., 2015)
Saponins	Legumes, oats, spinach	• Form insoluble complexes with cholesterol • Modulate immune function • Lower cholesterol levels • Reduce the risk of atherosclerosis	• Lower cholesterol levels • Reduce the risk of atherosclerosis	(Matsuura, 2001)

Table 3. *In Vitro* and *In Vivo* studies on nanophytoherbals: focus areas, components, findings

Study Type	Focus Area	Nanophytoherbal Components	Research Findings	Reference
In vitro	Antioxidant Activity	Quercetin, Resveratrol	Enhanced antioxidant properties, reduced oxidative stress in endothelial cells	(Yang et al., 2023; Zordoky et al., 2015)
	Anti-inflammatory Effects	Curcumin	Significant inhibition of pro-inflammatory cytokines and pathways (e.g., NF-kB)	(He et al., 2024)
	Lipid Metabolism Modulation	Phytosterols, Flavonoids	Inhibited LDL cholesterol oxidation, decreased foam cell formation	(Mansi et al., 2024; Plat et al., 2019)
	Endothelial Function	Green tea polyphenols	Improved nitric oxide production, enhanced endothelial cell function	(Jiang et al., 2024; Queiroz et al., 2024)
In vivo	Atherosclerosis Prevention	Resveratrol, Curcumin	Reduced development of atherosclerotic plaques, decreased lipid accumulation, reduced inflammation	(He et al., 2024; Zordoky et al., 2015)
	Blood Pressure Regulation	Garlic, Ginger extracts	Effectively lowered blood pressure, improved vasodilation, inhibited renin-angiotensin system	(Binka et al., 2023; He et al., 2024)
	Cholesterol Management	Phytosterols	Significantly reduced total and LDL cholesterol levels in hypercholesterolemic models	(Plat et al., 2019)
	Cardioprotective Effects	Epigallocatechin gallate (EGCG)	Reduced myocardial damage, improved cardiac function, decreased infarct size	(Bakun et al., 2023)
	Thrombolytic and Antiplatelet Activity	Gingerol, Flavonoids	Demonstrated antiplatelet and thrombolytic activities, reduced risk of clot formation	(Abdi Syahputra et al., 2024; Jikah & Edo, 2023)

Based on the results from existing clinical trials, nanophytoherbals generally exhibit good safety profiles and effectiveness. Safety data suggest overall tolerance, with only minor gastrointestinal discomfort reported in a small number of instances involving nano-encapsulated curcumin, which has shown substantial decreases in inflammatory markers and enhanced endothelial function. With few adverse effects, including minor headaches or gastrointestinal issues, nano-encapsulated resveratrol has been successful in reducing LDL cholesterol and improving lipid profiles (Firdous et al., 2021). Despite the potential for uncommon allergic responses and moderate gastrointestinal side effects, nano-encapsulated garlic extract has shown promise in lowering blood pressure and enhancing vasodilation. Nano-encapsulated flavonoids are safe, exhibit few side effects (such as allergic reactions or gastrointestinal issues), and improve endothelial function while reducing oxidative stress. Nano-encapsulated polyphenols from green tea have demonstrated cardioprotective benefits in long-term trials, including smaller myocardial infarcts and improved cardiac function, with very few adverse effects, such as headaches and mild nausea. With few adverse effects and minimal gastrointestinal problems, nano-encapsulated phytosterols have shown promise in reducing total and LDL cholesterol (Abid et al., 2024; du Toit et al., 2022; Plat et al., 2019).

Challenges and Future Directions

If nanophytoherbals are to make significant strides in cardiovascular treatment, several obstacles and opportunities for improvement must be addressed before they can enter clinical use (Jose et al., 2022). There are numerous regulatory hurdles. The regulatory process is complicated by the absence of a globally recognized methodology for analyzing nanophytoherbals. Thorough toxicity studies and long-term evaluations of nanoparticles are essential, given their distinct toxicity profiles and the associated safety concerns. Additionally, consistent synthesis and characterization procedures are needed, as nanoparticle design is complex, leading to heterogeneity in formulations that interact with biological systems in different ways. Nanophytoherbals also present regulatory classification challenges due to the potential for multiple classifications (e.g., medications, dietary supplements, or medical devices). Establishing transparent categorization criteria requires concerted efforts with regulatory bodies. Patent disputes and other intellectual property challenges further complicate the development process, underscoring the need for legal experts to safeguard discoveries (Alsaleh, 2021; Wang et al., 2024). Overcoming these obstacles is crucial for commercialization. Significant investment is required due to the high development costs associated with research, development, and clinical trials. Securing funding through grants, collaborations, and venture capital is essential to address this. Manufacturing scalability poses another challenge, as it is difficult to increase output without compromising quality or consistency. Developing quality control systems and scalable production methods may help address this issue. Additionally, the market's acceptance of nanophytoherbals remains uncertain, as consumer and healthcare provider reactions are still evolving. Gaining buy-in necessitates informing stakeholders of the therapies' advantages and safety. Pricing and reimbursement concerns may hinder commercialization, requiring partnerships with healthcare systems and insurers to establish effective reimbursement plans. Transparency and public engagement are critical in addressing ethical concerns and shaping the public perception of nanotechnology in medicine (Alsaleh, 2021; Amjad & Mahdi, 2023; Babazadeh et al., 2018; Chirazi, 2022). Several promising avenues exist for the future use of nanophytoherbals. Personalized medicine, which tailors treatments to individual genetic and phenotypic profiles, could enhance effectiveness and reduce adverse effects. Combining nanophytoherbals with conventional medications or other therapies may offer synergistic benefits, potentially improving overall treatment outcomes while allowing for lower medication doses. In preventive cardiovascular care, nanophytoherbals could help reduce the prevalence of CVDs and initiate preventive measures in at-risk populations earlier. Advanced nanoparticle systems for targeted drug delivery could optimize the effectiveness of phytochemicals and cardiovascular medications while minimizing side effects. Additionally, integrating nanophytoherbals into bioimaging and diagnostic technologies could enhance the early and accurate detection of CVDs, thereby improving identification and treatment strategies (Abdi Syahputra et al., 2024; Alsaleh, 2021).

Conclusion

Nanophytoherbals have the potential to significantly reduce side effects and enhance cardiovascular therapy outcomes, making it crucial to study their long-term safety and effectiveness in clinical trials. Investigating the targeted dispersion and regulated release of phytochemicals in cardiovascular treatments is essential to determine their therapeutic impact. Additionally, exploring the synergistic effects of combining nanophytoherbals with standard cardiovascular drugs could further improve treatment outcomes. Understanding the regulatory challenges and commercial constraints of nanophytoherbals is also important, including the need for clear classification standards and strategies for patent disputes and intellectual property protection. Innovative nanoparticle technologies for targeted drug delivery can enhance pharmaceutical efficacy and minimize side effects by precisely delivering both phytochemicals and cardiovascular medications. Although phytoherbals are increasingly recognized as therapeutic agents in cardiovascular studies, they face issues such as low solubility, poor bioavailability, limited stability, and low patient compliance. Combining nanoparticles like liposomes, nanomicelles, and solid lipid nanoparticles with phytochemical constituents such as tilianin, magnolol, and resveratrol can significantly improve bioavailability, solubility, and stability. Further research is needed to explore these improvements in depth.

References

Abdi Syahputra, R., Dalimunthe, A., Utari, Z. D., Halim, P., Sukarno, M. A., Zainalabidin, S., Salim, E., Gunawan, M., Nurkolis, F., Park, M. N., Luckanagul, J. A., Bangun, H., Kim, B., & Harahap, U. (2024). Nanotechnology and flavonoids: Current research and future perspectives on cardiovascular health. *Journal of Functional Foods*, *120*, 106355.

Abid, J., Khalil, F. M. A., Saeed, S., Khan, S. U., Iqbal, I., khan, S. U., Anthony, S., Shahzad, R., Koerniati, S., & Naz, F. (2024). Nano revolution in cardiovascular health: Nanoparticles (NPs) as tiny titans for diagnosis and therapeutics. *Current Problems in Cardiology*, *49*(5), 102466.

Akhileshwar Jha, L., Imran, M., Shrestha, J., Prasad Devkota, H., Bhattacharya, K., Alsayari, A., Wahab, S., Kumar Jha, S., Raj Paudel, K., & Kesharwani, P. (2024). Effectiveness of phytoconstituents and potential of phyto-nanomedicines combination to treat osteoarthritis. *European Polymer Journal*, *215*, 113243.

Alsaleh, N. B. (2021). Adverse cardiovascular responses of engineered nanomaterials: Current understanding of molecular mechanisms and future challenges. *Nanomedicine: Nanotechnology, Biology and Medicine*, *37*, 102421.

Amjad, S., & Mahdi, A. A. (2023). Application of phyto-nanomedicine for the treatment of different disease conditions such as diabetes, cardiovascular diseases, and neurodegenerative disorders. In *Nanotechnology in Herbal Medicine* (pp. 293-312). Woodhead Publishing.

Aschner, M. (2009). Nanoparticles: transport across the olfactory epithelium and application to the assessment of brain function in health and disease. *Progress in brain research*, *180*, 141-152.

Babazadeh, A., Zeinali, M., & Hamishehkar, H. (2018). Nano-Phytosome: A Developing Platform for Herbal Anti-Cancer Agents in Cancer Therapy. *Current Drug Targets*, *19*(2), 170–180.

Bakun, P., Mlynarczyk, D. T., Koczorowski, T., Cerbin-Koczorowska, M., Piwowarczyk, L., Kolasiński, E., Stawny, M., Kuźmińska, J., Jelińska, A., & Goslinski, T. (2023). Tea-break with epigallocatechin gallate derivatives – Powerful polyphenols of great potential for medicine. *European Journal of Medicinal Chemistry*, *261*, 115820.

Binka, E., Urbina, E. M., Manlhiot, C., Alsaied, T., & Brady, T. M. (2023). Association of Childhood Blood Pressure with Left Atrial Size and Function: Study of High Blood Pressure in Pediatrics–Adult Hypertension in Youth (SHIP AHOY). *The Journal of Pediatrics*, *255*, 190-197.e1.

Blumer, V., Januzzi, J. L., Lindenfeld, J., Solomon, S. D., Psotka, M. A., Carson, P. E., Bristow, M. R., Abraham, W. T., Gandotra, C., Saville, B. R., O'Connor, C., & Fiuzat, M. (2024). Heart Failure Drug Development Over the Eras. *JACC: Heart Failure*, S2213-1779(24)00416-5.

Chirazi, J. E. (2022). Commercialization journeys: Bringing biomimetic innovation to the market. In *Biomimicry for Materials, Design and Habitats* (pp. 393–436). Elsevier.

du Toit, L. C., Hulisani Demana, P., & Essop Choonara, Y. (2022). A nano-enabled biotinylated anti-LDL theranostic system to modulate systemic LDL cholesterol. *International Journal of Pharmaceutics*, *628*, 122258.

Dufort, S., Sancey, L., & Coll, J. L. (2012). Physico-chemical parameters that govern nanoparticles fate also dictate rules for their molecular evolution. *Advanced Drug Delivery Reviews*, *64*(2), 179–189.

Ezzeddine, F. M., Davis, N. E., & Pereira, N. L. (2024). Arrhythmogenic right ventricular cardiomyopathy masquerading as peripartum cardiomyopathy. *HeartRhythm Case Reports*, *10*(7), 486–489.

Farley, A., McLafferty, E., & Hendry, C. (2012). The cardiovascular system. *Nursing Standard*, *27*(9), 35–39.

Feng, D., Ye, Y., Li, Z., Zhang, B., Liu, Q., Wang, W., Zhao, Z., Zhou, Z., Zhao, Q., Yu, Z., Zhang, H., Duan, Z., Wang, B., Lv, J., Guo, S., Gao, R., Xu, H., & Wu, Y. (2023). Total Cholesterol Levels and Risk of Mortality or Heart Failure Rehospitalization in Patients with Valvular Heart Disease. *The American Journal of Cardiology*, *205*, 473–480.

Firdous, S. M., Hazra, S., Gopinath, S. C. B., El-Desouky, G. E., & Aboul-Soud, M. A. M. (2021). Antihyperlipidemic potential of diosmin in Swiss Albino mice with high-fat diet induced hyperlipidemia. *Saudi Journal of Biological Sciences*, *28*(1), 109–115.

Global, regional, and national age–sex specific all-cause and cause-specific mortality for 240 causes of death, 1990–2013: a systematic analysis for the Global Burden of Disease Study 2013. (2015). *The Lancet*, *385*(9963), 117–171.

He, J., Wu, X., Li, L., Chen, J., Liao, J., Wu, A., Zhang, M., Chen, Y., Mao, X., Shen, X., & Tao, L. (2024). Construction of curcumin-loaded macrophage and HUVECs membrane-derived vesicles for drug delivery in cardiovascular inflammatory. *Journal of Drug Delivery Science and Technology*, *95*, 105611.

Huang, L., Zhang, F., Xu, P., Zhou, Y., Liu, Y., Zhang, H., Tan, X., Ge, X., Xu, Y., Guo, M., & Long, Y. (2023). Effect of Omega-3 Polyunsaturated Fatty Acids on Cardiovascular Outcomes in Patients with Diabetes: A Meta-analysis of Randomized Controlled Trials. *Advances in Nutrition*, *14*(4), 629–636.

Jalili, A., Bagherifar, R., Nokhodchi, A., Conway, B., & Javadzadeh, Y. (2023). Current Advances in Nanotechnology-Mediated Delivery of Herbal and Plant-Derived Medicines. *Advanced Pharmaceutical Bulletin*, *13*(4), 712–722.

Jenkins, D. J. A., Kendall, C. W. C., & Sievenpiper, J. L. (2021). Plant Polyphenols Lignans and Cardiovascular Disease. *Journal of the American College of Cardiology*, *78*(7), 679–682.

Jiang, Y., Dong, B., Jiao, X., Shan, J., Fang, C., Zhang, K., Li, D., Xu, C., & Zhang, Z. (2024). Nano-selenium alleviates the pyroptosis of cardiovascular endothelial cells in chicken induced by decabromodiphenyl ether through ERS-TXNIP-NLRP3 pathway. *Science of The Total Environment*, *915*, 170129.

Jikah, A. N., & Edo, G. I. (2023). Mechanisms of action by sulphur compounds in Allium sativum. A review. *Pharmacological Research - Modern Chinese Medicine*, *9*, 100323.

Jose, A., K., S., & E. K., R. (2022a). Advancements in nanophyto formulations. In *Advances in Nanotechnology-Based Drug Delivery Systems* (pp. 103–132). Elsevier.

Karahmet Sher, E., Alebić, M., Marković Boras, M., Boškailo, E., Karahmet Farhat, E., Karahmet, A., Pavlović, B., Sher, F., & Lekić, L. (2024). Nanotechnology in medicine revolutionizing drug delivery for cancer and viral infection treatments. *International Journal of Pharmaceutics*, *660*, 124345.

Khan, S. U., Saeed, S., Alsuhaibani, A. M., Fatima, S., ur Rehman, K., Zaman, U., Ullah, M., Refat, M. S., & Lu, K. (2023). Advances and Challenges for GWAS Analysis in Cardiac Diseases: A Focus on Coronary Artery Disease (CAD). *Current Problems in Cardiology*, *48*(9), 101821.

Liu, Y., Han, F., Zhuang, J., Ou, Y., Qu, Y., Lin, Y., Zhang, W., Wang, H., & Huang, L. (2023). Maternal Vascular Dysfunction in Congenital Heart Defects. *Congenital Heart Disease*, *18*(5), 561–570.

Mansi, Garg, V., & Sahu, B. D. (2024). Carvacrol and its effect on cardiovascular diseases: From molecular mechanism to pharmacological modulation. *Food Bioscience*, *57*, 103444.

Matsushita, K., Gao, Y., Sang, Y., Ballew, S. H., Salameh, M., Allison, M., Selvin, E., & Coresh, J. (2022). Comparative mortality according to peripheral artery disease and coronary heart disease/stroke in the United States. *Atherosclerosis*, *354*, 57–62.

Matsuura, H. (2001). Saponins in Garlic as Modifiers of the Risk of Cardiovascular Disease. *The Journal of Nutrition*, *131*(3), 1000S-1005S.

Moissl, A., Delgado, G., Kleber, M., März, W., Krämer, B., Pilz, S., Scharnagl, H., Siekmeier, R., Silbernagel, G., Tomaschitz, A., Winklhofer-Roob, B., & Lorkowski, S. (2023). Associations of carotenoids, vitamin A and mortality: The Ludwigshafen Risk and Cardiovascular Health (LURIC) study. *Atherosclerosis*, *379*, S164–S165.

Pai, U. M., Prabhu, M. A., Devasia, D. T., Rao, D. S., V, R., Samanth, J., Prabhu, S., Mathias, H. L., & V, C. (2023). Prevalence of metabolic syndrome and its association with atrial arrhythmias in patients with implanted permanent pacemaker for cardiac conduction abnormality. *Indian Heart Journal*, *75*(6), 462–464.

Pebam, M., Buddhiraju, H. S., Verma, A., & Rengan, A. K. (2023). Nano Phyto-Phenols as potential immunomodulators: A review. *Food and Humanity*, *1*, 809–816.

Petersen, K. S., & Kris-Etherton, P. M. (2021). Diet Quality Assessment and the Relationship between Diet Quality and Cardiovascular Disease Risk. *Nutrients*, *13*(12), 4305.

Plat, J., Baumgartner, S., Vanmierlo, T., Lütjohann, D., Calkins, K. L., Burrin, D. G., Guthrie, G., Thijs, C., Te Velde, A. A., Vreugdenhil, A. C. E., Sverdlov, R., Garssen, J., Wouters, K., Trautwein, E. A., Wolfs, T. G., van Gorp, C., Mulder, M. T., Riksen, N. P., Groen, A. K., & Mensink, R. P. (2019). Plant-based sterols and stanols in health & disease: "Consequences of human development in a plant-based environment?" *Progress in Lipid Research*, *74*, 87–102.

Queiroz, M., Matos, P., Sena, C. M., Figueirinha, A., & Ramos, F. (2024). Role of phenolic acids in treatment and prevention of cardiovascular diseases. In *Advancement of Phenolic Acids in Drug Discovery* (pp. 367–391). Elsevier.

Sharma, G., Susmita, D., Kumar, P., & Stangar, U. L. (2024). Parametric effect of continuous synthesis of metal nanoparticles within microchannels and application: A review study. *Chemical Engineering Research and Design*, 209, 142-156.

Singh, A. K. (2016). Structure, Synthesis, and Application of Nanoparticles. In *Engineered Nanoparticles* (pp. 19–76). Elsevier.

Sun, L. R., & Lynch, J. K. (2023). Advances in the Diagnosis and Treatment of Pediatric Arterial Ischemic Stroke. *Neurotherapeutics*, *20*(3), 633–654.

Thijssen, C. G. E., Dekker, S., Bons, L. R., Geenen, L. W., Gökalp, A. L., Takkenberg, J. J. M., Mokhles, M. M., Bekkers, J. A., Boersma, E., Bouwens, E., van Kimmenade, R. R. J., & Roos-Hesselink, J. W. (2023). Novel biomarkers associated with thoracic aortic disease. *International Journal of Cardiology*, *378*, 115–122.

Wang, Y., Rehman, A., Jafari, S. M., Shehzad, Q., Yu, L., Su, Y., Wu, G., Jin, Q., Zhang, H., Suleria, H. A. R., & Wang, X. (2024). Micro/nano-encapsulation of marine dietary oils: A review on biomacromolecule-based delivery systems and their role in preventing cardiovascular diseases. *International Journal of Biological Macromolecules*, *261*, 129820.

Yang, X., Fu, Y., Zhang, J., Liu, J., Liu, X., Peng, Y., Kyin, S. L., Zhang, M., & Zhou, D. (2023). Preparation, characterization, and antioxidant and antiapoptotic activities of biosynthesized nano-selenium by yak-derived Bacillus cereus and chitosan-encapsulated chemically synthesized nano-selenium. *International Journal of Biological Macromolecules*, *242*, 124708.

Zhang, X., Chen, Z., Fang, A., Kang, L., Xu, W., Xu, B., Chen, J., & Zhang, X. (2024). Trends in prevalence, risk factor control and medications in atherosclerotic cardiovascular disease among US Adults, 1999–2018. *American Journal of Preventive Cardiology*, *17*, 100634.

Zordoky, B. N. M., Robertson, I. M., & Dyck, J. R. B. (2015). Preclinical and clinical evidence for the role of resveratrol in the treatment of cardiovascular diseases. *Biochimica et Biophysica Acta (BBA) - Molecular Basis of Disease*, *1852*(6), 1155–1177.

Chapter 8

Nanophytoherbals: Enhancing Cardiovascular Therapy with Herbal and Nanotechnology Integration

Parul Gupta
Shikha Kamboj
Rohit Kamboj
Kumar Guarve
and Sweta Kamboj*
Guru Gobind Singh College of Pharmacy, Yamuna Nagar, Haryana, India

Abstract

Given the rising prevalence of cardiovascular diseases (CVDs) as the leading cause of mortality, developing effective prevention and treatment strategies is crucial. Alternative therapies, such as natural products and medicinal herbs, are increasingly favored due to their lower toxicity, greater chemical diversity, and affordability compared to conventional treatments. Integrating herbal therapy with nanotechnology, known as nanophytoherbals, presents a novel approach to addressing the complex mechanisms underlying CVDs. This approach aims to evaluate the potential of phytoherbal components as cardiovascular therapeutics by exploring their effects on endothelial function, oxidative stress, inflammation, and lipid metabolism—key factors in the onset and progression of CVDs. Key phytoherbal compounds, including polyphenols, flavonoids, alkaloids, and terpenoids, are identified and extracted from medicinal plants traditionally used to treat CVDs. These bioactive components are then encapsulated into biocompatible nanoparticles to create nanophytoherbals, enhancing their bioavailability through targeted delivery and controlled release. Nanophytoherbals offer promising new avenues for CVD treatment by potentially reducing critical risk factors, paving the way for more personalized, targeted, and effective therapeutic strategies to combat cardiovascular disorders.

Keywords: nanophytoherbals, cardiovascular diseases, nanotechnology, bioactive compounds, targeted drug delivery, oxidative stress, endothelial function

---

* Corresponding Author's Email: swetakamboj20@gmail.com.

In: Phyto-Nanomedicine
Editors: Hitesh Chopra, Vinod Kumar Gauttam, Ajmer Singh Grewal et al.
ISBN: 979-8-89530-317-7

Introduction

Cardiovascular diseases (CVDs) encompass a wide range of disorders affecting the heart and coronary blood vessels (Alves-Silva et al., 2016). Among the various risk factors for CVD, high blood pressure is notably linked to strong causal evidence and a high prevalence of exposure (Fuchs & Whelton, 2020). Hyperlipidemia, characterized by abnormal lipid metabolism, often underlies many chronic conditions, including CVD (Islam et al., 2021). CVDs include conditions such as peripheral vascular diseases, hypertension, dyslipidemias, heart failure, heart attack, coronary heart disease, and stroke (Toth, 2007; Reiner et al., 2019). Representing a significant global source of mortality and morbidity, CVDs have emerged as a critical public health concern in recent years (Shaito et al., 2020) and have been the leading cause of death for decades (Hesari et al., 2021). Notably, women face a worse prognosis and higher mortality rates than men following acute cardiovascular events, including coronary heart disease, stroke, heart failure, and aortic diseases (Gao et al., 2019). The World Health Organization (WHO) predicts that CVD will be responsible for 22.2 million deaths by 2030 (WHO, 2014). Conventional medications prescribed for cardiovascular diseases often come with high costs and negative side effects. Therefore, there is an increasing need for more reliable, affordable, and effective alternatives. Medicinal herbs have emerged as a crucial therapeutic option for CVDs, as their potential benefits for health and quality of life become more recognized within the medical community (Panda et al., 2009). As illustrated in Figure 1, which depicts the structural diversity of key phytoconstituents, these herbal remedies have been employed to treat various conditions, including arrhythmia, congestive heart failure, cerebral and venous insufficiency, atherosclerosis, angina pectoris, and systolic hypertension. In addition to therapeutic herbs, physical exercise is also recognized for its cardioprotective effects (Hamer et al., 2019). Recent studies indicate that natural substances effectively prevent, control, or inhibit key risk factors for cardiovascular disease, such as oxidative stress and inflammatory mediators (Pop et al., 2018). The therapeutic qualities of medicinal plants are attributed to their bioactive compounds (Sangwan et al., 2004). Numerous plant-derived bioactive substances, including diosgenin, isoflavones, polyphenols, sulforaphane, quercetin, resveratrol, carotenoids, tocotrienols, and flavonoids, have demonstrated protective effects against CVD. Epidemiological studies and some clinical trials have shown that a healthy diet reduces the incidence of cardiovascular diseases. In particular, diets rich in monounsaturated and polyunsaturated fats are associated with a protective effect against CVD compared to those high in saturated fats (Kim et al., 2021). The complex interactions between bioactive substances and pathophysiological factors in cardiovascular disease are depicted in Figure 2, showcasing how these compounds enhance vascular health, reduce oxidative stress, and mitigate inflammation. However, scientific research on phytochemicals in nanoform is still limited. Existing studies suggest that natural-based nanoformulations are significantly effective in treating and preventing CVD, whether used alone or in combination with synthetic or herbal medications (Hesari et al., 2021).

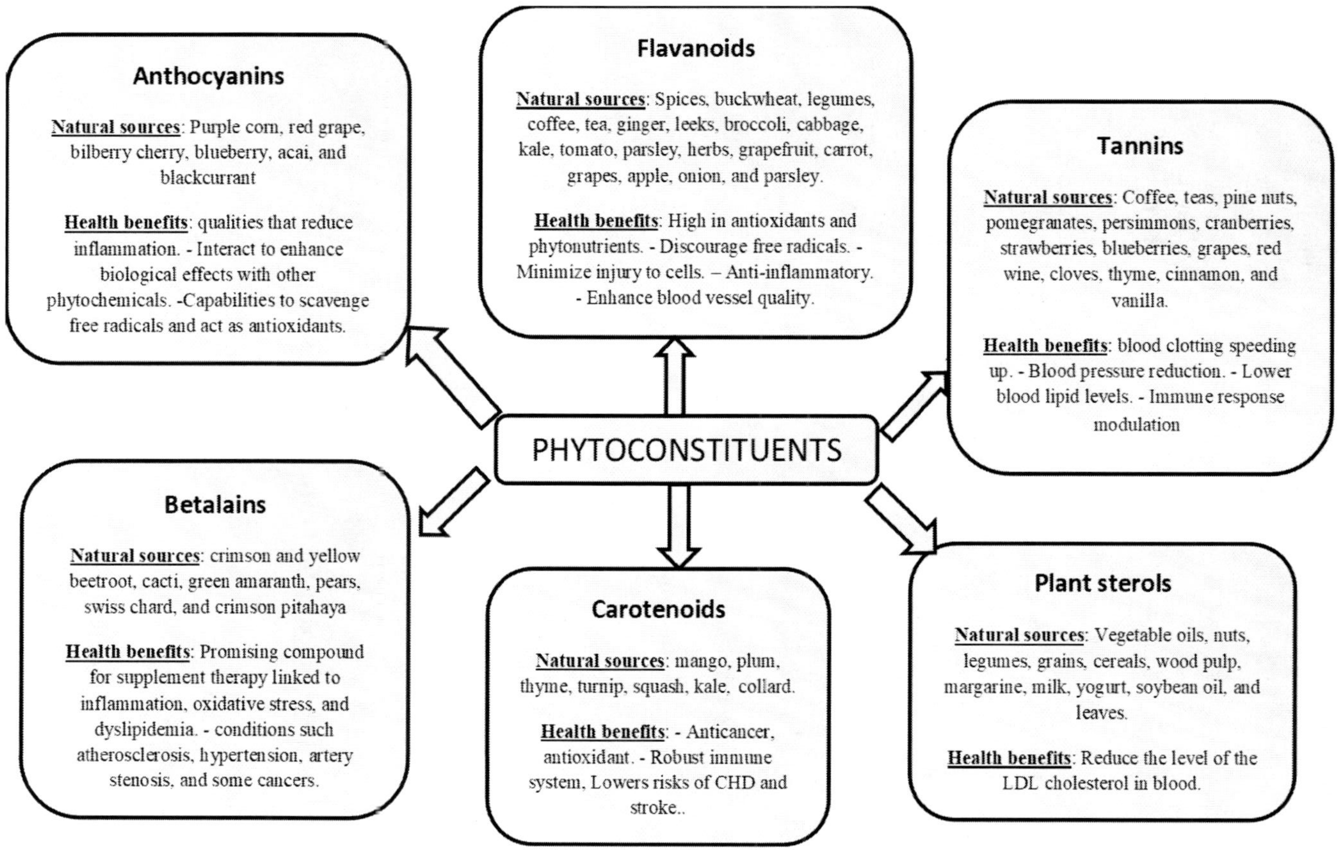

Figure 1. Specific phytoconstituents in natural sources with their health benefits.

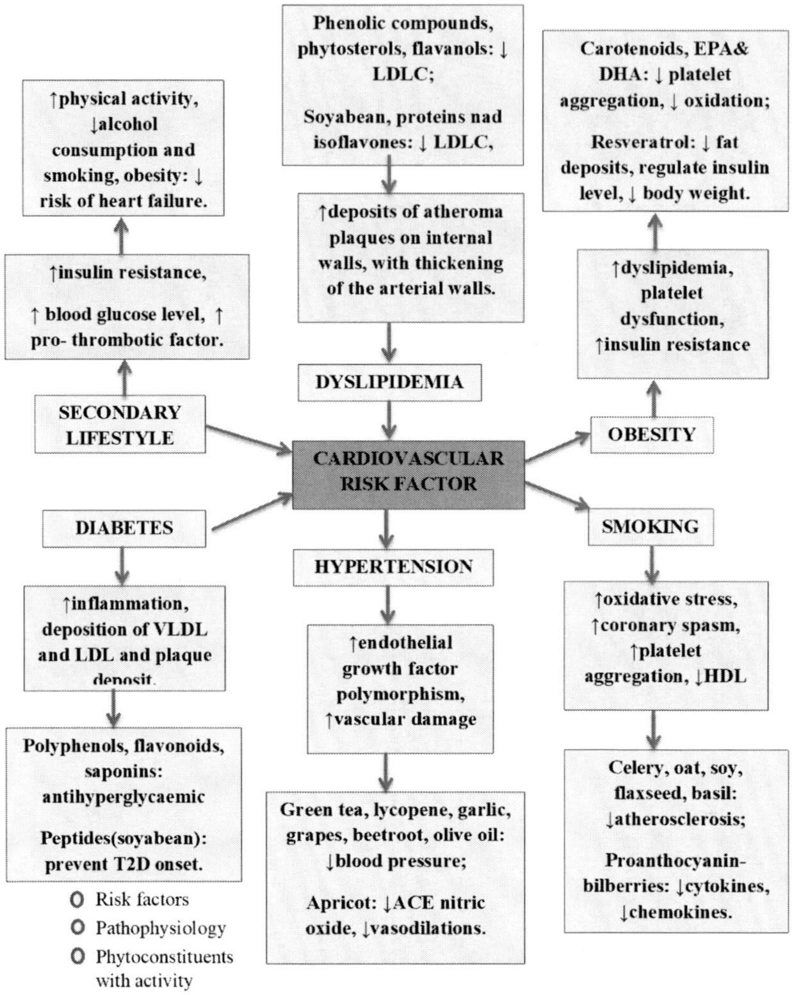

Figure 2. Pathophysiology and bioactive compounds with their action along with their risk factor in CVDs.

Herbal Drugs Used in Cardiovascular Diseases

The potential therapeutic effects of herbal medications, derived from various plant sources, have been extensively studied in relation to cardiovascular diseases. Herbal treatments have a long history of use in traditional medicine practices worldwide for addressing cardiovascular issues. Bioactive substances found in many plants may have beneficial effects on cardiovascular health. Phytoconstituents are medicinal compounds generated during primary or secondary metabolism. Carotenoids, triterpenes, flavonoids, cardiac glycosides, alkaloids, saponins, sapogenins, polyphenols, terpenoids, fatty acids, and other secondary metabolites have been suggested to mediate cardioprotective properties (Shah et al., 2019). Due to their well-established cardioprotective capabilities, medicinal plants such as *Terminalia arjuna* Linn, *Glycyrrhiza glabra* Linn, and *Albizia lebbeck* Linn are frequently used in herbal preparations intended to treat cardiovascular diseases. Reports indicate that Terminalia arjuna reduces myocardial superoxide dismutase levels, lowers glutathione, and causes focal dilation of the smooth endoplasmic reticulum, which has a positive ionotropic effect. *Glycyrrhiza glabra* promotes blood vessel regeneration by inducing the proliferation of vascular endothelial cells, while *Albizia lebbeck* rearranges the cytoskeleton, enhancing contractile function and reperfusion. Garlic (*Allium sativum*) is one of these natural treatments, used for centuries in various cultures. High in allicin, garlic has demonstrated antiplatelet and vasodilatory properties, which may help control blood pressure and lower cholesterol. Herbal remedies extend beyond specific plants; formulations containing green tea (*Camellia sinensis*) and turmeric (*Curcuma longa*) harness the antioxidant and anti-inflammatory qualities of these plants' bioactive compounds (Patel et al., 2018). Table 1 provides a comprehensive summary of the various plant components and their effects on the cardiovascular system, highlighting their potential use in the treatment or prevention of cardiovascular diseases.

Commercial Heart Drugs Derived from Plants

Synthetic medication treatment for heart disease does not reduce mortality by more than 30%, and cardiovascular risks still require careful consideration. As a result, the search for new cardioprotective drugs is shifting toward natural sources. The constant demand for novel medications with fewer side effects and lower costs is increasingly met by plants (Silva et al., 2021). Therefore, the pursuit of safe, effective, cost-efficient, and environmentally friendly medication candidates is crucial. It is widely recognized that medications used to treat heart problems are often derived from phenols, flavonoids, and polysaccharides found in medicinal plants. Particularly positive outcomes have been reported for plant-based medications concerning heart conditions such as hypertension, hyperlipidemia, atherosclerosis, and chronic heart failure (Chang et al., 2020). There is considerable optimism surrounding the development of green medications to treat various cardiac issues, especially with plant-derived isoflavonoids (Yanbei et al., 2021). Several commercially available medications that treat heart-related diseases are derived from plants, including warfarin, digitalis, aspirin, verapamil, and statins. Aspirin, which originates from the bark of the willow tree, has evolved from a folk remedy to a widely accepted pharmaceutical. Its primary ingredient, salicin, possesses anti-inflammatory and antiplatelet properties, making it a valuable tool in combating cardiovascular disease. Digoxin, derived from the foxglove plant, has a long history of use in treating arrhythmias and heart failure. Reserpine, extracted from the roots of *Rauvolfia serpentina*, has traditionally been used as an antihypertensive medication due to its ability to lower blood pressure by depleting neurotransmitters. Additionally, substances found in the venom of the Brazilian pit viper (*Bothrops jararaca*) have led to the development of ACE inhibitors, which are crucial in managing hypertension and heart failure (Shaito et al., 2020).

Nanoformulations as a Novel Drug Delivery Approach in Cardiovascular Diseases

Phytoconstituent nanoformulations represent a novel strategy for medication administration in cardiovascular disorders, offering enhanced accuracy and potency. By leveraging nanotechnology, these formulations improve the solubility, targeted distribution, and bioavailability of plant-based bioactive compounds. This innovative approach holds significant promise for addressing the complex challenges associated with cardiovascular disorders. For instance, antioxidant and anti-inflammatory agents such as flavonoids, terpenoids, and polyphenols can be engineered through nanotechnology to specifically target atherosclerotic or inflammatory regions within the cardiovascular system. By acting as carriers, nanoparticles maximize therapeutic effects while minimizing the risk of adverse reactions, resulting in a controlled and prolonged release of phytoconstituents. The precision in drug administration is particularly critical for cardiovascular disorders, as targeted therapies can substantially influence patient outcomes. Essential factors affecting a drug's effectiveness *in vivo* include stability, solubility, bioavailability, dissolution rate, and absorption (Patra & Das, 2018). Two primary types of nanostructured carrier systems are employed in drug delivery: organic nanocarriers (such as liposomes, polymeric nanogels, dendrimers, and micelle and vesicle nanocarriers) and inorganic nanoparticles (including carbon nanotubes, quantum dots (QDs), mesoporous silica nanoparticles, and metallic nanoparticles like iron oxide and gold) (Lombardo et al., 2019). In the context of CVDs following an ischemic episode, a variety of therapeutic options are available. Intracoronary catheterization or direct intramyocardial injection are commonly used methods for more reliable drug delivery to the myocardium. While intramyocardial injection offers several advantages, it is invasive and can pose significant risks to the heart. Additionally, embolization can occur with intracoronary catheterization. Therefore, systemic intravenous drug administration is often a better choice. This method is less invasive and provides an optimal environment for sufficient drug circulation within the cardiovascular system (Lundy et al., 2016). Non-functionalized medications are frequently eliminated by reticuloendothelial organs and cannot effectively target the heart. Consequently, encapsulating drugs within nanoparticles enhances their persistence and circulatory half-life compared to their free forms. For example, solid lipid nanoparticles (SLN) loaded with the calcium channel blocker nitrendipine have shown three to four times greater bioavailability than conventional formulations when administered intraduodenally in patients with hypertension (Kumar et al., 2007). Given that cardiomyocytes have limited regenerative capacity and poor self-healing ability, treatment for acute myocardial infarction often leads to irreversible heart damage. Therefore, stem cell therapy is a promising approach for treating CVDs; however, less than 10% of transplanted stem cells typically remain at the intended site (La Francesca, 2012). Iron oxide superparamagnetic nanoparticles have garnered increasing interest as a potential solution to these challenges. These nanoparticles can be utilized to track stem cell growth and orientation (Binsalamah et al., 2011). Research into nanoformulations of phytoconstituents targeting cardiovascular disease has investigated the encapsulation of key compounds, including curcumin, quercetin, and resveratrol, within polymeric nanoparticles. In *in vitro* studies using cardiac cell lines, these nanoformulations demonstrated improved absorption compared to free phytoconstituents. Additionally, the nanoformulations exhibited notable outcomes, such as enhanced antioxidant activity and protection against oxidative stress-induced damage. *In vivo* studies conducted on a rat model of cardiovascular disease revealed improved pharmacokinetics and a significant reduction in oxidative stress and inflammatory markers within heart tissues, as detailed in Table 2.

Table 1. Various plants having cardiovascular effect

Plant source	Phyto-constituents	Cardiovascular Activity	References
Stem of Amaranthus viridis (green amaranth) F. Amaranthaceae	Amino acids	Manages high cholesterol	Jayasuriya, & Sarveswaran, 2017
Wood, bark and leaf of Aniba canelilla (Kunth) F. Lauraceae	Essential oil, phenolic acids, and flavonoids	Controls the oxidative stress and blood pressure	Souza-Junior et al., 2020
Leaf of Aspalathus linearis (red tea) F. Fabaceae	Polyphenolic compounds	Controls inflammatory response and oxidative stress.	Smith & Swart, 2018
Aerial part of Baccharis trimera (Carqueja) F. Asteraceae	Flavonoids and phenolic compounds	Contributes to the function of reducing lipids and preventing the production of free radicals	Souza et al., 2020
Stem, bark of Berberis spp. (Common barberry) F. Berberidaceae	Berberine	Regulates oxidative responses, immunity, and metabolism.	Neag et al., 2018
Leaf of Camellia oleifera (Tea-Oil Camellia) F. Theaceae	Terpenoid and saponins	Increases cardioprotection against damage from ischemia-reperfusion	Singh & Chaudhuri, 2018
Leaf of Camellia sinensis (green tea) F. Theaceae	Catechins, sterols, alkaloids	Decreases apolipoprotein B, low-density lipoprotein cholesterol, nonhigh-density lipoprotein cholesterol, and total cholesterol levels.	Fürst & Zündorf, 2014
Flower of Carthamus tinctorius (Safflower) F. Asteraceae	Chalcone compounds	Reduced arterial pressure	Zhou et al., 2021
Fruit of Citrus bergamia (Bergamot) F. Rutaceae	Flavonoids	Controls cardiotoxicity because to its lipid-lowering and antioxidant properties.	Anwar et al., 2016
Stem, leaf, seeds and flower of (Cocos nucifera coconut tree) F. (Arecaceae)	Phenols, tannins, leucoanthocyanidins, flavonoids, triterpenes, steroids, and alkaloids	Reduces oxidative stress and damage to cells	Maiuolo et al., 2021
Seeds of Coriandrum sativum (Coriander) F. (Apiaceae)	Essential oils and polyphenols	Reduces dyslipidemia in diabetics to avoid cardiovascular problems	Jayaraman et al., 2021
Flower of crocus sativus (Saffron) F. Iridaceae	Essential oil, crocin, crocetin, and picrocrocin	Demonstrates positive effects against atherosclerosis and hypertension	Prachayasittikul et al., 2018
Leaf of Cudrania tricuspidata (Chinese Mulberry) F. Moraceae	Essential oil	Lowers hypertension patients' systolic blood pressure	Xin et al., 2017
Rhizomes of Curcuma longa (Turmeric) F. Zingiberaceae	Curcumin	Benefits for the heart by lowering oxidative stress	Wang et al., 2021
Seeds of Dracocephalum moldavica (Moldavian dragonhead) F. (Labiatae)	Flavonoids: tilianin, luteolin	Lowers TNF-α and IL-1β levels while enhancing the cardiac membrane's and its fibers' integrity	Hesari et al., 2021

Table 1. (Continued)

Plant source	Phyto-constituents	Cardiovascular Activity	References
Fruit of Eleocharis dulcis (Chinese water chestnut) F. Cyperaceae	Amino acids, carbohydrates, phenolics, sterols and saponins.	Crucial to maintaining cardiovascular homeostasis	Zhang et al., 2022
Fruit of Garcinia indica (Kokum) F. Clusiaceae	Phenolic compounds and flavanoids	Protective for the heart against myocardial damage	Kharadi et al., 2016
Leaf of Ginkgo biloba (Ginkgo) F. Ginkgoaceae	Flavonoids, terpenoids, glycosides.	Enhances the lifespan of cardiomyocytes and prevents their apoptosis via regulating the PI3K-AKT and NF-κB pathways.	Xiang et al., 2021
Seeds of Glycine max (soybean) F. Angiospermae	Beta-sitosterol	Enhances low-density lipoprotein oxidation resistance, prevents thrombus formation, and improves vascular reactivity.	Vasanthi et al., 2022
Aerial part of Gynostemma pentaphyllum Jiaogulan F. Cucurbitaceae	Gypenosides, saponins	Reactivity exhibits synergistic effects in reducing lipid synthesis and increasing oxidation. It also demonstrates inhibition against foam cell formation and intracellular lipid buildup caused by oxidized low-density lipoprotein. Finally, it regulates cholesterol metabolism.	Nguyen et al., 2021
Leaf of Moringa olifera (Moringa) F. Moringaceae	Quercetin, chlorogenic acid, beta-carotene, and other antioxidants	Reduces blood cholesterol levels	Adekanmi et al., 2020
Leaf of Moringa stenopetala (Moringa) F. Moringaceae	Quercetin (flavonoid)	Manage the hypertension	Castejón et al., 2020
Seeds of Nigella sativa (Kalonji) F. Ranunculaceae	Thymoquinone, cinnamaldehyde	Reduces oxidative stress and controls to prevent the development of hypertension	Shamlan, 2021
Leaf of Ocimum sanctum (Tulsi) F. Lamiaceae	Ursolic acid, eugenol	Demonstrates the substantial impact of reducing blood pressure on treating cardiovascular consequences	Pour et al., 2021
Leaf of Olea europaea (Olive) F. Oleaceae	Oleuropein, iridoids and secoiridoids	Plays a preventive role for the heart against lipid oxidation and cholesterol excess	Adekanmi et al., 2020
Root, berry and leaf of Panax spp. Ginseng) F. Araliaceae	Ginsenosides, protopanaxadiol, protopanaxatriol, and oleanan	Controls blood pressure and blood flow.	Shamlan, 2021
Seeds of Persea americana (Avocado) F. Lauraceae	Beta-sitosterol	Reduces the cardiotoxicity caused by doxorubicin	Shamlan, 2021
Fruit of Phoenix dactylifera (Date Palm) F. Arecaceae	Flavonoids and phenolic	Demonstrates a heart tissue's ability to withstand cardiotoxicity brought on by doxorubicin treatment.	Khalid et al., 2020

Plant source	Phyto-constituents	Cardiovascular Activity	References
Root, leaves of Potentilla reptans (Creeping Cinquefoil) F. Rosaceae	Tannins, triterpenoids	Numerous signaling pathways' up- or down-regulation in relation to their cardiovascular qualities	Enayati et al., 2022
Root of Rhodiola rosea (Arctic Root) F. Crassulaceae	Monoterpene alcohols and their glycosides, cyanogenic glycosides, and flavonoids	Preventing cardiovascular illnesses	Argyropoulou et al., 2013
Flowers of Rosa damascene (Damask Rose) F. Rosaceae	Flavonoids, glycosides, polyphenols	Preventing cardiovascular disease by controlling blood lipids and oxidative stress	Argyropoulou et al., 2013
Root, stem of Rumex obtusifolius (Bitter Dock) F. Polygonaceae	Anthracene derivatives, flavonoids, and procyanidins	Lowers the chance of developing cardiovascular disease by regulating obesity, oxidative stress, and blood lipid accumulation.	Feduraev et al., 2019
Seeds and flowers of Trifolium pratense (Red Clover) F. Fabaceae	Isoflavones: daidzein,genistein, formononetin	Lowers cholesterol to prevent cardiovascular illnesses	Ramos et al., 2011
Root and rhizome of Salvia miltiorrhiza (Danshen) F. Lamiaceae	Tanshinones, salvianolic acids	Increases plasminogen activator, anticoagulant thrombomodulin, eNOS-dependent NO generation, limits LDL oxidation and extravasation, and guarantees OxLDL-induced endothelial cell damage in order to modify endothelial hemostasis.	Li et al., 2018; Orgah et al., 2020
Fruit of Solanum lycopersicum (Tomato) F. Solanaceae	Lycopene	Lowers blood pressure to lessen the risk of cardiovascular illnesses in humans and keeps an eye on type 2 diabetes	Alseekh et al., 2020
Leaves, root of Sophora mollis (Mexican Mountain Laurel) F. Fabaceae	Matrine, rutin	Conventional treatment for the cardio protective effect	Kunwar et al., 2010
Fruit of Vaccinium myrtillus (Bilberry) F. Ericaceae	Anthocyanosides	Reduces LDL-C/TG and raises HDL-C levels	Danielewski et al., 2020
Rhizome and root of Veratrum grandiflorum (Green False Hellebore) F. Melanthiaceae	Jervine, resveratrol	Cardiovascular protection against oxidative stress and inflammation	Dull et al., 2019

Table 2. Nano formulation of some phytoconstituents with study of *in vitro/in vivo* experimental model and their respective results

Nano formulation	Bioactive Compound	Experimental Model	Results	References
Polyethylene glycol methyl ether-block-poly, D,L- lactide, Nanoparticles	Curcumin	Ehrlich ascites carcinoma and cardiomyocytes exposed to palmitate	Inhibiting the oxidative stress and cell death caused by NADPH	Alotaibi et al., 2021
Chitosan nanoparticles	Curcumin	Ehrlich ascites carcinoma and animal model (albino mice)	Reduction of EAC-induced cardiotoxicity, protection against myocardial damage	Li et al., 2017
Glyceryl mono-oleate oil phase and Nano emulsion	Curcumin	(3-hydroxy-3-methylglutaryl-coenzyme A) reductase assay	Increased levels of the angiotensin-converting enzyme as well as inhibition of antihyper cholesterolemic effect	Rachmawati et al., 2016
Micelles of F127	Curcumin, resveratrol	Embryonic rat Cardiomyocytes	Cardio protection, a decrease in ROS and apoptosis in cardiomyocytes under doxorubicin treatment.	Carlson et al., 2014
Mesoporous silica nanoparticles	Quercetin	*In vivo* rat model of myocardial ischemia reperfusion	Enhances the degree of oxidative stress and death in myocardial cells through control of the JAK2/STAT3 signaling pathway, which aids in the restoration of cardiac blood flow.	Zhang et al., 2019
PLGA Nanoparticles	Quercetin	H9c2 cells, a surrogate model of cardiac cells	Enhances the potential of PLGA-quercetin NP to protect against hypoxia-reoxygenation injury by maintaining mitochondrial function, making it more effective than free quercetin.	Xu et al., 2018
Nanoparticles of Albumin	Resveratrol Nanoparticles	*In vivo*/male Sprague–Dawley rats	Considerable reduction in oxidative stress as a result of longer blood circulation and sustained release pattern; improved neurological score and lowered infarct volume 24 hours after injection in a dose-dependent manner.	Lozano et al., 2019
Solid–lipid Nanoparticles/ glycerol monostearate oil phase	Resveratrol Nanoparticles	In-vivo pharmacodynamics study/*in vitro* male mice	Doxorubicin cardiotoxicity is inhibited, the myocardium is protected, the cardiomyocyte calcium cycling is improved, and reactive oxygen species generation is inhibited.	Liu et al., 2021
Soybean oil, egg lecithin surfactant, and nanoemulsion	Coenzyme Q10	*In vitro*/cardiomyocytes and fibroblasts model	Various molecular mechanisms of cardioprotection with trastuzumab and doxorubicin therapies; cardiac microenvironment modulation by anti-inflammatory actions.	Quagliariello et al., 2020

Applications of Phytoconstituents in Cardiovascular Diseases

Flavonoids

Flavonoids are bioactive compounds with significant biological effects that may aid in the prevention of chronic diseases, including CVDs. Numerous epidemiological and experimental studies have demonstrated a negative correlation between flavonoid consumption and cardiovascular events. Research indicates that various flavonoids present in foods, such as beverages, spices, fruits, vegetables, and medicinal plants, can help reduce the risk of CVDs (Hanafi & Amrani, 2007). Flavonoids are abundant in a wide range of foods, particularly in fruits and vegetables like onions and apples. One study found that higher flavonoid intake was significantly associated with a reduced incidence of stroke. Additionally, flavonoids positively influence the cardiovascular system by promoting vasodilation and inhibiting endothelial apoptosis (Keli et al., 1996). Polygonum minus is rich in methyl-flavonol, quercetin, and myricetin, all of which possess anti-inflammatory and antioxidant properties that contribute to the treatment of cardiovascular disease. Quercetin, which is also effective in managing CVD, is found in foods such as onions, apples, wine, and tea (Hollman et al., 1997).

Plant Sterols

Plant sterols function similarly to animal cholesterol and are found in various food sources, including vegetables, grains, bread, spreads and margarine, vegetable oils, and fruits. Together, these foods contribute to approximately 12% of the daily intake of plant sterols. The most abundant dietary sources of plant sterols come from oils, oil seeds, and oily fruits, with pistachios containing the highest percentage among fatty fruits. Additionally, corn, rapeseed, and wheat germ oils are particularly rich in sterols. Other sources include cereals and legumes (Wang et al., 2018). Key plant sterols include campesterol, β-sitosterol, and stigmasterol, all of which are essential for health (Paduch et al., 2007). Plant sterols are beneficial in managing cardiovascular disease as they reduce cholesterol absorption in the intestines.

Terpenoids

Terpenoids are a broad and diverse class of lipids found in nature, characterized by their structure, which consists of one or more isoprene units (Bachheti et al., 2022). Monoterpenes, diterpenes, and sesquiterpenes are produced by specialized organs such as cell schizogenous glands, lysigenous glands, and ducts. Plant terpenoids are widely valued for their aromatic properties, and their bioactivity has been studied, including notable compounds such as salvinorin-A, menthol, citral, and camphor. Several terpenoids have been explored for their potential therapeutic effects on CVDs. These include ceraserol, boswellic acid, 6β-OH-Betulinic acid, astragaloside IV, asiatic acid, triterpenic acid, ursolic acid, and β-sitosterol glycoside. Notably, corrosolinic acid has been shown to reduce the extent of atherosclerosis in the abdominal aorta.

Alkaloids

Alkaloids are an intriguing group of basic nitrogen atom-containing phytochemicals that exist naturally. They are members of the Solanaceae, Acanthaceae, Apocynaceae, and Papaveraceae plant families. Certain alkaloids are known to possess cardioprotective properties as they can decrease cholesterol levels and may exhibit antioxidant and anti-inflammatory effects. The most common alkaloids include morphine, propane, purine, acridone, indole, and imidazole. Historically, reserpine has been used as an antihypertensive drug. It works by depleting neurotransmitters from nerve terminals, such as norepinephrine, which causes vasodilation and a reduction in blood pressure. Although its adverse effects have led to a decrease in use, this has opened the door for research into other alkaloids that may positively affect heart health. Potential antioxidant qualities of alkaloids as phytoconstituents in cardiovascular health are being investigated. Certain alkaloids, such as theophylline and theobromine, found in green tea, may improve blood vessel function, lower oxidative stress, and reduce inflammation to promote cardiovascular health (Andraws et al., 2005). With their bioactive compounds displaying a variety of pharmacological actions, plants containing alkaloids have become significant players in managing cardiovascular disease. Specific alkaloids, such as reserpine from *Rauwolfia serpentina* and vincamine from *Vinca minor*, have shown promise in controlling blood pressure and enhancing cardiovascular health.

Quinones

Furthermore, traditional medicines are derived from the aforementioned classes of secondary metabolites. Quinones possess cardioprotective properties; in a rat experiment, pyrroloquinoline was shown to protect rat cardiac myocytes from oxidative damage while maintaining mitochondrial activity. Thymoquinone can be obtained from species such as *Satureja*, *Origanum*, *Eupatorium ayapana*, *Calocedrus decurrens*, *Thymus vulgaris*, *Nepeta distans*, and the seeds of *Nigella sativa.* An investigation involving rats revealed that these compounds exhibit cardioprotective properties by enhancing mitochondrial activity through increased ATP synthesis (Arauna et al., 2019). Plants containing quinones have garnered attention for their potential medicinal use in heart disease. Notable examples include the antioxidant coenzyme Q10 (CoQ10) and shikonin found in *Lithospermum erythrorhizon*, both of which demonstrate heart-protective qualities.

Plant Sulfur Compounds

The most well-known plants containing sulfur compounds associated with the prevention of CVDs include leeks, onions, garlic, and cruciferous vegetables such as kale, cauliflower, cabbage, and broccoli. The primary sulfur compound found in cruciferous vegetables is sulforaphane. Additionally, garlic has been shown to lower blood pressure, prevent platelet aggregation, and slow coagulation. Sulforaphane reduces CVD by activating Nrf2, while compounds such as diallyl disulfide and allicin inhibit atherosclerosis by lowering lipid levels and preventing cholesterol production (Bachheti et al., 2022). Some sulfur-rich plant extracts have demonstrated cardioprotective effects, particularly in blood pressure regulation, inflammatory modulation, and lipid metabolism.

Conclusion

In conclusion, utilizing nanophytoherbals as a therapeutic approach offers a promising pathway for treating cardiovascular disorders. The integration of herbal medicine and nanotechnology addresses the limitations of traditional therapies, presenting a novel strategy for managing cardiovascular conditions. By enhancing the absorption and bioavailability of phytochemicals from medicinal plants, nanoparticles facilitate effective drug delivery. This targeted approach not only minimizes the risk of side effects but also maximizes the therapeutic potential of phytoherbals. The compositions possess inherent anti-inflammatory, antioxidant, and vasorelaxant properties, contributing to their efficacy in preventing and treating cardiovascular ailments. As we explore this interdisciplinary field further, more research is needed to clarify the mechanisms, long-term effects, and overall safety profile of nanophytoherbals. Advances in this area could herald a new era of personalized, effective, and safer treatment options for patients with CVDs.

References

Adekanmi, A. A., Adekanmi, S. A., & Adekanmi, O. S. (2020). Qualitative and quantitative phytochemical constituents of moringa leaf. *International Journal of Engineering and Information Systems, 4*, 10–17.

Alotaibi, B., Tousson, E., El-Masry, T. A., Altwaijry, N., & Saleh, A. (2021). Ehrlich ascites carcinoma as a model for studying the cardiac protective effects of curcumin nanoparticles against cardiac damage in female mice. *Environmental Toxicology, 36*(1), 105–113.

Alseekh, S., Perez de Souza, L., Benina, M., & Fernie, A. R. (2020). The style and substance of plant flavonoid decoration: Towards defining both structure and function. *Phytochemistry, 174*, 1–15.

Alves-Silva, J. M., Zuzarte, M., Marques, C., Salgueiro, L., & Girao, H. (2016). Protective effects of terpenes on the cardiovascular system: Current advances and future perspectives. *Current Medicinal Chemistry, 23*(40), 4559–4600.

Andraws, R., Chawla, P., & Brown, D. L. (2005). Cardiovascular effects of ephedra alkaloids: a comprehensive review. *Progress in cardiovascular diseases*, *47*(4), 217-225.

Anwar, M. A., Al Disi, S. S., & Eid, A. H. (2016). Anti-hypertensive herbs and their mechanisms of action. *Frontiers in Pharmacology, 6*, 1–25.

Arauna, D., Furrianca, M., Espinosa-Parrilla, Y., Fuentes, E., Alarcón, M., & Palomo, I. (2019). Natural bioactive compounds as protectors of mitochondrial dysfunction in cardiovascular diseases and aging. *Molecules*, *24*(23), 4259.

Argyropoulou, A., Aligiannis, N., Trougakos, I. P., & Skaltsounis, A. (2013). Natural compounds with anti-ageing activity. *Natural Product Reports, 30*, 3099–3113.

Bachheti, R. K., Worku, L. A., Gonfa, Y. H., Zebeaman, M., Deepti, Pandey, D. P., & Bachheti, A. (2022). Prevention and Treatment of Cardiovascular Diseases with Plant Phytochemicals: A Review. *Evidence-Based Complementary and Alternative Medicine*, *2022*(1), 5741198.

Binsalamah, Z. M., Paul, A., Khan, A. A., Prakash, S., & Shum-Tim, D. (2011). Intramyocardial sustained delivery of placental growth factor using nanoparticles as a vehicle for delivery in the rat infarct model. *International Journal of Nanomedicine, 6*, 2667–2678.

Carlson, L. J., Cote, B., Alani, A. W., & Rao, D. A. (2014). Polymeric micellar co-delivery of resveratrol and curcumin to mitigate *in vitro* doxorubicin-induced cardiotoxicity. *Journal of Pharmaceutical Sciences, 103*(8), 2315–2322.

Castejón, M. L., Montoya, T., Alarcón-de-la-lastra, C., & Sánchez-Hidalgo, M. (2020). Potential protective role exerted by secoiridoids from *Olea europaea* L. in cancer, cardiovascular, neurodegenerative, aging-related, and immunoinflammatory diseases. *Antioxidants, 9*, 1–38.

Chang, X., Zhang, T., Zhang, W., Zhao, Z., & Sun, J. (2020). Natural drugs as a treatment strategy for cardiovascular disease through the regulation of oxidative stress. *Oxidative Medicine and Cellular Longevity, 2020*, 5430407.

Danielewski, M., Matuszewska, A., Nowak, B., Kucharska, A. Z., & Sozański, T. (2020). The effects of natural iridoids and anthocyanins on selected parameters of liver and cardiovascular system functions. *Oxidative Medicine and Cellular Longevity, 2020*, Article ID 2735790, 12 pages.

Dull, A. M., Moga, M. A., Dimienescu, O. G., Sechel, G., Burtea, V., & Anastasiu, C. V. (2019). Therapeutic approaches of resveratrol on endometriosis via anti-inflammatory and antiangiogenic pathways. *Molecules, 24*, 1–21.

Enayati, A., Salehi, A., Alilou, M., Stuppner, H., Mirzaei, H., Omraninava, A., Khori, V., & Yassa, N. (2022). Six new triterpenoids from the root of *Potentilla reptans* and their cardioprotective effects in silico. *Natural Product Research*, 36(10), 2504–2512.

Feduraev, P., Chupakhina, G., Maslennikov, P., Tacenko, N., & Skrypnik, L. (2019). Variation in phenolic compounds content and antioxidant activity of different plant organs from *Rumex crispus* L. and *Rumex obtusifolius* L. at different growth stages. *Antioxidants, 8*(1), 1–15.

Fuchs, F. D., & Whelton, P. K. (2020). High blood pressure and cardiovascular disease. *Hypertension, 75*(2), 285–292.

Fürst, R., & Zündorf, I. (2014). Plant-derived anti-inflammatory compounds: Hopes and disappointments regarding the translation of preclinical knowledge into clinical progress. *Mediators of Inflammation, 2014*, 9.

Gao, Z., Chen, Z., Sun, A., & Deng, X. (2019). Gender differences in cardiovascular disease. *Med. Novel Technol. Devices, 4*.

Hamer, M., O'Donovan, G., & Stamatakis, E. (2019). Association between physical activity and sub-types of cardiovascular disease death causes in a general population cohort. *European Journal of Epidemiology, 34*(5), 483–487.

Hanafi, H., & Amrani, S. (2007). Flavonoids as potent phytochemicals in cardiovascular diseases prevention. *Pharmacognosy Reviews, 1*(2), 193–202.

Hesari, M., Mohammadi, P., Khademi, F., et al. (2021). Current advances in the use of nanophytomedicine therapies for human cardiovascular diseases. *International Journal of Nanomedicine, 16*, 3293.

Hollman, P. C., Van Trijp, J. M., Buysman, M. N., van der Gaag, M. S., Mengelers, M. J., De Vries, J. H., & Katan, M. B. (1997). Relative bioavailability of the antioxidant flavonoid quercetin from various foods in man. *FEBS Letters, 418*(1–2), 152–156.

Islam, S. U., Ahmed, M. B., Ahsan, H., & Lee, Y. S. (2021). Recent molecular mechanisms and beneficial effects of phytochemicals and plant-based whole foods in reducing LDL-C and preventing cardiovascular disease. *Antioxidants, 10*(5), 784.

Jayaraman, M. J., Hanna, P., Balaji, A., Sadiya Banu, M., & Prathyusha, M. (2021). A comprehensive review of medicinal plants for cardioprotective potential. *International Journal of Advanced Pharmaceutics and Biotechnology, 7*, 24–29.

Jayasuriya, W. J. A., & Sarveswaran, B. R. (2017). *In vitro* assays to investigate the anti-inflammatory. *World Journal of Pharmacy, 6*, 131–141.

Keli, S. O., Hertog, M. G., Feskens, E. J., & Kromhout, D. (1996). Dietary flavonoids, antioxidant vitamins, and incidence of stroke: The Zutphen study. *Archives of Internal Medicine, 156*(6), 637-642.

Khalid, S., Arshad, M., Saad, B., Imran, M., Bader Ul Ain, H., Tufail, T., Shahid, M. Z., Atif, M., Ikram Ullah, M., & Ahmed, S. (2020). Cardioprotective effects of dates. *International Journal of Biosciences, 6655*, 110–123.

Kharadi, G. B., Patel, K. J., Purohit, B. M., Baxi, S. N., & Tripathi, C. B. (2016). Evaluation of cardioprotective effect of aqueous extract of *Allium cepa* Linn. bulb on isoprenaline-induced myocardial injury in Wistar albino rats. *Research in Pharmaceutical Sciences, 11*, 419–427.

Kim, Y., Youjin, J., & Giovannucci, E. L. (2021). Association between dietary fat intake and mortality from all causes, cardiovascular disease, and cancer: A systematic review and meta-analysis of prospective cohort studies. *Clinical Nutrition, 40*(3), 1060–1070.

Kumar, V. V., Chandrasekar, D., Ramakrishna, S., Kishan, V., Rao, Y. M., & Diwan, P. V. (2007). Development and evaluation of nitrendipine-loaded solid lipid nanoparticles: Influence of wax and glyceride lipids on plasma pharmacokinetics. *International Journal of Pharmaceutics, 335*(1–2), 167–175.

Kunwar, R. M., Burlakoti, C., Chowdhary, L., & Bussmann, R. W. (2010). Medicinal plants in Farwest Nepal: Indigenous uses and pharmacological validity. *Medicinal and Aromatic Plant Science and Biotechnology, 4*(1), 28–42.

La Francesca, S. (2012). Nanotechnology and stem cell therapy for cardiovascular diseases: Potential applications. *Methodist Debakey Cardiovascular Journal, 8*(1), 28–35.

Li, J., Zhou, Y., Zhang, W., Bao, C., & Xie, Z. (2017). Relief of oxidative stress and cardiomyocyte apoptosis by using curcumin nanoparticles. *Colloids and Surfaces B: Biointerfaces, 153*, 174–182.

Li, Z. M., Xu, S. W., & Liu, P. Q. (2018). *Salvia miltiorrhiza* Burge (Danshen): A golden herbal medicine in cardiovascular therapeutics. *Acta Pharmacologica Sinica, 39*, 802–824.

Liu, C. J., Yao, L., Hu, Y. M., & Zhao, B. T. (2021). Effect of quercetin-loaded mesoporous silica nanoparticles on myocardial ischemia-reperfusion injury in rats and its mechanism. *International Journal of Nanomedicine, 16*, 741–752.

Lombardo, D., Kiselev, M. A., & Caccamo, M. T. (2019). Smart nanoparticles for drug delivery application: Development of versatile nanocarrier platforms in biotechnology and nanomedicine. *Journal of Nanomaterials, 2019*, Article ID 3702518.

Lozano, O., Lázaro-Alfaro, A., Silva-Platas, C., Oropeza-Almazán, Y., Torres-Quintanilla, A., Bernal-Ramírez, J., Alves-Figueiredo, H., & García-Rivas, G. (2019). Nanoencapsulated quercetin improves cardioprotection during hypoxia-reoxygenation injury through preservation of mitochondrial function. *Oxidative Medicine and Cellular Longevity, 2019*, Article ID 7683051.

Lundy, D. J., Chen, K. H., Toh, E. K. W., & Hsieh, P. C. H. (2016). Distribution of systemically administered nanoparticles reveals a size-dependent effect immediately following cardiac ischaemia-reperfusion injury. *Scientific Reports, 6*, 25613.

Maiuolo, J., Carresi, C., Gliozzi, M., Musolino, V., Scarano, F., Coppoletta, A. R., Guarnieri, L., Nucera, S., Scicchitano, M., Bosco, F., Ruga, S., Zito, M. C., Macri, R., Cardamone, A., Serra, M., Mollace, R., Tavernese, A., & Mollace, V. (2021). Effects of bergamot polyphenols on mitochondrial dysfunction and sarcoplasmic reticulum stress in diabetic cardiomyopathy. *Nutrients, 13*, 1–20.

Neag, M. A., Mocan, A., Echeverría, J., Pop, R. M., Bocsan, C. I., Crişan, G., & Buzoianu, A. D. (2018). Berberine: Botanical occurrence, traditional uses, extraction methods, and relevance in cardiovascular, metabolic, hepatic, and renal disorders. *Frontiers in Pharmacology, 9*, 1–30.

Nguyen, N. H., Ha, T. K. Q., Yang, J. L., Pham, H. T. T., & Oh, W. K. (2021). Triterpenoids from the genus *Gynostemma*: Chemistry and pharmacological activities. *Journal of Ethnopharmacology, 268*, 113691.

Orgah, J. O., He, S., Wang, Y., Jiang, M., Wang, Y., Orgah, E. A., Duan, Y., Zhao, B., Zhang, B., Han, J., & Zhu, Y. (2020). Pharmacological potential of the combination of *Salvia miltiorrhiza* (Danshen) and *Carthamus tinctorius* (Honghua) for diabetes mellitus and its cardiovascular complications. *Pharmacological Research, 153*, 1–13.

Paduch, R., Kandefer-Szerszeń, M., Trytek, M., & Fiedurek, J. (2007). Terpenes: substances useful in human healthcare. *Archivum immunologiae et therapiae experimentalis*, *55*, 315-327.89.

Panda, V. S., & Naik, S. R. (2009). Evaluation of cardioprotective activity of Ginkgo biloba and Ocimum sanctum in rodents. *Alternative Medicine Review, 14*(2), 161.

Patel, R. V., Mistry, B. V., Shinde, S. K., Syed, R., Singh, V., & Shin, H.-S. (2018). Therapeutic potential of quercetin as a cardiovascular agent. *European Journal of Medicinal Chemistry, 155*, 889–904.

Patra, J. K., & Das, F. L. (2018). Nano-based drug delivery systems: Recent developments and future prospects. *Journal of Nanobiotechnology, 16*(1), 1–23.

Pop, R. M., Popolo, A., Trifa, A. P., & Stanciu, L. A. (2018). Phytochemicals in cardiovascular and respiratory diseases: Evidence in oxidative stress and inflammation. *Oxidative Medicine and Cellular Longevity, 2018*, 1603872.

Pour, M. P., Farzaei, M. H., Soleiman Dehkordi, E., Bishayee, A., & Asgary, S. (2021). Therapeutic targets of natural products for the management of cardiovascular symptoms of coronavirus disease 2019. *Phytotherapy Research, 35*, 2021.

Prachayasittikul, V., Prachayasittikul, S., Ruchirawat, S., & Prachayasittikul, V. (2018). Coriander (*Coriandrum sativum*): A promising functional food toward well-being. *Food Research International, 105*, 305–323.

Quagliariello, V., Vecchione, R., De Capua, A., Lagreca, E., Iaffaioli, R. V., Botti, G., Netti, P. A., & Maurea, N. (2020). Nano-encapsulation of coenzyme Q10 in secondary and tertiary nano-emulsions for enhanced cardioprotection and hepatoprotection in human cardiomyocytes and hepatocytes during exposure to anthracyclines and trastuzumab. *International Journal of Nanomedicine, 15*, 4859–4876.

Rachmawati, H., Soraya, I. S., Kurniati, N. F., & Rahma, A. (2016). *In vitro* study on antihypertensive and anti-hypercholesterolemic effects of a curcumin nanoemulsion. *Scientia Pharmaceutica, 84*(2), 131–140.

Ramos, G. P., Apel, M. A., de Morais, C. B., Ceolato, P. C., Schapoval, E. E. S., Dall'Agnol, M., & Zuanazzi, J. A. S. (2011). *In vivo* and *in vitro* anti-inflammatory activity of red clover *Trifolium pratense* dry extract. *Brazilian Journal of Pharmacognosy, 22*, 176–180.

Reiner, Z., Laufs, U., Cosentino, F., & Landmesser, U. (2019). The year in cardiology 2018: Prevention. *European Heart Journal, 40*(4), 336–344.

Sangwan, R. S., Chaurasiya, N. D., Misra, L. N., Lal, P., Uniyal, G. C., Sharma, R., Sangwan, N. S., Suri, K. A., Qazi, G. N., & Tuli, R. (2004). Phytochemical variability in commercial herbal products and preparations of *Withania somnifera* (Ashwagandha). *Current Science, 86*, 461–465.

Shah, S. M. A., Akram, M., Riaz, M., Munir, N., & Rasool, G. (2019). Cardioprotective potential of plant-derived molecules: A scientific and medicinal approach. *Dose-Response, 17*(2), 1559325819852243.

Shaito, A., Thuan, D. T. B., Phu, H. T., Nguyen, T. H. D., Hasan, H., Halabi, S., Abdelhady, S., Nasrallah, G. K., Eid, A. H., & Pintus, G. (2020). Herbal medicine for cardiovascular diseases: Efficacy, mechanisms, and safety. *Frontiers in Pharmacology, 11*, 422.

Shamlan, G. (2021). Ethanolic and aqueous extracts of avocado (*Persea americana*) seeds attenuate doxorubicin-induced cardiotoxicity in male albino rats. *Arabian Journal for Science and Engineering, 46*, 5265–5274.

Silva, H., Francisco, R., Saraiva, A., Francisco, S., Carrascosa, C., & Raposo, A. (2021). The cardiovascular therapeutic potential of propolis—a comprehensive review. *Biology, 10*(1), 1–20.

Singh, D., & Chaudhuri, P. K. (2018). Structural characteristics, bioavailability, and cardioprotective potential of saponins. *Integrative Medicine Research, 7*, 33–43.

Smith, C., & Swart, A. (2018). *Aspalathus linearis* (Rooibos)–a functional food targeting cardiovascular disease. *Food & Function, 9*, 5041–5058.

Souza, M. M. Q., Silva, G. R. D., Cola, I. M., Silva, A. O., Schaedler, M. I., Guarnier, L. P., Palozi, R. A. C., Barboza, L. N., Menetrier, J. V., Froelich, D. L., Auth, P. A., Veiga, A. A., Souza, L. M., Lovato, E. C. W., Ribeiro-Paes, J. T., Gasparotto Junior, A., & Lívero, F. A. D. R. (2020). *Baccharis trimera* (Less.) DC: An innovative cardioprotective herbal medicine against multiple risk factors for cardiovascular disease. *Journal of Medicinal Food, 23*, 676–684.

Souza-Junior, F. J. C., Luz-Moraes, D., Pereira, F. S., Barros, M. A., Fernandes, L. M. P., Queiroz, L. Y., Maia, C. F., Maia, J. G. S., & Fontes-Junior, E. A. (2020). *Aniba canelilla* (Kunth) Mez (Lauraceae): A review of ethnobotany, phytochemical, antioxidant, anti-inflammatory, cardiovascular, and neurological properties. *Frontiers in Pharmacology, 11*, 1–14.

Toth, P. P. (2007). Making a case for quantitative assessment of cardiovascular risk. *Journal of Clinical Lipidology, 1*(4), 234–241.

Vasanthi, H., Shrishrimal, N., & Das, D. (2012). Phytochemicals from plants to combat cardiovascular disease. *Current Medicinal Chemistry, 19*, 2242–2251.

Wang, M., Huang, W., Hu, Y., Zhang, L., Shao, Y., Wang, M., & Lu, B. (2018). Phytosterol profiles of common foods and estimated natural intake of different structures and forms in China. *Journal of Agricultural and Food Chemistry, 66*(11), 2669–2676.

Wang, Z., Mu, W., Li, P., Liu, G., & Yang, J. (2021). Anti-inflammatory activity of ortho-trifluoromethoxy-substituted 4-piperidione-containing mono-carbonyl curcumin derivatives *in vitro* and *in vivo*. *European Journal of Pharmaceutical Sciences, 160*, 105737.

World Health Organization. (2014). *Global status report on noncommunicable diseases*. WHO.

Xiang, K., Yang, J., Wu, X., Peng, J., Guo, J., & Fan, C. (2021). Advances in traditional Chinese medicine for cardiovascular disease therapy in 2020. *Traditional Medicine Research, 6*, 1–18.

Xin, L. T., Yue, S. J., Fan, Y. C., Wu, J. S., Yan, D., Guan, H. S., & Wang, C. Y. (2017). *Cudrania tricuspidata*: An updated review on ethnomedicine, phytochemistry, and pharmacology. *RSC Advances, 7*, 31807–31832.

Xu, H., Hua, Y., Zhong, J., Li, X., Xu, W., Cai, Y., Mao, Y., & Lu, X. (2018). Resveratrol delivery by albumin nanoparticles improved neurological function and neuronal damage in transient middle cerebral artery occlusion rats. *Frontiers in Pharmacology, 9*, 1403.

Yanbei, T., Ying, Y., Yanfang, L., & Chengwei, H. (2021). Naturally occurring coumestans from plants, their biological activities, and therapeutic effects on human diseases. *Pharmacological Research, 169*, 1–24.

Zhang, L., Zhu, K., Zeng, H., Zhang, J., Pu, Y., Wang, Z., Zhang, T., & Wang, B. (2019). Resveratrol solid lipid nanoparticles to trigger credible inhibition of doxorubicin cardiotoxicity. *International Journal of Nanomedicine, 14*, 6061–6071.

Zhang, Y., Xu, H., Hu, Z., Yang, G., Yu, X., Chen, Q., Zheng, L., & Yan, Z. (2022). *Eleocharis dulcis* corm: Phytochemicals, health benefits, processing, and food products. *Journal of the Science of Food and Agriculture*, 1–15.

Zhou, D. D., Luo, M., Shang, A., Mao, Q. Q., Li, B. Y., Gan, R. Y., & Li, H. B. (2021). Antioxidant food components for the prevention and treatment of cardiovascular diseases: Effects, mechanisms, and clinical studies. *Oxidative Medicine and Cellular Longevity, 2021*, 17.

Chapter 9

Applications of Nanophytoherbals in Diabetes Therapy

Sanchit Dhankhar[1,*]
Nitika Garg[1]
Samrat Chauhan[1]
Chander Parkash[1]
and Monika Saini[2]
[1]Chitkara College of Pharmacy, Chitkara University, Punjab, India
[2]M.M. College of Pharmacy, Maharishi Markandeshwar (Deemed to be University), Mullana, Ambala, Haryana, India

Abstract

Diabetes is becoming increasingly prevalent worldwide, necessitating innovative and effective therapeutic approaches. The field of nanophytoherbals is a promising intersection of nanotechnology and the medicinal properties of phytochemicals derived from plants. This chapter explores the potential of nanophytoherbals, focusing primarily on diabetes therapy. It comprehensively examines the synthesis, characterization, and application of nanophytoherbals in managing diabetes mellitus. A key aspect of this chapter is the various ways in which nanophytoherbals can be utilized for diabetes control. This includes investigating a wide range of phytochemicals known to possess anti-diabetic properties, encapsulating these phytochemicals in nanocarriers, and assessing their impact on therapeutic outcomes. The chapter provides a detailed and up-to-date review of the applications of nanophytoherbals in diabetes treatment. It targets researchers, clinicians, and pharmaceutical scientists interested in harnessing the potential of nanotechnology and herbal medicine to address the complex challenges posed by diabetes mellitus, aiming to serve as a valuable resource for all stakeholders involved.

Keywords: applications, nanophytoherbals, diabetes, plants, phytochemicals

* Corresponding Author's Email: sanchitdhankhar@gmail.com.

In: Phyto-Nanomedicine
Editors: Hitesh Chopra, Vinod Kumar Gauttam, Ajmer Singh Grewal et al.
ISBN: 979-8-89530-317-7

Introduction

Hyperglycemia is a hallmark of diabetes mellitus (DM) and can lead to various complications, including hyperlipidemia, hyperinsulinemia, obesity, atherosclerosis, and cardiovascular disease. Symptoms of severe hyperglycemia include polyuria, polydipsia, polyphagia, weight loss, and blurred vision (Arora et al., 2021; Chauhan et al., 2023; Corb Aron et al., 2021; Kumar et al., 2021; Testa et al., 2017). This syndrome is characterized by hyperglycemia, abnormal lipid metabolism, and the body's inability to effectively utilize consumed glucose, resulting from either insufficient insulin supply or inadequate insulin response (Chauhan et al., 2021; Giri et al., 2018; Shi et al., 2019). Diabetes disrupts glucose, lipid, and protein metabolism due to insulin's ineffective action on target tissues. The most common types of this chronic metabolic disease include type 1 (T1DM), type 2 (T2DM), gestational diabetes mellitus (GDM), and "other specific forms" (Forouhi & Wareham, 2019; Gollapalli et al., 2022). Overcoming hyperglycemia can be achieved by either increasing insulin sensitivity or decreasing hepatic glucose production. Predisposing factors for T2DM include an individual's genetic makeup and lifestyle choices. Additional risk factors for peripheral artery disease in diabetics encompass smoking, high blood pressure, and high cholesterol. GDM can complicate pregnancy and increase the risk of complications such as altered pregnancy duration, placental failure, hypertension/pre-eclampsia, and delivering a high-weight baby. This classification also includes various specific forms of diabetes mellitus (McIntyre et al., 2019). Monogenic diabetes, exocrine pancreatic pathology, other endocrine disorders, drug side effects, and other forms of secondary diabetes are frequently encountered in clinical practice. Diabetes is the most common metabolic disease, affecting an estimated 200 million people worldwide (Yang & Chan, 2016). In 2010, 285 million people were estimated to have T2DM, and this number is projected to rise to 438 million by 2030, marking a 65 percent increase (Singh, 2016). In developing countries, diabetes accounts for approximately 2 to 3 percent of the total death rate, while in industrialized nations such as the United States, Canada, and countries in the Middle East, the diabetic mortality rate exceeds 8 percent. Diabetes mellitus is responsible for 6 to 27 percent of all deaths among individuals aged 35 to 64. In 2010, the global prevalence of DM in individuals aged 20 to 79 years was estimated at approximately 7 percent (Aynalem & Zeleke, 2018), with projections indicating an increase of more than fifty percent over the next twenty years. Similarly, India's diabetic population is expected to rise from 51 million in 2010 to 87 million in 2030, reflecting a 58 percent increase (Ram & Ram, 2021). Diabetes medication presents a global health crisis, as many commercially available drugs have adverse effects. Researchers are actively seeking effective diabetes treatments with minimal side effects. Diabetes management typically involves dietary modifications focused on weight control, optimal glycemic management, and correcting blood lipid abnormalities, often combined with exercise. When dietary changes and physical activity are insufficient, oral hypoglycemic drugs are considered (Dhankhar et al., 2023). Biguanides, such as metformin, primarily affect fasting glycemia by suppressing hepatic glucose production but commonly cause gastrointestinal side effects, including diarrhea, nausea, stomach pain, and a metallic taste (Zhao et al., 2020). Thiazolidinediones enhance insulin sensitivity in muscle, fat, and liver cells, potentially leading to increased subcutaneous adiposity, fluid retention, peripheral edema, and weight gain. Sulphonylureas stimulate insulin secretion by preventing potassium ion outflow from pancreatic β-cells but can also contribute to increased body fat and hypoglycemia. Alpha-glucosidase inhibitors act as competitive inhibitors in the small intestine, delaying glucose absorption and often causing gastrointestinal disturbances such as gas, indigestion, flatulence, and diarrhea. Exenatide, similar to the GLP-1 hormone, promotes insulin secretion and inhibits glucagon but may cause gastrointestinal issues like constipation, nausea, and vomiting. Dipeptidyl peptidase 4 (DPP-4) inhibitors enhance insulin and suppress glucagon secretion by inhibiting the breakdown of insulinotropic polypeptides and GLP-1, with common side effects including headaches and, rarely, exacerbation of nasopharyngitis. Pramlintide, a synthetic form of amylin, slows gastric emptying and reduces hunger but may lead to digestive issues and hypoglycemia. Bromocriptine, a central dopamine agonist taken in the morning, helps control blood sugar levels in type 2 diabetics. Insulin, a longstanding treatment, becomes essential when other medications fail, particularly in managing type 1 diabetes through injections or pumps. Despite its effectiveness, insulin therapy carries risks such as hypoglycemia, lipohypertrophy, hypersensitivity, and various other complications (Okur et al., 2017; Padhi et al., 2020).

The Importance of Natural Products in DM Treatment

According to Ayurveda and various Indian texts, many human ailments can be alleviated through the use of medicinal plants. Phytotherapy has long been a viable treatment option for a range of illnesses and conditions in numerous Asian cultures and around the world. India boasts approximately 45,000 different plant species, with thousands believed to have therapeutic uses. However, the mechanisms by which bioactive plants and compounds exert their effects are still largely unknown. Traditional antidiabetic herbs may offer a pathway to novel oral hypoglycemic lead compounds, addressing the high costs and limited accessibility of modern medications (Ahmed et al., 2023; Lalit et al., 2014; Patle et al., 2021; Rohilla et al., 2023; Saharan et al., 2024). This approach could be especially beneficial for rural communities in developing nations. WHO's Expert Committee on Diabetes has advocated for increased research into traditional medicinal herbs, as they are generally considered safe and free from negative side effects. Ethnobotanical data suggest that approximately 800 plants and their active extracts may possess antidiabetic properties. Utilizing plants with traditional medicinal uses presents an alternative strategy for managing diabetes. Despite their mention in historical texts, the efficacy of plants and their components in treating diabetes has been the focus of significant research in recent decades. Herbal formulations have gained widespread acceptance as diabetes treatments (Blahova et al., 2021). The simplification of chemical principles derived from natural sources has greatly facilitated the discovery of novel medications from medicinal plants. For example, the chemical foundation of metformin, guanidine, which exhibits blood glucose-lowering effects, was found to be abundant in Galega officinalis, leading to the development of this insulin sensitizer in 1957. Plants with antidiabetic properties can be categorized based on their diverse phytochemicals, which appear to be the active hypoglycemic agents (Dhankar et al., 2024; Xu et al., 2018). It is possible to classify the reported plant antidiabetics according to their potential mechanisms of action (Figure 1).

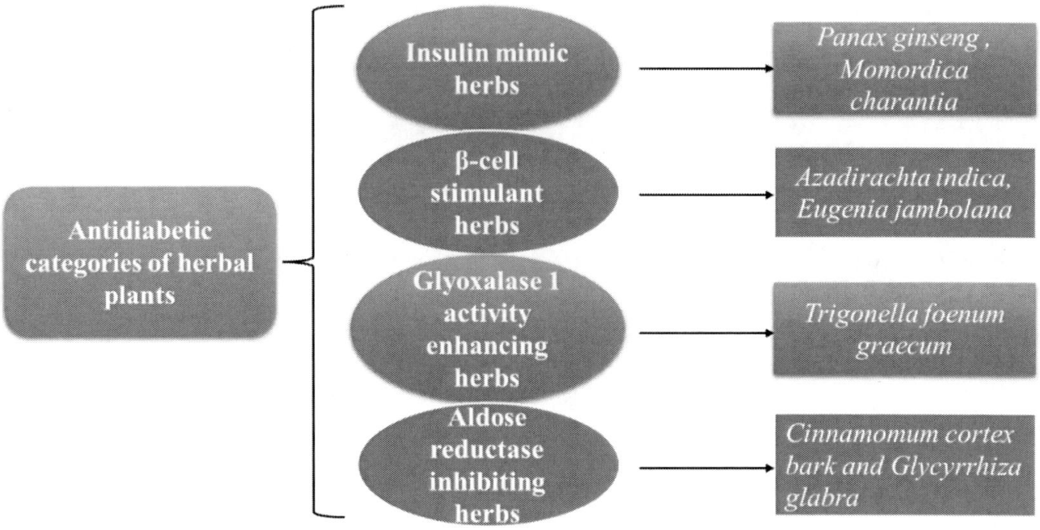

Figure 1. Antidiabetic categories of herbal plants.

Insulin Mimicing Herbs

Numerous plant parts, including onions, green bean leaves, and lettuce, have been identified as containing insulin-like proteins and compounds. Notably, significant hypoglycemic effects were observed *in vivo* for both ginseng polypeptide, derived from the root of *Panax ginseng*, and a pure protein extract from *Momordica charantia* (bitter gourd), which exhibited effects comparable to animal insulin. The ginseng polypeptide was isolated from the root of *Panax ginseng* (Manukumar et al., 2017).

β-Cell Stimulant Herbs

In a glucose-mediated insulin secretion inhibitory assay, *Azadirachta indica* leaf extract significantly inhibited serotonin. Additionally, oral treatment with *Eugenia jambolana* extract not only enhanced insulin secretion but also blocked insulinase activity in the liver and kidneys. A petroleum ether extract of dried onions demonstrated hypoglycemic activity and effectively treated alloxan-induced diabetes in rats, positioning it as a viable alternative to tolbutamide (Wickramasinghe et al., 2021).

β-Cell Regenerating Herbs

Isolated epicatechin from *Pterocarpus marsupium* heartwood exhibited regenerative effects on the islet β-cell population, which had been damaged by alloxan. In alloxan-induced rabbits, *Tinospora cordifolia* significantly reduced blood glucose levels without affecting lipid levels, demonstrating insulin-like activity (Wickramasinghe et al., 2021).

Glyoxalase 1 Activity Enhancing Herbs

In diabetic rats, powdered *Trigonella foenum-graecum* seeds restored all general metabolic parameters and normalized glyoxalase 1 activity to control values (Xue et al., 2016).

Glucagon Inhibiting Herbs

Ke-Tang-Ling is an Eastern antidiabetic drug that works by suppressing glucagon secretion from alpha cells in the pancreas, leading to a reduction in blood glucose levels in diabetic patients (Xue et al., 2016).

Glucose Absorption Reducing Herbs

The level of HbA1c gradually decreased with the petroleum extract of *Cyamopsis tetragonoloba*. Additionally, treatment with an alcoholic extract of *Ocimum sanctum* Linn leaves reduced glycemia in rats, regardless of whether they were streptozotocin-induced, glucose-fed hyperglycemic, or normoglycemic (Iid et al., 2020).

Aldose Reductase Inhibiting Herbs

Both *Cinnamomum cortex* bark and *Glycyrrhiza glabra* roots and rhizomes suppressed aldose reductase activity in rat lenses (Grewal et al., 2020).

Glucose Utility Enhancing Herbs

According to reports, the Gowar plant (*Cyamopsis tetragonolobus*) and phalsa (*Grewia asiatica*) may induce hypoglycemia through altered utilization. Additionally, pectin derived from *Coccinia indica* fruits demonstrated hypoglycemic effects, potentially due to impaired glucose absorption from the intestines (Hasanpour et al., 2020).

Glycogen Metabolic Enzyme Inhibiting Herbs

Trihydroxy octadecadienoic acids produced by *Bryonia alba* influenced the activity of hexokinase, glycogen phosphorylase, and phosphoprotein phosphatase in the liver and muscle tissues of alloxan-induced diabetic rats (Oyenihi et al., 2019).

Creatine Kinase Increasing Herbs

In experimental diabetic rats, *Trigonella foenum-graecum* restored normoglycemic conditions by normalizing the decreased levels of creatine kinase in the heart, skeletal muscle, and liver (Ghanbari-Niaki et al., 2019).

Need For Nanotechnology

To enhance patient compliance and eliminate the need for repeated administration, phytotherapeutics require a scientific approach to herbal medication delivery, particularly through innovative drug delivery systems. Nanotechnology presents a promising solution by improving therapeutic efficacy, reducing adverse effects, and enhancing bioavailability, thereby minimizing the need for multiple dosages. Nanotechnology-based drug delivery systems facilitate uniform distribution of medications throughout the body via the bloodstream and effectively target specific areas (Verma & Pandey, 2021). These systems offer several advantages, including the ability to traverse the smallest capillary vessels due to their minute size, penetrate cellular and tissue gaps to reach organs such as the liver, spleen, lungs, spinal cord, and lymph nodes, and provide prolonged, regulated release of medications. Animal studies have shown that nanoparticles (NPs) can enter the bloodstream, accumulate in various organs like the kidneys and liver, prevent drug degradation in the gastrointestinal tract, deliver medications in a controlled manner, and reduce side effects (Nikolova et al., 2020).

Nanoparticles in Drug Designing

To alleviate some of the symptoms and consequences of diabetes, there is an urgent need for new medication formulations based on existing phytochemicals with traditional uses. While conventional medicines typically exhibit a faster onset of action than herbal remedies, the high concentrations of phyto-antioxidants found in these herbs warrant further research to enhance their efficacy and bioavailability in targeting specific organs or systems. The effectiveness of herbal treatments is often more pronounced with long-term use (Mittal et al., 2023; Narwal et al., 2023; Panchal et al., 2024; Tzvetkov et al., 2023). NPs and materials at the nanoscale are appealing for use in biomedicine due to their favorable physical, chemical, and biological properties. Most NPs range in size from 100 to 1000 nm, though some are less than 100 nm in diameter and possess the unique ability to attract and repel water (Khan et al., 2019). These NPs release their medicinal content upon entering the bloodstream, responding to the pH of the blood. Their applications include delivering small-molecule and macromolecular therapies (such as DNA, RNA, and proteins), as well as disease diagnosis and progression monitoring. A particularly popular and environmentally friendly method for synthesizing NPs is through plant extraction (Tyagi & Santos, 2018). This approach offers several advantages over physical and chemical methods, such as availability, safety, and compatibility with pharmaceutical and biomedical applications, given the absence of toxic chemicals in the synthesis process. Consequently, nanodrugs can utilize the original drug material more efficiently and cost-effectively. Their enhanced ability to permeate cells results in a more rapid action compared to conventional medications. Moreover, nanodrugs are non-toxic, biocompatible, and biodegradable (Bhatia, 2016).

Nanoforumulations of Antidiabetic Herbal Drugs

Herbal medicine remains the cornerstone of diabetes management, despite the emergence of numerous novel treatment methods and the identification of new therapeutic targets. Plants serve as an excellent choice for the large-scale synthesis of NPs due to their cost-effectiveness, environmental friendliness, and rich variety of secondary metabolites (Sharma et al., 2023). For instance, a tablet containing NPs has been shown to help diabetic pigs regulate their post-meal blood sugar levels. Given that many medicinal plants and their phyto-compounds often exhibit poor water solubility, investigating their biological activity through nanosuspension formulations may prove beneficial. To facilitate their transition into pharmacy, nanoformulations must be characterized prior to preclinical and clinical investigations. Consequently, nanoformulations have demonstrated significantly greater anti-diabetic efficacy compared to commercially available drugs (Ioannidis et al., 2018).

Non-Metals

A lipid-based nanoemulsion significantly enhanced the oral antidiabetic efficacy of *Tinospora cordifolia* phytochemicals, while encapsulation confirmed the antihyperglycemic effects of *Phaleria macrocarpa* leaf extract (Dewanjee et al., 2020). Extensive research indicated that PLGA nanoencapsulated *Syzygium jambolanum* and *Gymnema sylvestre* demonstrated greater effectiveness in lowering blood sugar levels compared to their unencapsulated counterparts, suggesting potential new treatments for diabetes (Vargas et al., 2023). Furthermore, diabetic rats induced by streptozotocin and fed a high-fat diet exhibited strong antidiabetic benefits after receiving a lipid-based nanoformulation of the ethanolic extract of *Talinum portulacifolium*, administered at a dosage of 250 mg/kg body weight. The tannins and flavonoids in the extract were once believed to be responsible for its therapeutic effects (Bahloul et al., 2023).

Silver NPs (AgNPs)

Reproducing *Costus pictus* leaves in an environmentally friendly manner through the synthesis of silver nanoparticles (AgNPs) presents an innovative approach to diabetes treatment. AgNPs are recognized for their low toxicity, cost-effectiveness, and stability, making them a promising alternative to existing therapies. In diabetes-induced animal models, *Sphaeranthus amaranthoides* has been explored for AgNP production, demonstrating its potential by inhibiting α-amylase and enhancing the effects of acarbose. The ethanolic extract of *Sphaeranthus amaranthoides* primarily contains compounds that inhibit α-amylase, which contributes to its effectiveness in managing diabetes (Yazdanian et al., 2022).

Au-Ag NPs

Another method for assessing sun-dried *Cinnamomum camphora* leaves under ambient conditions involved the production of nanosized noble metals, such as gold and silver. Additionally, NPs were synthesized using the floral and leaf components of *Ocimum basilicum* (Chen et al., 2017).

Copper NPs (CuNPs)

The antioxidant and anti-diabetic characteristics of CuNPs synthesized from *Dioscorea bulbifera* extract were discovered for the first time. The inhibitory action of CuNPs on pig pancreatic α-amylase and crude mouse pancreatic and intestinal amylase indicates their potential as antidiabetic agents (Bhuvaneswari et al., 2023). This evidence supports the antidiabetic potential of biogenic CuNPs as a possible treatment to halt free radical-induced DM and its complications (Bhagwat et al., 2018; Saini et al., 2022; Chauhan et al., 2015). An enhanced antidiabetic medication with improved bioavailability is anticipated from nanoforming stevioside extracted from *Stevia rebaudiana* leaves. Nanoformulated *Momordica charantia*, containing active antidiabetic compounds, effectively inhibited α-glucosidase and α-amylase enzymes in laboratory tests (Jampílek & Kráľová, 2019). In studies comparing diabetic controls, mice with type 2 diabetes receiving encapsulated Chinese propolis—derived from the buds of various medicinal plants—exhibited significantly lower fasting blood glucose levels. Furthermore, encapsulated propolis reduced triglyceride levels in these rats, likely due to its effects on insulin sensitivity and lipoprotein lipase activity. To investigate the potential anti-diabetic, antioxidant, and wound-healing properties of curcumin, male C57/B6 mice were administered various doses of nanoencapsulated curcumin (Hamilton & Gilbert, 2023). Additionally, AuNPs were used to encapsulate propanoic acid, a bioactive component from *Cassia auriculata*, to evaluate its therapeutic potential for diabetes. Diabetic rats treated with 0.5 mg/kg of this formulation showed reductions in blood glucose, triglycerides, and cholesterol levels, alongside improved insulin levels (Marella & Tollamadugu, 2018).

Toxicity Studies

The toxic effects and brain distribution profiles of NPs should be evaluated based on their surface charges. Neutral and anionic NPs, when tested at low concentrations, do not disrupt the blood-brain barrier, whereas cationic NPs can exhibit toxicity at higher concentrations (Bahadar et al., 2016). Specifically, cationic NPs have been shown to induce hemolysis and blood coagulation, while anionic NPs do not demonstrate these harmful effects. However, current research reveals a significant gap in comprehensive information regarding the safety of NPs in medical applications. Additionally, the long-term environmental impacts of NPs require further investigation (Kalpana & Devi Rajeswari, 2018).

Future Prospective

Recent advances in nanotechnology have generated optimism for developing treatments for various devastating diseases, including diabetes. Over the past three decades, nanotechnology has significantly impacted pharmacology, particularly in drug delivery systems. Engineered nanomaterials are now being utilized in diverse applications, such as food packaging, therapeutic interventions, and biosensors. A key objective of nanotechnology in drug delivery is to enhance the bioavailability of drugs at targeted sites while reducing overall medication use, treatment costs, and side effects. Nanodevices, which offer greater sensitivity and faster action compared to conventional systems, are crucial for achieving these goals. Nanomedicine-based drug delivery relies on three main factors: effective drug encapsulation, precise delivery to the intended site, and controlled drug release. Research has shown that NPs can significantly alter biomarkers based on their molecular mechanisms and the dosage required for encapsulation. Notably, insulin encapsulated in NPs has demonstrated promise in enhancing oral bioavailability, improving glycaemic control, and increasing blood insulin levels in diabetic rats.

Conclusion

Herbal medicine has been an integral part of human history for centuries and plays a crucial role in the evolution of contemporary medical practices. It is widely acknowledged that nanotechnology can enhance drug performance, dosage, and efficacy. By improving efficiency and safety, nanotechnology has the potential to reduce healthcare expenditures in the long run. Recent research on the toxicity of NPs in healthcare products has revealed a significant lack of comprehensive data regarding the effects of currently used NPs. To understand the long-term negative impacts of these materials, further research is essential. The intersection of nanomaterials and biology has led to the development of various applications, including physiological therapeutic interventions, diagnostic tools, analytical instruments, contrast agents, and drug delivery vehicles. Given that conventional medications for chronic diseases like diabetes are notoriously challenging to administer, nanotechnology presents a promising alternative for drug delivery mechanisms. However, the potential harmful effects of nanoscale medications cannot be overlooked, as they depend on the timing, method, and dosages of administration.

References

Ahmed, M. S., Khan, I. J., Aman, S., Chauhan, S., Kaur, N., Shriwastav, S., Goel, K., Saini, M., Dhankar, S., Singh, T. G., Dev, J., & Mujwar, S. (2023). Phytochemical investigations, *in-vitro* antioxidant, antimicrobial potential, and *in-silico* computational docking analysis of Euphorbia milii Des Moul. *Journal of Experimental Biology and Agricultural Sciences*, 11(2), 380-393.

Arora, A., Behl, T., Sehgal, A., Singh, S., Sharma, N., Bhatia, S., Sobarzo-Sanchez, E., and Bungau, S. (2021). Unravelling the involvement of gut microbiota in type 2 diabetes mellitus. *Life sciences,* 273, 119311.

Aynalem, S. B., and Zeleke, A. J. (2018). Prevalence of diabetes mellitus and its risk factors among individuals aged 15 years and above in Mizan-Aman town, Southwest Ethiopia, 2016: a cross sectional study. *International Journal of Endocrinology,* 2018, 9317987.

Bahadar, H., Maqbool, F., Niaz, K., and Abdollahi, M. (2016). Toxicity of nanoparticles and an overview of current experimental models. *Iranian biomedical journal*, 20(1), 1.

Bahloul, B., Castillo-Henríquez, L., Jenhani, L., Aroua, N., Ftouh, M., Kalboussi, N., Vega-Baudrit, J., and Mignet, N. (2023). Nanomedicine-based potential phyto-drug delivery systems for diabetes. *Journal of Drug Delivery Science and Technology,* 104377.

Bhagwat, T. R., Joshi, K. A., Parihar, V. S., Asok, A., Bellare, J., and Ghosh, S. (2018). Biogenic copper nanoparticles from medicinal plants as novel antidiabetic nanomedicine. *World Journal of Pharmaceutical Research,* 7(4), 183-196.

Bhatia, S. (2016). *Natural Polymer Drug Delivery Systems: Nanoparticles, Plants, and Algae*. Springer International Publishing, Switzerland.

Bhuvaneswari, K., Nisha, K., Kalimuthu, K., Kiruthika, M., and Priya, E. (2023). *In vitro* anti-inflammatory, anti-diabetic and anticancer properties of copper nanoparticles synthesized by medicinal plant *Leucas aspera* (Willd). *Advances in Pharmacology and Pharmacy*, 11(1), 57–65.

Blahova, J., Martiniakova, M., Babikova, M., Kovacova, V., Mondockova, V., and Omelka, R. (2021). Pharmaceutical drugs and natural therapeutic products for the treatment of type 2 diabetes mellitus. *Pharmaceuticals,* 14(8), 806.

Chauhan, S., Chalotra, R., Rathi, A., Saini, M., Deol, S., Lard, M., and Gupta, S. (2023). Current Approaches in Healing of Wounds in Diabetes and Diabetic Foot Ulcers. *Current Bioactive Compounds*, 19(3), 104-121.

Chauhan, S., Gupta, S., Yasmin, S., and Saini, M. (2021). Antihyperglycemic and Antioxidant Potential of Plant Extract of Litchi chinensis and Glycine max. International Journal of Nutrition, Pharmacology, *Neurological Diseases*, 11(3), 225-233.

Chen, Y., Wang, Y., Li, W., Yang, Q., Hou, Q., Wei, L., Liu, L., Huang, F., and Ju, M. (2017). Enhancement of photocatalytic performance with the use of noble-metal-decorated TiO2 nanocrystals as highly active catalysts for aerobic oxidation under visible-light irradiation. *Applied Catalysis B: Environmental,* 210, 352-367.

Corb Aron, R. A., Abid, A., Vesa, C. M., Nechifor, A. C., Behl, T., Ghitea, T. C., Munteanu, M. A., Fratila, O., Andronie-Cioara, F. L., and Toma, M. M. (2021). Recognizing the benefits of pre-/probiotics in metabolic syndrome and type 2 diabetes mellitus considering the influence of akkermansia muciniphila as a key gut bacterium. *Microorganisms*, 9(3), 618.

Dewanjee, S., Chakraborty, P., Mukherjee, B., and De Feo, V. (2020). Plant-based antidiabetic nanoformulations: the emerging paradigm for effective therapy. *International journal of molecular sciences,* 21(6), 2217.

Dhankar, S., Mujwar, S., Garg, N., Chauhan, S., Sharma, P., Kumar Sharma, S., Kamal, M. A., Rani, D. N., Kumar, S., and Saini, M. (2024). Artificial Intelligence in The Management of Neurodegenerative Disorders. *CNS and Neurological Disorders - Drug Targets*, 23, 1-10.

Dhankhar, S., Chauhan, S., Mehta, D. K., Nitika, Saini, K., Saini, M., Das, R., Gupta, S., and Gautam, V. (2023). Novel targets for potential therapeutic use in Diabetes mellitus. *Diabetology and Metabolic Syndrome,* 15(1), 17.

Forouhi, N. G., and Wareham, N. J. (2019). Epidemiology of diabetes. *Medicine,* 47(1), 22-27.

Ghanbari-Niaki, A., Saeidi, A., Kolahdouzi, S., Aliakbari-Baydokhty, M., Ardeshiri, S., Abderrahman, A., Rhibi, F., Malekian, F., and Zouhal, H. (2019). Effect of Crocus Sativus Linnaeus (saffron) supplementations combined with circuit resistance training on total creatine kinase, lactate dehydrogenase and creatine kinase MB levels in young untrained men. *Science and Sports,* 34(1), e53-e58.

Giri, B., Dey, S., Das, T., Sarkar, M., Banerjee, J., and Dash, S. K. (2018). Chronic hyperglycemia mediated physiological alteration and metabolic distortion leads to organ dysfunction, infection, cancer progression and other pathophysiological consequences: an update on glucose toxicity. *Biomedicine and Pharmacotherapy,* 107, 306-328.

Gollapalli, M., Alansari, A., Alkhorasani, H., Alsubaii, M., Sakloua, R., Alzahrani, R., Al-Hariri, M., Alfares, M., AlKhafaji, D., and Al Argan, R. (2022). A novel stacking ensemble for detecting three types of diabetes mellitus using a Saudi Arabian dataset: Pre-diabetes, T1DM, and T2DM. *Computers in Biology and Medicine,* 147, 105757.

Grewal, A. S., Thapa, K., Kanojia, N., Sharma, N., and Singh, S. (2020). Natural compounds as source of aldose reductase (AR) inhibitors for the treatment of diabetic complications: A Mini Review. *Current Drug Metabolism,* 21(14), 1091-1116.

Hamilton, A. E., and Gilbert, R. J. (2023). Curcumin release from biomaterials for enhanced tissue regeneration following injury or disease. *Bioengineering,* 10(2), 262.

Hasanpour, M., Iranshahy, M., and Iranshahi, M. (2020). The application of metabolomics in investigating anti-diabetic activity of medicinal plants. *Biomedicine and Pharmacotherapy*, 128, 110263.

Iid, I. I., Kumar, S., Shukla, S., Kumar, V., and Sharma, R. (2020). Putative antidiabetic herbal food ingredients: Nutra/functional properties, bioavailability and effect on metabolic pathways. *Trends in Food Science and Technology*, 97, 317-340.

Ioannidis, J. P., Kim, B. Y., and Trounson, A. (2018). How to design preclinical studies in nanomedicine and cell therapy to maximize the prospects of clinical translation. *Nature Biomedical Engineering*, 2(11), 797-809.

Jampílek, J., and Kráľová, K. (2019). Beneficial effects of metal-and metalloid-based nanoparticles on crop production. In *Nanotechnology for Agriculture: Advances for Sustainable Agriculture* (pp. 161-219). Springer, Singapore.

Kalpana, V., and Devi Rajeswari, V. (2018). A review on green synthesis, biomedical applications, and toxicity studies of ZnO NPs. *Bioinorganic Chemistry and Applications,* 2018, 3569758.

Khan, I., Saeed, K., and Khan, I. (2019). Nanoparticles: Properties, applications and toxicities. *Arabian Journal of Chemistry*, 12(7), 908-931.

Kumar, S., Behl, T., Sachdeva, M., Sehgal, A., Kumari, S., Kumar, A., Kaur, G., Yadav, H. N., and Bungau, S. (2021). Implicating the effect of ketogenic diet as a preventive measure to obesity and diabetes mellitus. *Life Sciences,* 264, 118661.

Lalit, K., Navpreet, K., Samrat, C., and Randhir, S. (2014). Phyto-pharmacological review of Coccinia indica. *World Journal of Pharmacy and Pharmaceutical Sciences,* 3(2), 1734-1745.

Manukumar, H., Shiva Kumar, J., Chandrasekhar, B., Raghava, S., and Umesha, S. (2017). Evidences for diabetes and insulin mimetic activity of medicinal plants: present status and future prospects. *Critical Reviews in Food Science and Nutrition,* 57(12), 2712-2729.

Marella, S., and Tollamadugu, N. V. K. V. P. (2018). Nanotechnological approaches for the development of herbal drugs in treatment of diabetes mellitus–a critical review. *IET Nanobiotechnology*, 12(5), 549-556.

McIntyre, H. D., Catalano, P., Zhang, C., Desoye, G., Mathiesen, E. R., and Damm, P. (2019). Gestational diabetes mellitus. *Nature reviews Disease primers,* 5(1), 47.

Mittal, P., Dhankhar, S., Chauhan, S., Garg, N., Bhattacharya, T., Ali, M., Chaudhary, A. A., Rudayni, H. A., Al-Zharani, M., and Ahmad, W. (2023). A Review on Natural Antioxidants for Their Role in the Treatment of Parkinson's Disease. *Pharmaceuticals*, 16(7), 908.

Narwal, S., Dhanda, T., Sharma, P., Sharma, V., Dhankhar, S., Garg, N., Ghosh, S. N., and Rani, N. (2023). Current Therapeutic Strategies for Chagas Disease. *Anti-Infective Agents,* 21, 1-11.

Nikolova, M., Slavchov, R., and Nikolova, G. (2020). Nanotechnology in medicine. In *Drug discovery and Evaluation: Methods in Clinical Pharmacology* (pp. 533-546). Springer, Cham.

Okur, M. E., Karantas, I. D., and Siafaka, P. I. (2017). Diabetes mellitus: A review on pathophysiology, current status of oral medications and future perspectives. *ACTA Pharmaceutica Sciencia,* 55, 61-82.

Oyenihi, A. B., Langa, S. O., Mukaratirwa, S., and Masola, B. (2019). Effects of Centella asiatica on skeletal muscle structure and key enzymes of glucose and glycogen metabolism in type 2 diabetic rats. *Biomedicine and Pharmacotherapy*, 112, 108715.

Padhi, S., Nayak, A. K., and Behera, A. (2020). Type II diabetes mellitus: a review on recent drug based therapeutics. *Biomedicine and Pharmacotherapy,* 131, 110708.

Panchal, M., Rana, P., Garg, N., Dhankhar, S., Chauhan, S., and Sharma, H. (2024). A Comprehensive Review of Alternative Therapeutic Approaches for Nausea and Vomiting Relief in Pregnancy. *New Emirates Medical Journal,* 5, 1-8.

Patle, D., Vyas, M., and Khatik, G. L. (2021). A review on natural products and herbs used in the management of diabetes. *Current Diabetes Reviews,* 17(2), 186-197.

Ram, U., and Ram, F. (2021). Demographic transition in India: insights into population growth, composition, and its major drivers. In *Oxford Research Encyclopedia of Global Public Health*. Oxford University Press.

Rohilla, M., Bansal, S., Garg, A., Dhiman, S., Dhankhar, S., Saini, M., Chauhan, S., Alsubaie, N., Batiha, G. E. S., and Albezrah, N. K. A. (2023). Discussing pathologic mechanisms of Diabetic retinopathy and therapeutic potentials of curcumin and β-glucogallin in the management of Diabetic retinopathy. *Biomedicine and Pharmacotherapy,* 169, 115881.

Saharan, R., Kaur, J., Dhankhar, S., Garg, N., Chauhan, S., Kumar, S., and Sharma, H. (2024). Hydrogel-based Drug Delivery System in Diabetes Management. *Pharmaceutical Nanotechnology,* 12, 1-11.

Saini, M., Das, R., Mehta, D. K., and Chauhan, S. (2022). Styrylquinolines Derivatives: SAR study and Synthetic Approaches. *Medicinal Chemistry,* 18, 859-870.

Chauhan, S., Kishore, L., Kaur, N., & Singh, R. (2015). Potential anti-arthritic agents from Indian medicinal plants. *Research and Reviews: Journal of Pharmacy and Pharmaceutical Sciences*, 4(3), 10-22.

Sharma, N., Bora, K. S., and Kumar, A. (2023). Holistic care management for diabetes mellitus: A futuristic approach. *Journal of Medical Pharmaceutical and Allied Sciences,* 12, 4588.

Shi, J., Fan, J., Su, Q., and Yang, Z. (2019). Cytokines and abnormal glucose and lipid metabolism. *Frontiers in Endocrinology,* 10, 703.

Singh, U. (2016). Prevalence of diabetes and other health related problems across India and worldwide: An overview. *Journal of Applied and Natural Science,* 8(1), 500-505.

Testa, R., Bonfigli, A. R., Prattichizzo, F., La Sala, L., De Nigris, V., and Ceriello, A. (2017). The "metabolic memory" theory and the early treatment of hyperglycemia in prevention of diabetic complications. *Nutrients*, 9(5), 437.

Tyagi, P., and Santos, J. L. (2018). Macromolecule nanotherapeutics: approaches and challenges. *Drug Discovery Today,* 23(5), 1053-1061.

Tzvetkov, N. T., Kirilov, K., Matin, M., and Atanasov, A. G. (2023). Natural product drug discovery and drug design: two approaches shaping new pharmaceutical development. *Nephrology Dialysis Transplantation*, 39, 375-378.

Vargas, J., García, L., and Baena, Y. (2023). Nanotechnology and herbal products: Advances and perspectives in the treatment of diabetes and some of its complications. *Journal of Applied Pharmaceutical Science*, 13(12), 001-014.

Verma, S., and Pandey, A. K. (2021). Improving Bioavailability of Nutrients Through Nanotechnology. Sustainable Agriculture Reviews 55: *Micro and Nano Engineering in Food Science,* 1, 135-170.

Wickramasinghe, A. S. D., Kalansuriya, P., and Attanayake, A. P. (2021). Herbal medicines targeting the improved β-cell functions and β-cell regeneration for the management of diabetes mellitus. *Evidence-based Complementary and Alternative Medicine*, 2021, 2920530.

Xu, L., Li, Y., Dai, Y., and Peng, J. (2018). Natural products for the treatment of type 2 diabetes mellitus: Pharmacology and mechanisms. *Pharmacological Research,* 130, 451-465.

Xue, M., Weickert, M. O., Qureshi, S., Kandala, N. B., Anwar, A., Waldron, M., Shafie, A., Messenger, D., Fowler, M., and Jenkins, G. (2016). Improved glycemic control and vascular function in overweight and obese subjects by glyoxalase 1 inducer formulation. *Diabetes*, 65(8), 2282-2294.

Yang, Y., and Chan, L. (2016). Monogenic diabetes: what it teaches us on the common forms of type 1 and type 2 diabetes. *Endocrine Reviews,* 37(3), 190-222.

Yazdanian, M., Rostamzadeh, P., Rahbar, M., Alam, M., Abbasi, K., Tahmasebi, E., Tebyaniyan, H., Ranjbar, R., Seifalian, A., and Yazdanian, A. (2022). The potential application of green-synthesized metal nanoparticles in dentistry: a comprehensive review. *Bioinorganic Chemistry and Applications,* 2022, 2311910.

Zhao, R., Lu, Z., Yang, J., Zhang, L., Li, Y., and Zhang, X. (2020). Drug delivery system in the treatment of diabetes mellitus. *Frontiers in Bioengineering and Biotechnology*, 8, 880.

Chapter 10

Nano-Phytoformulations: Enhancing Herbal Efficacy in Diabetes Management

Gagandeep Kaur*
Parul Sood
and Lovish Sharma
Chitkara University School of Pharmacy, Chitkara University, Himachal Pradesh, India

Abstract

Diabetes mellitus (DM) is a chronic metabolic disorder characterized by its persistent and complex nature. It affects millions of individuals worldwide and represents a significant and unresolved health challenge in the 21st century. While conventional medications are effective, they can also lead to undesirable side effects in diabetic patients. Consequently, there is a growing emphasis on exploring natural substances due to their minimal adverse effects, cost efficiency, and convenient availability. Despite the advantages of bioactive herbal components, many face challenges such as inadequate absorption and limited stability, which hinder their efficacy. The integration of nanotechnology with herbal medicine, known as nano-phytoformulation, has introduced innovative approaches for managing DM. These formulations are designed to enhance the absorption, solubility, stability, and targeted delivery of herbal components. As a result, lower doses are required, and the onset of adverse effects is delayed. This chapter aims to provide a comprehensive overview of nanotechnology-based herbal formulations for the treatment of diabetes that have been documented to date, highlighting their potential to revolutionize the management of this condition.

Keywords: health, formulation, nanotechnology, diabetes, disease, wellbeing

Introduction

Nanoscale refers to dimensions measuring one billionth of a meter (10^{-9} m). The emergence of nanotechnology as a scientific discipline arose from the understanding that products and

---

* Corresponding Author's Email: gagandeepkaur@chitkarauniversity.edu.in.

In: Phyto-Nanomedicine
Editors: Hitesh Chopra, Vinod Kumar Gauttam, Ajmer Singh Grewal et al.
ISBN: 979-8-89530-317-7

devices derived from nanosized particles exhibit distinct characteristics compared to their larger-scale counterparts. Nanomedicine, a multidisciplinary field, encompasses a broad spectrum of medical applications, including pain management, disease prevention, diagnostics, therapeutic interventions, human health enhancement, trauma treatment, and disease management strategies. This multidisciplinary approach integrates findings from biotechnology, nanomaterials science, biomedical robotics, and genetic engineering. The application of nanoscale medical technologies enhances efficiency, accelerates response times, and optimizes functionality in various biological and chemical processes involved in the production of medical materials. Ongoing research continues to inspire optimism for advancements in nanomedicine. By manipulating matter at the nanoscale, nanotechnology facilitates the development of innovative and enhanced products, particularly within the medical domain, yielding unique and improved actions as well as physicochemical properties. Various categories of nanocarriers, as depicted in Figure 1, including lipophilic nanoparticles, polymer-based nanoparticles, and inorganic nanoparticles, have been employed for drug delivery in phytoherbal medicine (Bhushan, 2017).

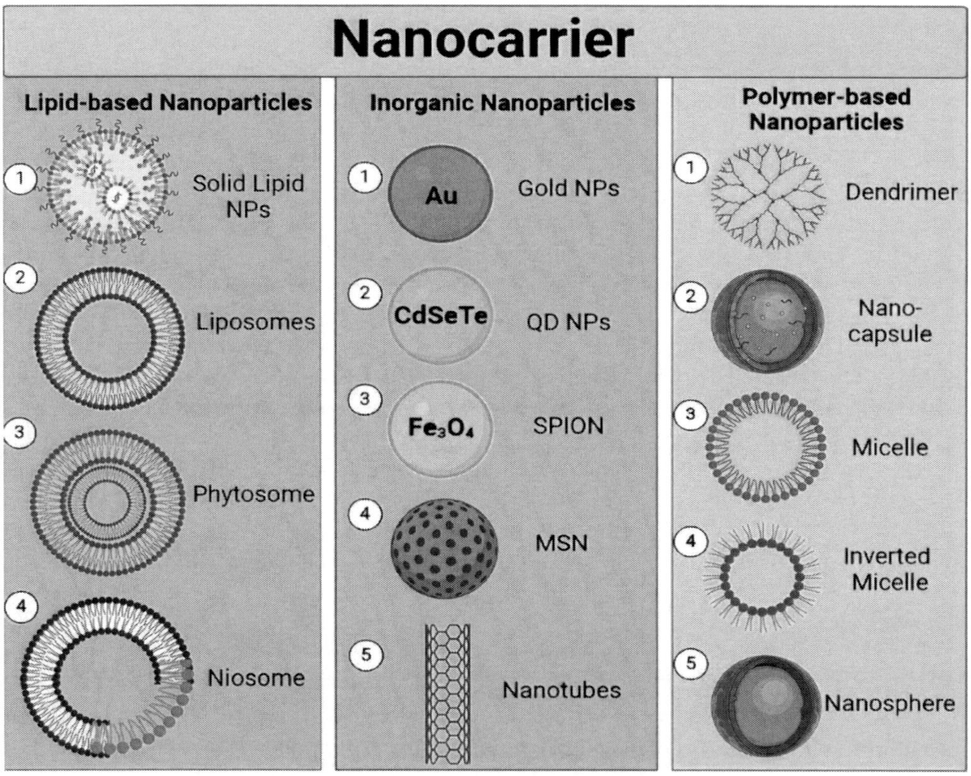

Figure 1. Various categories of nanocarriers formulated for phytoherbals.

Lipophile Nano Vehicle for Phytoherbal Drug Delivery

Lipid-based nanoparticles (NPs), such as rigid lipid nanoparticles, phytosomes, and liposomes, offer advantages in biocompatibility and the ability to enhance the solubility of phytoherbal medications with low water solubility. When selecting a preparation method, it is essential to consider challenges like aggregation and physical instability. After the creation of NPs, evaluating factors such as shape, size, and surface characteristics is crucial, as these significantly influence the pharmacological effects and cellular uptake of NPs. Liposomes are nanoscale vesicles composed of concentric lipid bilayers formed by amphipathic phospholipid molecules. These molecules aggregate to create circular formations in aqueous environments, enclosing a portion of the surrounding solvent (Van Der Vorm et al., 2020). Liposomes serve as effective carriers for herbal delivery, as they can enhance the solubility of the loaded drug and accommodate both hydrophilic and lipophilic pharmaceuticals. Additionally, they improve bioavailability and therapeutic efficacy. Phytosomes, also known as phyto-lipids, are delivery systems that demonstrate greater stability compared to liposomes. Unlike liposomes, phytosomes have a chemical linkage within their structure. They enhance the bioavailability of phytoherbals with low solubility by improving their absorption in the gastrointestinal tract. Solid lipid NPs (SLNs) provide several benefits, including superior physicochemical stability and enhanced protection compared to other nanoparticles like liposomes and polymeric nanoparticles. Moreover, the biocompatibility and compact size (ranging from 50 to 1000 nm) of SLNs allow for their utilization in various drug delivery methods.

Polymeric Nano Vehicle for Phytoherbal Drug Delivery

Recently, there has been increased interest in using polymeric NPs as a drug delivery mechanism in the field of phytomedicine. These nanoparticles, which include nanospheres and nanocapsules, range in size from 10 to 1000 nm and are classified into two categories based on their structural differences. Polymeric nanoparticles are made from either synthetic or natural polymers that are biodegradable and biocompatible, allowing for precise and targeted delivery of medications to specific locations in the body. Among polymers, dendrimers have garnered significant attention for their application in herbal delivery due to their unique properties, including poly-valency, monodispersity, and controlled structure (Sharabati et al., 2021). Dendrimers consist of three components: a central nucleus, terminal groups, and generational moieties. The medication can be attached to the terminal groups through either covalent or non-covalent interactions, while it can be encapsulated within the hydrophobic core (Hwang et al., 2020). Polymeric micelles, another type of polymeric nanoparticle, typically range in size from 10 to 100 nm. They are formed through the self-assembly of block copolymers in an aqueous medium and generally exhibit greater stability compared to surfactant micelles.

Inorganic Nanoparticles

Recently, a range of inorganic NPs has emerged as significant players in drug delivery (Huang et al., 2020). This includes various types of metal nanoparticles, magnetic nanoparticles, carbon nanotubes, and mesoporous silica nanoparticles. Metal nanoparticles, such as quantum dots, zinc oxide, gold, iron (II, III) oxide, platinum, titanium dioxide, and silver, were first identified in the early 1900s. Due to their unique characteristics—such as a high surface-to-volume ratio, multiple coordination sites, the ability to transition between metallic and molecular forms, and high surface energy—metal NPs have gained attention for herbal drug delivery. Mesoporous silica NPs (MSNs) possess substantial surface area and porosity, enabling them to transport significant quantities of cargo. They are widely utilized in both oral and parenteral medication administration due to their exceptional chemical stability and biocompatibility. Carbon nanotubes (CNTs), characterized by their tubular morphology, are formed by rolling graphite sheets and can be categorized into two types: multi-walled carbon nanotubes (MWCNTs) and single-walled carbon nanotubes (SWCNTs). SWCNTs, in particular, can enhance the absorption and solubility of herbal products. Their capacity for surface functionalization and hollow structure further contributes to improved chemical and physical properties of phytoherbal medicines. Among these nanoparticles, iron oxide configured as superparamagnetic NPs is less prone to oxidation compared to other magnetic NPs like nickel and cobalt. This characteristic makes it particularly suitable for future applications in biomedicine, especially in targeted drug delivery.

Mechanisms and Pathophysiology of Diabetes Mallitus

β-Cell Physiology

To maintain appropriate β-cell activity, it is crucial to preserve cell integrity and regulate physiological processes and pathways. These cells produce pre-proinsulin, which undergoes structural changes in the endoplasmic reticulum during maturation with the assistance of various proteins, resulting in the formation of pro-insulin. Once matured, insulin is stored in granules until it is released. High glucose levels trigger insulin secretion, although fatty acids, hormones, and amino acids can also enhance insulin production. The primary mechanism by which β-cells take up glucose is through the glucose transporter 2 (GLUT2) protein, which functions as a glucose sensor as circulating glucose levels rise. Upon glucose entry, catabolism initiates, leading to an increase in the intracellular ATP/ADP ratio. This increase causes the closure of ATP-sensitive potassium channels in the plasma membrane. Consequently, the cell membrane depolarizes, resulting in the opening of voltage-dependent Ca^{2+} channels and allowing Ca^{2+} to flow into the cell (Tan et al., 2021).

β-Cell Dysfunction

Historically, β-cell failure has been linked to increased mortality. Recent studies suggest that β-cell dysfunction in T2DM is associated with a complex network of cellular and metabolic interactions influenced by environmental factors (Sun et al., 2020). Elevated blood sugar levels and free fatty acids (FFAs) can lead to β-cell failure by inducing endoplasmic reticulum (ER) stress and activating apoptotic pathways related to the unfolded protein response (Ikegami et al., 2021). Obesity exacerbates oxidative stress and metabolic abnormalities, contributing to β-cell destruction through mechanisms such as lipotoxicity, glucotoxicity, and glucolipotoxicity. In severe cases, these processes may disrupt islet structure and organization, hindering communication between pancreatic cells. Consequently, the regulation of glucagon and insulin release becomes impaired, further exacerbating hyperglycemia. Insufficient insulin secretion may arise from deficits in insulin production, precursor availability, and the release mechanisms (Rachdaoui et al., 2020).

Pathological Factors Maintaining T2DM

Dietary Elements

High-calorie Western diets, rich in fats and carbohydrates, increase the production of reactive oxygen species and excessive inflammatory molecules. Following a large meal, oxidative stress and inflammation mutually reinforce each other, exacerbating postprandial effects. Chronically elevated levels of reactive oxygen species are associated with the development of T2DM and insulin resistance.

Exercise/Physical activity

Increasing sedentary behavior and decreasing physical activity contribute to the link between obesity and T2DM. These factors also elevate long-term, low-grade systemic inflammatory markers. Inflammatory compounds, such as interleukin-1 (IL-1), C-reactive protein (CRP), interleukin-6 (IL-6), and tumor necrosis factor-alpha (TNF-α), are released into the bloodstream and specific organs, leading to metabolic inflammation. Preclinical studies suggest that reducing inflammation in obese and prediabetic individuals may help delay the onset of T2DM. Weight loss is considered the primary intervention for improving insulin sensitivity and preventing type 2 diabetes in prediabetic and overweight patients (Boland et al., 2017). Individuals who engage in regular exercise show lower levels of IL-6, IL-18, and CRP, along with reduced leptin and antioxidant enzymes, which in turn decreases harmful free radicals over time (Rorsman et al., 2018).

Imbalance of Gut Microbiota

The gut microbiota comprises various bacteria that significantly influence human physiology and biological processes (Thursby et al., 2017). These bacteria affect the immune system and inflammatory response, produce metabolites, and regulate both the intestinal barrier and metabolism. Gut bacteria generate several compounds essential for maintaining normal physiological functions in healthy individuals. Dysbiosis, or imbalance in the gut microbiota, plays a key role in the development of T2DM and insulin resistance. The exploration of the gut microbiome's practical effects is a growing area of research, with more studies needed to fully understand the connection between gut bacteria and T2DM (Li et al., 2021).

Current Treatment Approaches and Limitations

DM poses a significant global health challenge, compounded by the adverse effects linked to many available treatments. Finding effective DM medications with minimal side effects remains a top priority. Key elements of diabetic management include a carefully structured nutritional regimen, often supported by physical activity. Diabetic individuals should focus on weight management and adhere to diets that promote near-normal blood glucose levels while addressing any related lipid abnormalities. When diet and exercise prove insufficient, oral hypoglycemic agents may be introduced (Handschin et al., 2008). Biguanides, such as metformin, are commonly prescribed to reduce hepatic glucose production, primarily influencing fasting glucose levels, though gastrointestinal side effects like diarrhea and stomach discomfort may occur. Sulphonylureas function by inhibiting potassium ion efflux from pancreatic β-cells, leading to depolarization and insulin release. Common side effects include weight gain and hypoglycemia (Park et al., 2013). Dipeptidyl peptidase-4 inhibitors slow the degradation of glucose-dependent insulinotropic polypeptide and GLP-1. Pramlintide, a synthetic form of amylin, targets postprandial blood glucose by suppressing glucagon secretion, delaying gastric emptying, and reducing appetite, with nausea and hypoglycemia being common side effects (Shan et al., 2017). Insulin therapy, one of the oldest treatments for diabetes, is typically reserved for later stages of T2DM, once other therapies become ineffective. As T2DM progresses, beta-cell dysfunction and deterioration make achieving HbA1c targets increasingly difficult, emphasizing the need for innovative drug delivery systems to improve treatment outcomes (Rosenstock et al., 2020).

Phytoherbals in Diabetes Management

Overview of Herbal Remedies for Diabetes

Herbal medicine has experienced rapid and significant growth in recent years. Indian traditional healthcare systems, such as Ayurveda, have long utilized rasayana, a category of therapeutic plants with a history spanning millennia, in their herbal formulations. Of the 2,500 species of medicinal plants found in India, 150 are economically significant and widely used. Several conventional medications have their origins in compounds found in medicinal plants. A prime example is metformin, a highly effective oral glucose-lowering drug, which was developed based on the traditional use of *Galega officinalis* for treating diabetes. *Galega officinalis* contains guanidine, the active compound responsible for its hypoglycemic effects. However, due to its high toxicity, guanidine was deemed unsuitable for clinical use. Through scientific advancements, safer derivatives like metformin were developed. Recent studies have confirmed that certain herbal extracts demonstrate significant potential in lowering blood sugar levels in both humans and animals with T2DM, reinforcing the therapeutic value of herbal medicine in diabetes management.

Mechanisms of Phytochemicals

The physiological mechanisms governing glucose metabolism and the pathological changes that lead to diabetes have been thoroughly investigated. Key peripheral tissues involved in glucose regulation include adipose tissue, skeletal muscle, and the liver. Botanical compounds may influence glucose metabolism by modulating these tissues, impacting processes that are central to the abnormalities seen in T2DM. In adipose tissue, botanical compounds can regulate the hormones involved in insulin sensitivity, thereby improving insulin efficiency in skeletal muscle. For example, some plant-derived compounds are known to affect hepatic processes, such as gluconeogenesis, which influences glucose production in the liver. Metformin, a biguanide derived from plant sources, specifically *Galega officinalis*, is a prime example of how botanical compounds can regulate liver processes to reduce blood sugar levels. T2DM is often characterized by irregularities in insulin secretion. Extensive research in both laboratory and clinical settings continues to explore the development of drugs that can enhance islet tissue growth or modulate apoptosis, offering potential advancements in diabetes treatment. While some botanicals are believed to improve insulin sensitivity and glucose metabolism, there is no conclusive evidence that any botanical supplement consistently delivers the anticipated benefits. Botanicals may also directly impact insulin activity in peripheral tissues such as adipose tissue and skeletal muscle, enhancing their potential as supportive treatments in T2DM management (Sindhu et al., 2021).

Phytochemicals Reduce Blood Sugar Levels in Subjects Diagnosed with T2DM

Dysregulation of blood glucose homeostasis is central to the development and progression of T2DM. Clinically, fasting blood glucose, postprandial blood sugar, fructosamine, and glycated hemoglobin (HbA1c) are common biomarkers used to assess blood glucose control in diabetic patients. Numerous studies have demonstrated the potential of various phytochemicals in lowering these markers in individuals with T2DM. Several compounds, including genistein, silybin, berberine, curcumin, and resveratrol, have been shown to reduce both fasting blood glucose and HbA1c levels, which are critical indicators of long-term glycemic control. Additional studies have shown that compounds such as puerarin, rutin, and anthocyanins also decrease fasting blood glucose in T2DM patients. Ellagic acid has been identified as potentially effective in lowering HbA1c levels, while anthocyanins may help reduce HbA1c in early-stage untreated diabetes or prediabetes (Gupta et al., 2020). Phytochemicals like berberine, puerarin, and quercetin have been found to lower postprandial blood glucose levels, while hesperidin has shown efficacy in reducing fructosamine, another marker of blood glucose. These findings suggest that berberine and curcumin, in particular, may help manage blood glucose levels in T2DM patients, thereby reducing the risk of complications associated with poor glycemic control. The root cause of T2DM is largely insulin resistance. Many studies have highlighted that improving insulin sensitivity and reducing resistance can lead to better diabetes management. For example, in a 12-week randomized, double-blind, placebo-controlled trial, postmenopausal women with T2DM who supplemented with genistein exhibited improved insulin sensitivity, as evidenced by increased QUICKI (Quantitative Insulin Sensitivity Check Index) levels. Furthermore, puerarin was shown to enhance insulin sensitivity and lower insulin resistance in T2DM patients by reducing HOMA-IR (Homeostasis Model Assessment of Insulin Resistance) and increasing ISI (Insulin Sensitivity Index).

Beneficial Effects of Phytochemicals on Blood Lipid Problems in Subject with T2DM

Dyslipidemia, characterized by abnormal lipid levels, is a common condition associated with T2DM. Key lipid markers, such as triglycerides (TG), low-density lipoprotein cholesterol (LDL-C), high-density lipoprotein cholesterol (HDL-C), and total cholesterol, are important predictors of cardiovascular risk in T2DM patients. HDL-C is primarily composed of apolipoprotein A-1, while LDL-C is rich in apolipoprotein B, both of which provide a comprehensive view of the body's lipid profile. Several phytochemicals have been shown to improve lipid profiles in individuals with T2DM. Compounds such as berberine, curcumin, ellagic acid, resveratrol, and silybin have demonstrated efficacy in reducing total cholesterol and triglyceride levels. In addition, anthocyanins and genistein have been found to specifically lower triglycerides, helping to mitigate dyslipidemia and the associated cardiovascular risks in T2DM patients (Engerman et al., 2012).

Phytochemicals Have a Beneficial Effect in Reducing Inflammation in Individuals with T2DM

T2DM is closely linked to chronic low-grade inflammation, which plays a critical role in the progression of the disease. Reducing inflammation has been shown to improve outcomes in T2DM patients (Simmons et al., 2018). Several inflammatory biomarkers, including interleukin-6 (IL-6), high-sensitivity C-reactive protein (hs-CRP), nuclear factor-κB (NF-κB), and tumor necrosis factor-α (TNF-α), are associated with the development and progression of T2DM. These markers can serve as early predictors of the disease. Recent studies highlight the anti-inflammatory effects of certain phytochemicals. For example, ellagic acid treatment at a dosage of 180 mg per day for eight weeks significantly reduced levels of CRP, TNF-α, and IL-6 in patients with T2DM. Additionally, compounds like curcumin, hesperidin, and silybin have been shown to lower hs-CRP, further emphasizing their potential role in managing inflammation and improving diabetic outcomes.

Phytochemicals Enhance the Reduction of Oxidative Strain within Individuals Diagnosed T2DM

Oxidative stress is a key factor in the onset and progression of T2DM, similar to inflammation. It also plays a significant role in the development of T2DM-related complications, such as microvascular dysfunction. Therefore, suppressing oxidative stress can be highly beneficial in improving both T2DM and its associated complications. Several biomarkers are commonly used to assess oxidative stress levels. These include malondialdehyde (MDA), which is a marker of lipid peroxidation, glutathione peroxidase (GPx), superoxide dismutase (SOD), and total antioxidant capacity (TAC). By monitoring and addressing oxidative stress through the regulation of these markers, it may be possible to alleviate oxidative damage and improve outcomes in individuals with T2DM (Arabshomali et al., 2023).

Integration of Nanotechnology and Phytoherbals in Diabetes Therapy

To enhance patient compliance and reduce the need for frequent dosing, a scientific approach to sustained herbal drug delivery is crucial. This goal can be achieved by developing innovative drug delivery systems in the field of phytotherapeutics. One promising method is nanotechnology, which offers numerous benefits in terms of therapeutic efficiency. Nanotechnology improves drug bioavailability, minimizes toxicity, and reduces the frequency of dosing by enabling precise and sustained delivery. Nanostructured drug delivery systems present several advantages. Their tiny size enables them to navigate even the smallest capillaries, allowing for easy distribution throughout the body via the bloodstream. Additionally, these systems can cross tissue barriers and reach specific organs, such as lymph nodes, the liver, spleen, lungs, and spinal cord. One of the most significant advantages is the ability to provide prolonged and controlled drug release, enhancing therapeutic outcomes over time. Compared to traditional drug administration, nanostructured delivery systems offer unique properties that make them superior. For instance, nanoparticles (NPs) protect drugs from degradation in the gastrointestinal tract, ensuring controlled and efficient release at targeted sites. This targeted and controlled delivery mechanism also helps reduce the likelihood of adverse side effects, making nanotechnology-based systems a preferred choice in modern phytomedicine.

Development of Nanoscale Formulations for Herbal Medicines Used in Diabetes Treatment

Despite the emergence of various treatment methods over the years and the discovery of novel therapeutic targets, herbal therapy remains the primary approach for managing diabetes. Plants serve as a valuable reservoir of secondary metabolites that have proven to be economical and environmentally safe for the effective synthesis of NP) (Lapierre et al., 2017). When NPs-containing formulations were administered to diabetic pigs, their blood glucose levels were successfully regulated post-meal. Enhancing the limited water solubility of medicinal plants or their phyto-compounds may be achievable through nanosuspension formulation. This methodology can be utilized to investigate the biological properties of therapeutic plants or their phyto-compounds. Before conducting preclinical and clinical research, it is essential to characterize nanoformulations for optimal pharmacy applications. Consequently, nanoformulations have shown significant improvements in their efficacy against diabetes when compared to other commercially available medications. Several therapeutic plants and extracts have been employed to produce gold NPs (AuNPs) biologically. For instance, the extract of the Mirabilis jalapa flower was utilized to generate AuNPs, resulting in spherical particles with a characteristic size of 100 nm. When nanoformulated Cassia fistula stem bark was administered to streptozotocin-induced diabetic rats, it produced superior reversal of renal dysfunction, along with significant improvements in weight, serum blood sugar levels, lipid profile, and transaminase activity compared to using aqueous extracts alone. The antidiabetic efficacy of AuNPs derived from the potent antidiabetic plant *Gymnema sylvestre* R. Br has been evaluated in Wistar albino rats (Ofori et al., 2017). Furthermore, copper NPs (CuNPs) were synthesized from Dioscorea bulbifera extract, demonstrating both antioxidant and antidiabetic effects (Latreille et al., 2014). The potential of CuNPs as antidiabetic agents was evidenced by their ability to effectively inhibit porcine pancreatic α-amylase, as well as crude murine pancreatic and intestinal amylase.

Table 1. Various nanoformulations of plant extract reported for the treatment of T2DM

Plant	Plant family	Plant part	Plant extract	Nano formulation	Reference
Lawsonia inermis L	Lythraceae	Leaves	Aqueous	Silver NPs and cerium oxide NPs	Kalakotla et al., 2019
Morus indica L	Moraceae	Leaves	Aqueous	ZnO NPs	Anandan et al., 2019
Musa paradisiaca L	Musaceae	Stem	Aqueous	Silver NPs	Anbazhagan et al., 2017
Pouteria sapota (Jacq) HE Moore & Stearn	Sapotaceae	Leaves	Aqueous	Silver NPs	Prabhu et al, 2018
Punica granatum L	Punicaceae	Peel fruit	Methanol	Gold NPs	Manna et al., 2019
Sambucus nigra L	Adoxaceae	Fruit	Aqueous	Gold NPs	Opris et al., 2017
Smilax glabra Roxb	Smilacaceae	Rhizomes	Aqueous	Gold NPs	Ansari et al., 2019
Syzygium cumini (L)	Myrtaceae	Seeds	Aqueous	Poly-ɛ-caprolactone NPs	Bitencourt et al., 2017
Zingiber officinale Roscoe	Zingiberaceae	Rhizomes	Ethanol	Silver NPs	Garg et al., 2017

Promising Nanophytoherbal Formulations

Various nanoherbal formulations of different plant extracts reported for the treatment of T2DM are presented in Table 1.

Conclusion

Extensive research has been conducted on natural products and herbal remedies worldwide. Numerous institutes are currently developing herbal medicines for drug delivery, both in basic research and clinical trials. The primary goal is to create improved methods for delivering these medications to targeted areas of the body while ensuring that the dosage aligns with the existing treatment plans. There is a strong demand for therapies that enhance the patient's internal strength while minimizing side effects, including toxicity and hypersensitivity reactions. In the future, some research organizations may explore the concept of using herbal nanoparticles to deliver cancer treatments, potentially yielding significant results. Incorporating "herbal remedies" into nanocarriers may enhance their effectiveness in treating various chronic conditions and contribute to overall health benefits. Numerous successful nano research initiatives are supported by a wealth of data from knowledgeable sources. Herbal remedies are rich in antioxidants and functional food ingredients, serving as important sources of therapeutic compounds. The integration of modern drug delivery techniques, such as nanotechnology, with traditional herbal remedies has paved the way for exciting new pharmacological treatments. These advancements are expected to significantly improve health outcomes in the near future. The use of nanocarriers in combination with natural and phytoherbal remedies is anticipated to greatly enhance the significance and efficacy of current drug delivery systems.

References

Al Sharabati, M., Abokwiek, R., Al-Othman, A., Tawalbeh, M., Karaman, C., Orooji, Y., & Karimi, F. (2021). Biodegradable polymers and their nano-composites for the removal of endocrine-disrupting chemicals (EDCs) from wastewater: A review. *Environmental Research*, *202*, 111694.

Anandan, S., Mahadevamurthy, M., Ansari, M. A., Alzohairy, M. A., Alomary, M. N., Farha Siraj, S., Halugudde Nagaraja, S., Chikkamadaiah, M., Thimappa Ramachandrappa, L., Naguvanahalli Krishnappa, H. K., Ledesma, A. E., Nagaraj, A. K., & Urooj, A. (2019). Biosynthesized ZnO-NPs from Morus indica attenuates methylglyoxal-induced protein glycation and RBC damage: *in-vitro*, *in-vivo* and molecular docking study. *Biomolecules*, *9*(12), 882.

Anbazhagan, P., Murugan, K., Jaganathan, A., Sujitha, V., Samidoss, C. M., Jayashanthani, S., Amuthavalli, P., Higuchi, A., Kumar, S., Wei, H., Nicoletti, M., Canale, A., & Benelli, G. (2017). Mosquitocidal, antimalarial and antidiabetic potential of Musa paradisiaca-synthesized silver nanoparticles: *in vivo* and *in vitro* approaches. *Journal of Cluster Science*, *28*, 91-107.

Ansari, S., Bari, A., Ullah, R., Mathanmohun, M., Veeraraghavan, V. P., & Sun, Z. (2019). Gold nanoparticles synthesized with Smilax glabra rhizome modulates the anti-obesity parameters in high-fat diet and streptozotocin induced obese diabetes rat model. *Journal of Photochemistry and Photobiology B: Biology*, *201*, 111643.

Arabshomali, A., Bazzazzadehgan, S., Mahdi, F., & Shariat-Madar, Z. (2023). Potential benefits of antioxidant phytochemicals in type 2 diabetes. *Molecules*, *28*(20), 7209.

Bhushan, B. (2017). Introduction to nanotechnology. In *Springer Handbook of Nanotechnology* (pp. 1-19). Springer.

Bitencourt, P. E., Cargnelutti, L. O., Stein, C. S., Lautenchleger, R., Ferreira, L. M., Sangoi, M., Denardi, L., Borges, R. M., Boligon, A., Moresco, R. N., Cruz, L., Zanette, R. A., Alves, S. H., & Moretto, M. B. (2017). (2017). Nanoparticle formulation increases Syzygium cumini antioxidant activity in Candida albicans-infected diabetic rats. *Pharmaceutical Biology*, *55*(1), 1082-1088.

Boland, B. B., Rhodes, C. J., & Grimsby, J. S. (2017). The dynamic plasticity of insulin production in β-cells. *Molecular Metabolism*, *6*(9), 958-973.

Engerman, R. L. (1989). Pathogenesis of diabetic retinopathy. *Diabetes*, *38*(10), 1203-1206.

Garg, V., Kaur, P., Singh, S. K., Kumar, B., Bawa, P., Gulati, M., & Yadav, A. K. (2017). Solid self-nanoemulsifying drug delivery systems for oral delivery of polypeptide-k: formulation, optimization, in-vitro and in-vivo antidiabetic evaluation. *European Journal of Pharmaceutical Sciences*, *109*, 297-315.

Gupta, A., Behl, T., Kumar, A., Singh, S., Bhardwaj, S., & Goyal, A. (2020). Unexplored Potential of Traditional Chinese Medicine in Diabetes Mellitus. *International Journal of Pharmaceutical Investigation*, *10*(1), 1-7.

Handschin, C., & Spiegelman, B. M. (2008). The role of exercise and PGC1α in inflammation and chronic disease. *Nature*, *454*(7203), 463-469.

Huang, H., Feng, W., Chen, Y., & Shi, J. (2020). Inorganic nanoparticles in clinical trials and translations. *Nano Today*, *35*, 100972.

Hwang, D., Ramsey, J. D., & Kabanov, A. V. (2020). Polymeric micelles for the delivery of poorly soluble drugs: From nanoformulation to clinical approval. *Advanced Drug Delivery Reviews*, *156*, 80-118.

Ikegami, H., Babaya, N., & Noso, S. (2021). β-Cell failure in diabetes: Common susceptibility and mechanisms shared between type 1 and type 2 diabetes. *Journal of Diabetes Investigation*, *12*(9), 1526-1539.

Kalakotla, S., Jayarambabu, N., Mohan, G. K., Mydin, R. B. S., & Gupta, V. R. (2019). A novel pharmacological approach of herbal mediated cerium oxide and silver nanoparticles with improved biomedical activity in comparison with Lawsonia inermis. *Colloids and Surfaces B: Biointerfaces*, *174*, 199-206.

LaPierre, M. P., & Stoffel, M. (2017). MicroRNAs as stress regulators in pancreatic beta cells and diabetes. *Molecular Metabolism*, *6*(9), 1010-1023.

Latreille, M., Hausser, J., Stützer, I., Zhang, Q., Hastoy, B., Gargani, S., Kerr-Conte, J., Pattou, F., Zavolan, M., Esguerra, J. L., Eliasson, L., Rülicke, T., Rorsman, P., & Stoffel, M. (2014). MicroRNA-7a regulates pancreatic β cell function. *The Journal of clinical investigation*, *124*(6), 2722-2735.

Li, G. D., Milani, D., Dunne, M. J., Pralong, W. F., Theler, J. M., Petersen, O. H., & Wollheim, C. B. (1991). Extracellular ATP causes $Ca^{2(+)}$-dependent and-independent insulin secretion in RINm5F cells. Phospholipase C mediates Ca^{2+} mobilization but not Ca^{2+} influx and membrane depolarization. *Journal of Biological Chemistry*, *266*(6), 3449-3457.

Manna, K., Mishra, S., Saha, M., Mahapatra, S., Saha, C., Yenge, G., Gaikwad, N., Pal, R., Oulkar, D., Banerjee, K., & Das Saha, K. (2019). Amelioration of diabetic nephropathy using pomegranate peel extract-stabilized gold nanoparticles: assessment of NF-κB and Nrf2 signaling system. *International Journal of Nanomedicine*, 14, 1753–1777.

Ofori, J. K., Salunkhe, V. A., Bagge, A., Vishnu, N., Nagao, M., Mulder, H., Wollheim, C. B., Eliasson, L., & Esguerra, J. L. S. (2017). Elevated miR-130a/miR130b/miR-152 expression reduces intracellular ATP levels in the pancreatic beta cell. *Scientific Reports*, *7*(1), 44986.

Opris, R., Tatomir, C., Olteanu, D., Moldovan, R., Moldovan, B., David, L., Nagy, A., Decea, N., Kiss, M. L., & Filip, G. A. The effect of Sambucus nigra L. extract and phytosinthesized gold nanoparticles on diabetic rats. *Colloids and Surfaces B: Biointerfaces*, *150*, 192-200.

Park, K. H., Zaichenko, L., Brinkoetter, M., Thakkar, B., Sahin-Efe, A., Joung, K. E., Tsoukas, M. A., Geladari, E. V., Huh, J. Y., Dincer, F., Davis, C. R., Crowell, J. A., & Mantzoros, C. S. (2013). Circulating irisin in relation to insulin resistance and the metabolic syndrome. *The Journal of Clinical Endocrinology & Metabolism*, 98(12), 4899-4907.

Prabhu, S., Vinodhini, S., Elanchezhiyan, C., & Rajeswari, D. (2018). Evaluation of antidiabetic activity of biologically synthesized silver nanoparticles using Pouteria sapota in streptozotocin-induced diabetic rats. *Journal of Diabetes*, *10*(1), 28–42.

Rachdaoui, N. (2020). Insulin: the friend and the foe in the development of type 2 diabetes mellitus. *International Journal of Molecular Sciences*, *21*(5), 1770.

Rorsman, P., and Frances, M. A. (2018). Pancreatic β-cell electrical activity and insulin secretion: of mice and men. *Physiological Reviews*, 98, 117-214.

Rosenstock, J., Bajaj, H. S., Janež, A., Silver, R., Begtrup, K., Hansen, M. V., Jia, T., Goldenberg, R., & NN1436-4383 Investigators (2020). Once-Weekly Insulin for Type 2 Diabetes without Previous Insulin Treatment. *New England Journal of Medicine*, 383(22), 2107-2116.

Shan, Z., Sun, T., Huang, H., Chen, S., Chen, L., Luo, C., Yang, W., Yang, X., Yao, P., Cheng, J., Hu, F. B., & Liu, L. (2017). Association between microbiota-dependent metabolite trimethylamine-N-oxide and type 2 diabetes. *American Journal of Clinical Nutrition*, 106(3), 888–894.

Simmons, R. (2011). Epigenetics and maternal nutrition: nature v. nurture. *Proceedings of the Nutrition Society*, 70(1), 73-81.

Rosen, E. D., Kaestner, K. H., Natarajan, R., Patti, M. E., Sallari, R., Sander, M., & Susztak, K. (2018). Epigenetics and epigenomics: implications for diabetes and obesity. *Diabetes*, *67*(10), 1923-1931.

Sindhu, R. K., Saini, B., Kaur, P., & El-Saber Batiha, G. (2021). The Role of Ethnomedicinal Plants for Treatment and Management of Diabetes Mellitus: An Updated Review. *J. Univ. Shanghai Sci. Technol*, *23*, 1014-1049.

Sun, Y., Lu, Y., Saredy, J., Wang, X., Drummer Iv, C., Shao, Y., Saaoud, F., Xu, K., Liu, M., Yang, W. Y., Jiang, X., Wang, H., & Yang, X. (2020). ROS systems are a new integrated network for sensing homeostasis and alarming stresses in organelle metabolic processes. *Redox Biology*, *37*, 101696.

Tan, S., Kennedy, B., & Wong, E. (2021). Mitochondrial biogenesis and mitophagy. In *Mitochondrial Physiology and Vegetal Molecules* (pp. 35-90). Academic Press.

Thursby, E., & Juge, N. (2017). Introduction to the human gut microbiota. *Biochemical Journal*, *474*(11), 1823-1836.

Van Der Vorm, S., Hansen, T., Van Hengst, J. M., Overkleeft, H. S., Van Der Marel, G. A., & Codée, J. D. (2019). Acceptor reactivity in glycosylation reactions. *Chemical Society Reviews*, *48*(17), 4688-4706.

Chapter 11

Applications of Nanophytoherbals in Wound Care Therapy

Purav Gupta
Jasmine Chaudhary
Akash Jain
and Kirti Goel*
M.M. College of Pharmacy, Maharishi Markandeshwar (Deemed to be University), Mullana, Ambala, Haryana, India

Abstract

Nanomedicine introduces innovative solutions to the complex challenges of wound healing and scar reduction, representing a promising frontier in this field. Research highlights various applications of nanotechnology in wound management and scar minimization, focusing on the unique physicochemical properties of nanomaterials like nanofibers and nanoparticles. These materials aid tissue regeneration, regulate inflammation, and enable targeted drug delivery. The role of nanocarriers in delivering therapeutic agents directly to wound sites is explored, helping to minimize systemic side effects. Additionally, the integration of controlled-release systems and nanotechnology-based scaffolds with anti-scar treatments, such as growth factors and extracellular matrix modifiers, is examined for their combined effects. Nanocarriers' ability to simultaneously carry multiple drugs enhances infection control and tissue healing. Combining nanotechnology-based scaffolds with gels or other anti-scar approaches further improves scar healing outcomes. Overall, nanomedicine offers a transformative approach to scar prevention and treatment, effectively addressing challenges like drug solubility, controlled release, and scarless wound healing. Significant advancements in scar removal and tissue remodeling are highlighted, paving the way for more targeted treatments and better patient outcomes. Future developments and challenges in nanomedicine are also considered, with attention to the evolving landscape of wound healing and scar reduction.

Keywords: wound healing, scar reduction, nanomedicine, nanocarriers, nanofibers

* Corresponding Author's Email: kirtijain2727@gmail.com.

In: Phyto-Nanomedicine
Editors: Hitesh Chopra, Vinod Kumar Gauttam, Ajmer Singh Grewal et al.
ISBN: 979-8-89530-317-7

Abbreviations

ECM	extracellular matrix
FGF	fibroblast growth factor
IL	interleukin
PDGF	platelet-derived growth factor
TNF	tumor necrosis factor
VEGF	vascular endothelial growth factor
ROS	reactive oxygen species
SOD	superoxide dismutase
CAT	catalase
WBC	white blood cells
MTT	3-(4, 5-dimethylthiazolyl-2)-2, 5-diphenyltetrazolium bromide

Introduction

Wounds are an inevitable part of life, caused by physical trauma, chemical exposure, or microbial infections. The primary goal of wound healing is to restore damaged tissues to a condition that closely resembles their pre-injury state. All organisms, including humans, have an innate ability to repair and regenerate tissues through continuous tissue repair. However, several factors can hinder this process, including the patient's age, stress levels, obesity, gender, habits such as smoking or alcohol use, overall health, the type and severity of the wound, medication regimen, environmental factors, and the risk of severe microbial infection. The global prevalence of chronic wounds is estimated to be 1.52 to 2.22 cases per thousand individuals (Zhu et al., 2022). In wealthier countries, around 1 to 2 percent of the population may experience a chronic wound at some point in their lives (Järbrink et al., 2016). Despite significant advances in chemistry and pharmacology, finding effective screening methods and developing drugs to heal wounds remains an ongoing challenge. The continued use of indigenous plants in therapeutics offers hope for the discovery of anti-inflammatory agents (Handa & Kaul, 2006). The use of plants and plant-derived extracts or pure compounds to treat diseases is a well-established medicinal practice. According to the WHO, approximately 75% of people rely on traditional remedies, primarily herbal, for their healthcare needs (Ansari & Inamdar, 2010). With the advancement of nanotechnology, nanoparticles have become widely used in drug delivery. Nanoparticles, such as liposomes, have several beneficial properties, making them valuable for drug administration. These advantages include the ability to provide sustained and controlled drug release, protect drugs from degradation, exhibit biocompatibility, enhance drug penetration into the bloodstream, and improve therapeutic efficacy (Arias, 2014; Benita, 2005). Nanophytoherbs, which combine nanotechnology with herbal therapy, have a broad range of potential applications, including the treatment of neurodegenerative diseases and wound healing. Research into the therapeutic potential of nanophytomedicines has focused primarily on neurodegenerative disorders, particularly Parkinson's disease. In addition to their neuroprotective properties, they can also modulate the molecular pathways associated with these conditions (Bhattacharya et al., 2022; Burns et al., 2023). The antibacterial, anti-inflammatory, and antioxidant properties of nanophytoherbs have demonstrated promise in wound healing. Their ability to promote cell proliferation, angiogenesis, and granulation tissue formation may lead to improved wound healing outcomes.

Mechanisms of Action of Nanophytoherbs in Wound Healing

Nanophytoherbs improve wound healing through multiple mechanisms, offering essential properties such as antifungal, anti-inflammatory, and antioxidant effects. A key factor in tissue regeneration is their ability to induce angiogenesis and promote cell proliferation. The use of nanophytoherbs also enhances the physical properties of wound dressings, improving their effectiveness in the healing process. These properties include the ability to absorb moisture and increased mechanical durability. Wound healing involves the activation of angiogenesis and epithelialization, where growth factors such as PDGF (platelet-derived growth factor), FGF (fibroblast growth factor), and VEGF (vascular endothelial growth factor) play significant roles. Studies have shown that nanoformulations of herbal extracts can boost the levels of these growth factors, further enhancing the healing process. Additionally, nanophytoherbs show potential in alleviating neurodegenerative disorders by modulating the activity of brain enzymes such as cytochrome P450 and Heat Shock Protein 70, which help limit lipid peroxidation (Bhattacharya et al., 2022; Burns et al., 2023; Nouri et al., 2020).

Nanophytoherbs in Wound Healing

Nanophytoherbs, which are nano-sized formulations of plant-derived compounds, have gained attention for their potential in wound healing. These nanostructures can enhance the availability and efficacy of phytoconstituents, leading to improved wound healing properties. Research suggests that formulations containing nanophytoherbs exhibit significant antioxidant, anti-inflammatory, and antibacterial activities, all of which are essential for promoting wound healing.

Table 1. Various nano phytoherb formulation and their action

Nano Phytoherb	Main Components	Potential Benefits	References
Nano Aloe Vera	Aloe vera extract	Anti-inflammatory, wound healing, antimicrobial	(Balaji et al., 2015)
Nano Curcumin	Curcumin extract	Anti-inflammatory,antioxidant, promotes tissue repair	(Hussain et al., 2017)
Nano Green Tea	Green tea extract	Antioxidant, antimicrobial, supports collagen synthesis	(Sadri et al., 2015)
Nano Chamomile	Chamomile oil	Anti-inflammatory,soothing, accelerates wound healing	(Gad et al., 2019)
Nano Honey	Honey extract	Antimicrobial, promotes tissue regeneration	(Salvo et al., 2023)
Nano Echinacea	Echinacea extract	Immunomodulatory, supports wound healing	(Fahimirad et al., 2023)
Nano Neem	Neem extract	Antimicrobial, anti-inflammatory, promotes healing	(Ramakrishnan et al., 2020)
Nano Propolis	Propolis extract	Antimicrobial, anti-inflammatory, promotes healing	(Al-saggaf, 2021)
Nano Ginseng	Ginseng extract	Immunomodulatory, promotes collagen synthesis	(Yang et al., 2023)

In addition, nanophytoherbs can stimulate cell proliferation and aid in tissue regeneration. Various nanophytoherbal formulations that have already been developed are shown in Table 1.

Nanoparticle-Based Therapeutic Approaches for Wound Healing

- *Biocompatible gold nanoparticles (AuNPs):* Nanophytoherbs have been extensively utilized due to their ability to interact effectively with living organisms. Unlike silver (Ag), AuNPs do not release toxic chemicals upon contact with biological tissues. This makes AuNPs particularly valuable in wound management. They have been used in treating diabetic foot ulcers and pressure ulcers, demonstrating improved wound healing outcomes (Kushwaha et al., 2022).
- *Silver nanoparticles (AgNPs):* AgNPs have been used to treat burn wounds, showing the ability to accelerate the healing process by stimulating the growth of new skin cells.

Innovative Drug Administration Techniques, Incorporating Herbal Ingredients, Aimed at Promoting the Healing of Wounds

Current research and development efforts are centered on incorporating herbal components into modern drug delivery systems for wound healing. These systems aim to enhance the therapeutic effectiveness of herbal extracts by improving their bioavailability and delivering them in a controlled manner, ultimately optimizing the wound healing process. Below are some key elements and methodologies related to advanced drug delivery systems that integrate herbal components for wound healing:

- *Nanoparticles:* Nanoparticles, including liposomes, polymeric nanoparticles, and micelles, can encapsulate herbal extracts. This encapsulation enhances the stability, solubility, and bioavailability of the extracts while allowing for targeted release at the wound site.
- *Nanoemulsions:* Nanoemulsions, which are emulsions at the nanoscale, can incorporate herbal components. They offer advantages such as enhanced stability, increased surface area, and improved skin penetration.
- *Hydrogels and scaffolds*: Herbal-loaded hydrogels can serve as drug carriers to promote wound healing. By incorporating herbal extracts into hydrogels, prolonged release can be achieved, creating a moist environment that supports the healing process.
- *Scaffolds:* Scaffolds, often in conjunction with nanotechnology, can serve as a structural support framework for herbal constituents. The utilisation of these three-dimensional structures may improve the process of tissue regeneration and facilitate the closure of wounds.
- *Microencapsulation*: Techniques such as spray drying and coacervation can be used to microencapsulate herbal extracts. These advanced methods help preserve the herbal components, regulate their release, and facilitate their incorporation into various formulations.

- *Herbal antimicrobial agents:* Certain plant preparations exhibit intrinsic antibacterial activity. Incorporating these extracts into drug delivery systems helps prevent the spread of infections, which is a crucial aspect of the wound healing process.
- *Anti-inflammatory and antioxidant herbs:* Herbal ingredients with anti-inflammatory and antioxidant properties can be utilized to reduce inflammation and oxidative stress at the site of an injury. Controlled release mechanisms ensure a prolonged therapeutic effect.
- *Bioactive compounds:* Enhancing the effectiveness of wound healing can be accomplished by identifying and isolating specific bioactive components from herbs and incorporating them into delivery systems.
- *Clinical applications*: Scientists and drug manufacturers are conducting preclinical and clinical investigations to verify the safety and efficacy of these innovative drug delivery systems for promoting wound healing.

Wound Healing Properties of Natural Products and Medicinal Plants

A comprehensive investigation has been conducted on the wound healing effects of natural products and medicinal plants. These substances contain bioactive components such as flavonoids, alkaloids, phenolic compounds, tannins, and terpenes, which contribute to their medicinal benefits. Natural products exert their effects on wound healing through various mechanisms, including reducing inflammation, combating microbial growth, and providing antioxidant properties. Additionally, they facilitate tissue regeneration and stimulate collagen production (Criollo-Mendoza et al., 2023). Several natural products have been identified to promote wound healing, including:

- *Aloe vera*: Aloe vera is renowned for its anti-inflammatory and antibacterial properties, making it a valuable resource for promoting wound healing and minimizing scar formation (Sivamani et al., 2012).
- *Curcuma longa*: Curcumin, a compound found in turmeric, possesses properties that reduce inflammation and oxidative stress, potentially enhancing its ability to promote wound healing (Sivamani et al., 2012).
- *Honey:* Honey possesses antibacterial and antiviral properties, which are beneficial for the wound healing process (Liu et al., 2022).
- *Chamomile:* Chamomile has gained attention for its ability to reduce inflammation and decrease oxidative stress, leading researchers to explore its potential in supporting wound recovery (Liu et al., 2022).
- *Banana Leaf*: It comprises bioactive compounds that have been studied for their ability to promote wound healing (Sivamani et al., 2012).

Plant Bioactives: Accelerating Wound Healing with Antimicrobial and Antioxidant Power

Phytochemicals derived from plants have demonstrated diverse therapeutic properties, including the ability to facilitate wound healing (Criollo-Mendoza et al., 2023). These compounds stimulate blood coagulation, combat infection, and accelerate the healing process. Here's how they work:

- *Blood coagulation*: Bioactive compounds enhance hemostasis, the physiological process that leads to the formation of a blood clot to stop bleeding. This attribute helps mitigate excessive hemorrhaging during wound healing (Ti et al., 2022).
- *Fight infection*: These compounds exhibit both antibacterial and antioxidant activities. Their antimicrobial properties help counter infections, while antioxidants protect healthy cells from damage caused by free radicals, particularly those involved in the wound healing process (Vitale et al., 2022).
- *Wound healing*: Bioactive substances promote the synthesis of collagen, an essential protein in the wound healing process. They also stimulate angiogenesis, a crucial aspect of healing, by inducing the formation of new blood vessels (Ti et al., 2022).
- *Accelerate wound healing*: These compounds enhance blood coagulation, resist infection, and speed up the healing process. This acceleration is particularly beneficial in situations where wound healing needs to be expedited, such as during surgical interventions or when managing chronic wounds (Vitale et al., 2022).

Stages of Wound Healing

Wound healing is a complex and dynamic process that typically occurs in several distinct phases. The four primary stages of wound healing are as follows:

- *Homeostasis stage*: The homeostasis stage is the initial phase of the wound healing process, where the body aims to stop bleeding. This phase typically lasts approximately 48 hours. During this stage, vasoconstriction occurs, causing blood vessels in the injured area to narrow and reduce blood flow. Concurrently, hemostatic substances are released at the injury site to combine with fibrin, forming a thrombus that serves as a barrier to prevent further blood leakage. This initial stage is crucial for preparing the wound for the subsequent stages of healing (Rodrigues et al., 2019).
- *Inflammatory Stage*: The inflammatory stage is the body's intrinsic reaction to injury, beginning with hemostasis and chemotaxis. Blood vessels contract to form a clot that halts bleeding. Once equilibrium is achieved, blood vessels dilate to facilitate the transport of essential cells, immunoglobulins, white blood cells (WBCs), growth factors, enzymes, and nutrients to the injured area. This results in increased exudate levels and the typical signs of inflammation, including redness, warmth, swelling, pain, and impaired function. The inflammatory phase usually lasts up to 2 weeks in normal wounds; however, it can be prolonged in chronic wounds, leading to tissue fibrosis and the development of non-healing ulcers. This phase is critical for managing

hemorrhage, preventing infection, and initiating the subsequent stages of wound healing, including proliferation and remodeling.

- *Proliferative Stage:* The proliferative stage is characterized by the formation of granulation tissue, restoration of epithelial cells, and the creation of new blood vessels. This phase can extend for several weeks, typically occurring within 3 to 21 days after the initial injury. During this stage, the wound undergoes reconstruction, forming new tissue composed of collagen and extracellular matrix (ECM). The primary objective of this stage is to replenish the wound defect and restore the basic integrity of the damaged tissue. Angiogenesis, the formation of new blood vessels, is crucial in this phase, as it enhances the supply of oxygen and nutrients to the healing tissue. Additionally, the migration and rapid proliferation of cells at the wound edges lead to the development of an epithelial layer, which is essential for wound closure. The entire process can conclude within 48 to 72 hours in a sterile wound. The increase in type I collagen concentration directly correlates with enhanced wound strength, allowing the skin to regain up to 80% of its initial tensile strength. The proliferative stage is vital as it lays the groundwork for the later maturation phase, during which the wound achieves maximum strength (Landén et al., 2016).
- *Remodelling Stage*: The remodeling stage represents the final phase of the healing process, during which granulation tissue matures into scar tissue, enhancing the tensile strength of the tissue. This stage typically begins around 21 days after the initial injury and can persist for one year or longer. During this phase, the extracellular matrix (ECM) undergoes remodeling, replacing initial scar tissue with ECM that closely resembles normal skin. Fibroblast and capillary density decrease, while the wound site reorganizes to optimize tensile strength. Collagen fibers are remodeled to align with the direction of stress, further enhancing the tensile strength of the healed tissues. The remodeling phase is a decisive stage in the overall wound healing process, as it establishes the foundation for the maturation phase, during which the wound reaches its maximum strength (Landén et al., 2016).

The Role of Nanophytoherbs in Each Phase of Wound Healing

Nanophytoherbs play a crucial role in all stages of the wound healing process. They enhance healing by reducing inflammation, exhibiting antioxidant and antifungal effects, and stimulating collagen production and deposition (Mirrezaei et al., 2020). The incorporation of nanotechnology amplifies these effects, improving the effectiveness and bioavailability of specific treatments (Hajialyani et al., 2018). Various nanomaterials, including metal and metal oxide nanoparticles, lipid vehicles, ceramic nanoparticles, and carbon nanomaterials, contribute to all four stages of wound healing. Additionally, natural compounds derived from alkaloids, flavonoids, retinoids, volatile oils, terpenes, carotenoids, and polyphenolic compounds have been shown to accelerate the wound healing process (Salimi et al., 2021). Notably, the discovery of a nanoparticle-in-nanofiber system that releases growth factors has been demonstrated to significantly expedite wound healing by stimulating new blood vessel growth, enhancing the regeneration of the outer skin layer, and regulating granulation tissue production

(Xie et al., 2013). The actions of nanophytoherbs in various phases of wound healing (Figure 1) are detailed below:

- *Inflammatory phase*: Nanophytoherbs possess the ability to mitigate inflammation, a crucial component of the healing process. They achieve this by suppressing the synthesis of inflammatory cytokines and chemokines. Curcumin, quercetin, and resveratrol are examples of nanophytoherbs that have demonstrated efficacy in reducing inflammation.
- *Proliferative phase*: Nanophytoherbs can also enhance cell proliferation, an essential process for the development of new tissue. This is accomplished by stimulating the proliferation of fibroblasts, the cells responsible for collagen synthesis. Notable nanophytoherbs that have shown effectiveness in promoting cell proliferation include aloe vera, honey, and gotu kola.
- *Remodeling phase*: Nanophytoherbs have the capability to facilitate wound remodeling, which is the final stage of wound healing. They do this by enhancing collagen production and minimizing the formation of fibrous tissue. *Centella asiatica* and turmeric are examples of nanophytoherbs that have demonstrated efficacy in wound remodeling.

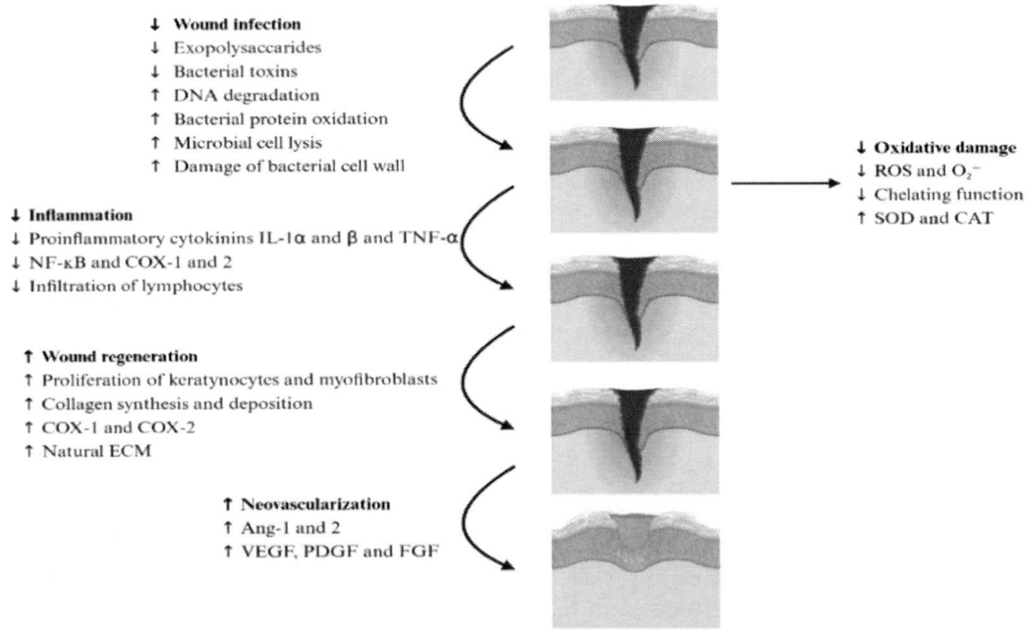

Figure 1. The role of nanophytoherb in different phases of wound healing (Hajialyani et al., 2018).

The Role of Disinfection, Debridement, and Providing a Moist Atmosphere for Wound Healing

- *Moist wound healing*: Maintaining a moist wound environment offers numerous benefits that contribute to faster and more effective healing. It aids in the natural breakdown of dead tissue, alleviates pain, minimizes scarring, stimulates collagen production, promotes the movement of skin cells over the wound, and ensures the availability and effectiveness of essential nutrients and growth factors (Nuutila & Eriksson, 2021).

- *Debridement:* Debridement involves the removal of necrotic tissue and any foreign substances from a lesion. Thorough removal of dead tissue is crucial for optimal wound healing. Scientific evidence has shown that proper cleaning can significantly impact the rate of wound healing. The choice of debridement technique should be guided by factors such as the amount of exudate, the presence of infection, the volume of non-viable tissue, and the moisture level in the ulcer (Nowak et al., 2022).
- *Disinfection:* Disinfection is vital for effective wound management. An ideal wound dressing should provide protection for the wound while creating a conducive moist environment to facilitate healing. Maintaining a wet atmosphere is essential for promoting healing and preventing infection (BATAVIA, 2006).

Clinical Studies of Nanophytoherbs for Wound Healing

In Vitro and *In Vivo* Experiments for Wound Healing Studies

In vitro and *in vivo* studies are essential for evaluating the efficacy of wound healing therapeutics, including those based on nanomaterials and natural products. The findings provide valuable insights into the methodologies and frameworks employed in these assessments.

In Vivo

The studies are conducted on living organisms, including both animals and humans. They demonstrate superior fidelity compared to in vitro tests when it comes to replicating real-world conditions. Common *in vivo* tests include:

- *Wound healing models:*
  - Incisional or excisional wound models: Develop consistent wounds to evaluate the progress of healing.
  - Burn models: Simulate burn injuries to investigate the processes of tissue regeneration and inflammation.
- *Nanomaterial-based therapy:*
  - Conducting *in vivo* assays to assess the impact of nanomaterials, such as nanophytoherbs, on the wound healing process is crucial for evaluating their effectiveness and safety. These studies offer valuable information on the capacity of nanomaterials to enhance cellular and molecular mechanisms that contribute to the wound microenvironment, facilitating antifungal, anti-inflammatory, and vasculogenic actions (Kushwaha et al., 2022; Naskar & Kim, 2020).
- *Macroscopic and Microscopic Analysis:*
  - Macroscopic evaluation: Measures wound closure, contraction, and overall appearance.

- Histological analysis: Analyzes tissue sections to identify different cell types, evaluate collagen deposition, and detect any other histopathological alterations.

- *Animal models:*
  - Animal models, specifically mice, have been employed to assess the effectiveness of natural products and bioactive components in promoting wound healing. These models offer significant insights into the impact of putative medicines on the wound healing process (Masson-Meyers et al., 2020; Sofrona et al., 2020).
- *Microbial assessment:*
  - Microbiological Cultures: Evaluates wound infections by culturing microbes from the wound site.

In Vitro

These assays are conducted on skin samples or cells in a laboratory environment, replicating the *in vivo* settings without the need for living beings. Common *in vitro* tests comprise:

- *Wound healing assays:*
  - *In vitro* wound healing tests replicate the later steps of the wound healing process, specifically the inflammatory and proliferative phases. These assays utilize both 2D and 3D models, with the 2D cell monolayer format being the most commonly used due to its ease, cost-effectiveness, and ability to accurately measure wound healing in both qualitative and quantitative terms (Ahmad, 2022).
- *Cell-culture models:*
  - The selection of commonly used cell lines and the justification for their use are essential in conducting *in vitro* studies on wound healing. These models offer valuable insights into the molecular mechanisms involved in the healing process, as well as the impact of interactions between cells and the extracellular matrix. They also suggest prospective strategies for enhancing wound healing through therapeutic interventions (Ahmad, 2022).
- *Cell viability and proliferation assays*:
  - MTT Assay: This method assesses cell vitality by measuring their capacity to transform a yellow tetrazolium salt into a purple formazan dye.
  - Cell Counting Kit (CCK) Assay: This assay determines cell viability through the reduction of WST-8 tetrazolium salt.
- *Collagen gel contraction assay:*
  - Purpose: To assess the contractile capacity of fibroblasts, a crucial mechanism involved in the healing of wounds.
  - Example: Fibroblast-populated collagen lattice assay.

Well-Controlled Clinical Trials of Nanophytoherbal Treatments for Wound Healing

Nanomaterials are being extensively studied for their prospective applications and advantages in wound healing, making it a rapidly advancing area of research. Here are several attributes of effectively regulated clinical trials:

- *Define the endpoint*: The primary objective should be the complete restoration of the wound. The statistical power of this endpoint is low due to the heterogeneity of wounds and the variability in their healing trajectories (Bull et al., 2023).
- *Design a robust trial*: To overcome the limitations of inadequate statistical power, a carefully designed randomized controlled trial should be utilized. Ensure that the trial has sufficient statistical power to identify a meaningful difference in wound healing (Dorai, 2012).
- *Inclusion and exclusion criteria*: To maintain the integrity of the trial, it is imperative to establish well-defined inclusion and exclusion criteria that ensure the participation of only appropriate individuals. By ensuring the homogeneity of the study population, the trial's internal validity will be enhanced (Patino & Ferreira, 2018).
- *Randomization*: Implement a reliable and trustworthy randomization mechanism to ensure an impartial allocation of subjects to the various treatment groups. This measure will mitigate any potential bias that may influence the study results (Lim & In, 2019).
- *Placebo-controlled arm*: Incorporate a placebo-controlled group to evaluate the distinct impacts of the nanophytoherbal treatment compared to a placebo while accounting for the placebo effect (Nair, 2019).
- *Blinding:* To minimize bias, it is crucial to ensure that participants, treatment providers, and outcome assessors are blinded. This can be accomplished by employing placebo or active control groups (Monaghan et al., 2021).
- *Data collection and analysis*: Utilize validated and reliable methods for gathering and reviewing data. This will help ensure the accuracy and consistency of the collected information.

Conclusion

In conclusion, the application of nanophytoherbs in wound therapy shows significant promise for advancing wound healing practices. Integrating nanotechnology with herbal extracts offers multiple benefits that could surpass traditional methods. Key advantages include enhanced therapeutic efficacy, as nanophytoherb formulations improve the effectiveness of herbal extracts by addressing issues such as limited bioavailability and controlled release. Nanocarriers enable precise targeting of bioactives to injury sites, optimizing their therapeutic impact and ensuring sustained effects on tissue regeneration. By enhancing the solubility and stability of herbal constituents, nanotechnology boosts bioavailability, allowing for a higher concentration of active substances at the wound site. Nanophytoherbs also modulate the inflammatory response, fostering a healing environment while minimizing inflammation, and exhibit antimicrobial properties essential for infection prevention during the early healing stages. Additionally, they may promote angiogenesis, supporting new blood vessel formation crucial for tissue repair, and stimulate collagen synthesis, aiding tissue regeneration and reducing scar formation. The potential for combining various herbal extracts into a single product allows for a synergistic approach to wound healing. Despite these advancements, further research, including rigorous preclinical and clinical studies, is needed to validate the safety, efficacy, and practical applications of nanophytoherb formulations. Future research directions include investigating the mechanisms of interaction between nanophytoherbs and cellular processes, assessing long-term safety, exploring combination therapies, developing patient-specific approaches, employing advanced imaging techniques, conducting clinical trials, and addressing economic and environmental considerations.

References

Ahmad, N. (2022). *In vitro* and *in vivo* characterization methods for evaluation of modern wound dressings. *Pharmaceutics*, 15(1), 42.

Al-saggaf, M. S. (2021). Formulation of Insect Chitosan Stabilized Silver Nanoparticles with Propolis Extract as Potent Antimicrobial and Wound Healing Composites. *International Journal of Polymer Science*, 2021, 1–9.

Ansari, J. A., & Inamdar, N. N. (2010). The Promise of Traditional Medicines. *International Journal of Pharmacology*, *6*(6), 808–812.

Arias JL. (2014). *Nanotechnology and drug delivery* (Vol. 1).

Balaji, A., Vellayappan, M. V., John, A. A., Subramanian, A. P., Jaganathan, S. K., SelvaKumar, M., Mohd Faudzi, A. A. bin, Supriyanto, E., & Yusof, M. (2015). Biomaterials based nano-applications of Aloe vera and its perspective: a review. *RSC Advances*, *5*(105), 86199–86213.

BATAVIA, M. (2006). Wound Care. In *Contraindications in Physical Rehabilitation* (pp. 510–527). Elsevier.

Benita S. (2005). *Microencapsulation: methods and industrial applications*. CRC Press.

Bhattacharya, T., Soares, G. A. B. e, Chopra, H., Rahman, Md. M., Hasan, Z., Swain, S. S., & Cavalu, S. (2022). Applications of Phyto-Nanotechnology for the Treatment of Neurodegenerative Disorders. *Materials*, 15(3), 804.

Bull, R. H., Clements, D., Collarte, A. J., & Harding, K. G. (2023). A Novel Randomized Trial Protocol for Evaluating Wound Healing Interventions. *Advances in Wound Care*, 12(12), 671–679.

Burns, J., Buck, A. C., D' Souza, S., Dube, A., & Bardien, S. (2023). Nanophytomedicines as Therapeutic Agents for Parkinson's Disease. *ACS Omega*, 8(45), 42045–42061.

Criollo-Mendoza, M. S., Contreras-Angulo, L. A., Leyva-López, N., Gutiérrez-Grijalva, E. P., Jiménez-Ortega, L. A., & Heredia, J. B. (2023). Wound Healing Properties of Natural Products: Mechanisms of Action. *Molecules*, 28(2), 598.

Dorai, A. A. (2012). Wound care with traditional, complementary and alternative medicine. *Indian Journal of Plastic Surgery*, 45(02), 418–424.

Fahimirad, S., Satei, P., Ganji, A., & Abtahi, H. (2023). Wound healing capability of the double-layer Polycaprolactone/Polyvinyl alcohol-Chitosan lactate electrospun nanofiber incorporating Echinacea purpurea extract. *Journal of Drug Delivery Science and Technology*, 87, 104734.

Gad, H. A., Abd El-Rahman, F. A. A., & Hamdy, G. M. (2019). Chamomile oil loaded solid lipid nanoparticles: A naturally formulated remedy to enhance the wound healing. *Journal of Drug Delivery Science and Technology*, 50, 329–338.

Hajialyani, M., Tewari, D., Sobarzo-Sánchez, E., Nabavi, S. M., Farzaei, M. H., & Abdollahi, M. (2018). Natural product-based nanomedicines for wound healing purposes: therapeutic targets and drug delivery systems. *International Journal of Nanomedicine, Volume* 13, 5023–5043.

Handa SS, & Kaul MK. (2006). Supplement to Cultivation and Utilization of Medicinal Plants, Jammu-Tawi. *Regional Research Laboratory*, 566.

Hussain, Z., Thu, H. E., Ng, S. F., Khan, S., & Katas, H. (2017). Nanoencapsulation, an efficient and promising approach to maximize wound healing efficacy of curcumin: A review of new trends and state-of-the-art. *Colloids and Surfaces B: Biointerfaces*, 150, 223–241.

Järbrink, K., Ni, G., Sönnergren, H., Schmidtchen, A., Pang, C., Bajpai, R., & Car, J. (2016). Prevalence and incidence of chronic wounds and related complications: a protocol for a systematic review. *Systematic Reviews*, 5(1), 152.

Kushwaha, A., Goswami, L., & Kim, B. S. (2022). Nanomaterial-Based Therapy for Wound Healing. *Nanomaterials*, 12(4), 618.

Landén, N. X., Li, D., & Ståhle, M. (2016). Transition from inflammation to proliferation: a critical step during wound healing. *Cellular and Molecular Life Sciences*, 73(20), 3861–3885.

Lim, C. Y., & In, J. (2019). Randomization in clinical studies. *Korean Journal of Anesthesiology*, 72(3), 221–232.

Liu, E., Gao, H., Zhao, Y., Pang, Y., Yao, Y., Yang, Z., Zhang, X., Wang, Y., Yang, S., Ma, X., Zeng, J., & Guo, J. (2022). The potential application of natural products in cutaneous wound healing: A review of preclinical evidence. *Frontiers in Pharmacology*, 13.

Masson-Meyers, D. S., Andrade, T. A. M., Caetano, G. F., Guimaraes, F. R., Leite, M. N., Leite, S. N., & Frade, M. A. C. (2020). Experimental models and methods for cutaneous wound healing assessment. *International Journal of Experimental Pathology*, 101(1–2), 21–37.

Mirrezaei, N., Yazdian-Robati, R., Oroojalian, F., Sahebkar, A., & Hashemi, M. (2020). Recent Developments in Nano-Drug Delivery Systems Loaded by Phytochemicals for Wound Healing. *Mini-Reviews in Medicinal Chemistry*, 20(18), 1867–1878.

Monaghan, T. F., Agudelo, C. W., Rahman, S. N., Wein, A. J., Lazar, J. M., Everaert, K., & Dmochowski, R. R. (2021). Blinding in Clinical Trials: Seeing the Big Picture. *Medicina*, 57(7), 647.

Nair, B. (2019). Clinical Trial Designs. *Indian Dermatology Online Journal*, *10*(2), 193.

Naskar, A., & Kim, K. (2020). Recent Advances in Nanomaterial-Based Wound-Healing Therapeutics. *Pharmaceutics*, 12(6), 499.

Nouri, Z., Hajialyani, M., Izadi, Z., Bahramsoltani, R., Farzaei, M. H., & Abdollahi, M. (2020). Nanophytomedicines for the Prevention of Metabolic Syndrome: A Pharmacological and Biopharmaceutical Review. *Frontiers in Bioengineering and Biotechnology*, 8.

Nowak, M., Mehrholz, D., Barańska-Rybak, W., & Nowicki, R. (2022). Wound debridement products and techniques: clinical examples and literature review. *Advances in Dermatology and Allergology*, 39(3), 479–490.

Nuutila, K., & Eriksson, E. (2021). Moist Wound Healing with Commonly Available Dressings. *Advances in Wound Care*, 10(12), 685–698.

Patino, C. M., & Ferreira, J. C. (2018). Inclusion and exclusion criteria in research studies: definitions and why they matter. *Jornal Brasileiro de Pneumologia*, 44(2), 84–84.

Ramakrishnan, A., Gokul, R., & Pandimadevi, M. (2020). Preparation and characterisation of nanofibres from bio cellulose and neem-AgNP bio composites for wound healing. *International Journal of Biomedical Nanoscience and Nanotechnology*, 4(1/2), 80.

Rodrigues, M., Kosaric, N., Bonham, C. A., & Gurtner, G. C. (2019). Wound Healing: A Cellular Perspective. *Physiological Reviews*, 99(1), 665–706.

Sadri, M., Arab-Sorkhi, S., Vatani, H., & Bagheri-Pebdeni, A. (2015). New wound dressing polymeric nanofiber containing green tea extract prepared by electrospinning method. *Fibers and Polymers*, 16(8), 1742–1750.

Salimi, F., & Mohammadipanah, F. (2021). Nanomaterials Versus the Microbial Compounds with Wound Healing Property. *Frontiers in Nanotechnology*, 2.

Salvo, J., Sandoval, C., Schencke, C., Acevedo, F., & del Sol, M. (2023). Healing Effect of a Nano-Functionalized Medical-Grade Honey for the Treatment of Infected Wounds. *Pharmaceutics*, 15(9), 2187.

Sivamani, R. K., Ma, B. R., Wehrli, L. N., & Maverakis, E. (2012). Phytochemicals and Naturally Derived Substances for Wound Healing. *Advances in Wound Care*, 1(5), 213–217.

Sofrona, E., Tziveleka, L. A., Harizani, M., Koroli, P., Sfiniadakis, I., Roussis, V., Rallis, M., & Ioannou, E. (2020). *In Vivo* Evaluation of the Wound Healing Activity of Extracts and Bioactive Constituents of the Marine Isopod Ceratothoa oestroides. *Marine Drugs*, 18(4), 219.

Ti, Y. L., Song, F., Fang, Z., & Zhang, P. (2022). Plants and phytochemicals inhibit scar formation: A systematic review. *Industrial Crops and Products*, 185, 115113.

Vitale, S., Colanero, S., Placidi, M., Di Emidio, G., Tatone, C., Amicarelli, F., & D'Alessandro, A. M. (2022). Phytochemistry and Biological Activity of Medicinal Plants in Wound Healing: An Overview of Current Research. *Molecules*, 27(11), 3566.

Xie, Z., Paras, C. B., Weng, H., Punnakitikashem, P., Su, L. C., Vu, K., Tang, L., Yang, J., & Nguyen, K. T. (2013). Dual growth factor releasing multi-functional nanofibers for wound healing. *Acta Biomaterialia*, 9(12), 9351–9359.

Yang, S., Lu, S., Ren, L., Bian, S., Zhao, D., Liu, M., & Wang, J. (2023). Ginseng-derived nanoparticles induce skin cell proliferation and promote wound healing. *Journal of Ginseng Research*, 47(1), 133–143.

Zhu, X., Olsson, M. M., Bajpai, R., Järbrink, K., Tang, W. E., & Car, J. (2022). Health-related quality of life and chronic wound characteristics among patients with chronic wounds treated in primary care: A cross-sectional study in Singapore. *International Wound Journal*, 19(5), 1121–1132.

Chapter 12

Nanophytoherbals: Advanced Formulations for Enhanced Wound Healing

Shikha Baghel Chauhan*
Indu Singh
Aiman Usmani
and Astha Singh
Amity Institute of Pharmacy, Amity University, Noida, Uttar Pradesh, India

Abstract

The integration of nanotechnology and herbal medicine has paved the way for innovative approaches in wound care therapy. This chapter explores the promising field of nanophytoherbals, where nanoscale formulations of phytochemicals derived from medicinal plants are employed for enhanced wound healing. It begins by elucidating the principles of wound healing and the challenges associated with conventional wound care methods. It then delves into the potential of nanophytoherbals in overcoming these challenges, discussing the unique properties of nanomaterials that enable targeted delivery, sustained release, and improved bioavailability of phytoconstituents. Furthermore, the chapter provides an overview of various medicinal plants and their bioactive compounds that have demonstrated therapeutic efficacy in wound healing. The synthesis and characterization of nanophytoherbals are explored, shedding light on the nanotechnological tools and techniques employed in the process. It also reviews pre-clinical and clinical studies that demonstrate the effectiveness of nanophytoherbals in promoting tissue regeneration, reducing inflammation, and preventing microbial infections. Additionally, safety considerations and potential challenges associated with the application of nanophytoherbals in wound care are addressed. The chapter concludes by highlighting the prospects and emerging trends in this interdisciplinary field, emphasizing the need for further research and development to harness the full therapeutic potential of nanophytoherbals in wound care therapy. Overall, this chapter serves as a comprehensive resource for researchers, clinicians, and professionals interested in the intersection of nanotechnology and herbal medicine for advancing wound healing strategies.

* Corresponding Author's Email: shikha.pharma@gmail.com.

In: Phyto-Nanomedicine
Editors: Hitesh Chopra, Vinod Kumar Gauttam, Ajmer Singh Grewal et al.
ISBN: 979-8-89530-317-7

Keywords: nanophytoherbals, nanomedicine, herbal medicine, phytochemicals, wound therapy

Abbreviations

HPLC	High Performance Liquid Chromatography
DLS	Dynamic Light Scattering
GC-MS	Gas chromatography-Mass Spectrometry

Introduction

Wound healing is a complex phenomenon that requires the coordinated action of various cells, cytokines, and growth factors. Chronic wounds, however, pose a significant challenge to the healthcare system due to their delayed healing and high morbidity. Conventional wound care therapies often have limitations, such as poor bioavailability, inadequate targeting, and potential side effects (Gorain et al., 2022a). Nanophytoherbals have emerged as a promising approach to address the challenges associated with conventional wound care therapies. These are nanocarriers loaded with bioactive phytochemicals derived from medicinal plants. These nanocarriers offer several advantages over conventional therapies, including:

- *Enhanced bioavailability*: Nanoparticles can bypass biological barriers and deliver phytochemicals directly to the target site, improving their absorption and efficacy.
- *Targeted delivery*: By using ligands that bind selectively to receptors present on target cells, nanoparticles can be functionalized to ensure that phytochemicals are delivered precisely to the intended cells, thereby minimizing peripheral effects.
- *Controlled release*: Nanoparticles can be engineered to release phytochemicals gradually over an extended period, prolonging the therapeutic effect and reducing the frequency of administration.
- *Antimicrobial properties*: Many phytochemicals exhibit inherent antimicrobial activity, which can help combat wound infections and promote healing.
- *Anti-inflammatory properties*: Phytochemicals can modulate the inflammatory response, reducing inflammation and promoting tissue regeneration.
- *Biocompatibility and safety*: Nanophytoherbals are often composed of natural materials and are generally well-tolerated by the body.

This chapter aims to comprehensively explore the application of nanophytoherbals in wound care therapy. It will delve into the synergistic effects of nanotechnology and phototherapeutic agents, elucidating their mechanisms of action in promoting wound healing, combating infections, reducing inflammation, and accelerating tissue regeneration. Furthermore, it will discuss the various formulations and delivery systems employed in nanophytoherbal-based wound care products, highlighting their efficacy and safety profiles (Qadir et al., 2021a).

Principles of Wound Healing

Wound healing is a complex biological process that occurs in several overlapping stages: hemostasis, inflammation, proliferation, and remodeling. Each stage is characterized by specific cellular and molecular events that work in concert to restore tissue integrity and functionality.

Hemostasis

The initial stage of wound healing is termed hemostasis, which aims to stop bleeding. When a blood vessel is damaged, vasoconstriction occurs to reduce blood flow. Platelets are then recruited to the injury site, aggregating to form a temporary platelet plug. The activated platelets release clotting factors, such as fibrinogen, which polymerize into a fibrin meshwork. This meshwork, along with entrapped platelets and red blood cells, forms a stable blood clot, preventing further blood loss (Mirrezaei et al., 2020a).

Inflammation

The inflammatory stage begins immediately after an injury, clearing debris, pathogens, and damaged cells present at the wound site. The key players in this stage are immune cells, particularly neutrophils and macrophages. The earliest immune cells to reach the wound site are neutrophils, which use phagocytosis to eliminate bacteria. Macrophages then replace neutrophils, continuing the phagocytic activity while releasing cytokines and growth factors that initiate the next stage of wound healing.

Proliferation

The formation of new tissue to cover the wound gap occurs during the proliferation stage. The main processes in this stage include angiogenesis, fibroplasia, and reepithelialization.

- *Angiogenesis*: The formation of new blood vessels is essential to supply oxygen and nutrients to the healing tissue. Endothelial cells sprout from existing blood vessels and form capillary buds that grow into the wound bed, ultimately establishing a new network of blood vessels.
- *Fibroplasia*: In this stage, fibroblasts play a crucial role by synthesizing and depositing extracellular matrix (ECM) components, such as collagen and elastin. Collagen provides tensile strength to the wound, while elastin offers flexibility. Fibroblasts also secrete growth factors that promote cell proliferation and tissue remodeling.
- *Reepithelialization:* A new layer of epithelium forms through the migration of epithelial cells from the wound edges across the wound bed. This migration is driven by a specialized subset of epithelial cells known as keratinocytes. These cells proliferate, migrate, and differentiate, eventually sealing the wound.

Remodeling

The remodeling stage involves the maturation and reorganization of the newly formed tissue. During this phase, collagen fibers undergo remodeling, becoming more organized and cross-linked, which significantly increases the tensile strength of the wound. Excess collagen is also removed, allowing the wound to gradually regain strength. This process can take months to years, and the final scar tissue may differ in appearance and texture from the original tissue (Qadir et al., 2021b). Several key principles influence the overall outcome of the wound healing process:

- *Oxygenation:* Adequate oxygen supply is critical for wound healing. Oxygen is necessary for cellular metabolism, collagen synthesis, and angiogenesis. Poor oxygenation, as seen in chronic wounds or in patients with compromised blood flow, can impair the healing process.
- *Infection control*: Preventing and managing infections is vital, as infections can lead to delayed healing, increased tissue damage, and complications.
- *Moist wound environment*: Maintaining a moist wound environment promotes faster healing, reduces pain, and minimizes scarring by supporting the natural breakdown of dead tissue and encouraging cell migration.
- *Nutritional support:* Proper nutrition, including adequate protein intake, vitamins, and minerals, supports the various cellular processes involved in wound healing.
- *Systemic factors:* Individual characteristics such as age, underlying health conditions, and medication use can impact the healing process. Comorbidities like diabetes or vascular diseases can significantly hinder healing.
- *Mechanical factors*: The physical forces acting on a wound, including tension and pressure, can affect tissue integrity and healing, highlighting the importance of appropriate wound care and management techniques.

Nanophytoherbals: A Conceptual Framework

The convergence of nanotechnology and herbal medicine has blossomed into the exciting field of nanophytoherbals, holding immense potential to revolutionize wound care therapy. This conceptual framework aims to delve into the core principles and mechanisms by which these botanical-infused nanoparticles act, providing a deeper understanding and allowing further development of this revolutionary approach (Mirrezaei et al., 2020b).

Phytochemicals as Therapeutic Weapons

Phyto herbal therapy, the use of plant-based substances for therapeutic purposes, has been practiced for centuries and continues to be a valuable tool in modern medicine. In this essay, we will elaborate on the various ways in which phyto herbal therapy serves as a therapeutic weapon, its mechanisms of action, and its potential benefits.

- *Anti-inflammatory properties*: Many phytoherbal constituents possess potent anti-inflammatory properties. For example, curcumin, a compound found in turmeric, has been extensively studied for its anti-inflammatory effects. It inhibits inflammatory mediators and enzymes, reducing inflammation in various conditions such as arthritis, inflammatory bowel disease, and skin disorders. Other herbs like ginger, Boswellia, and green tea also exhibit anti-inflammatory properties, making them valuable in managing inflammatory conditions.
- *Antioxidant effects*: Phyto herbal constituents are often rich in antioxidants. Free radicals contribute to aging, chronic diseases, and tissue damage. Herbs such as green tea, grape seed extract, and resveratrol from red grapes have potent antioxidant properties. These antioxidants scavenge free radicals, reduce oxidative stress, and help prevent or manage conditions such as cardiovascular diseases, neurodegenerative disorders, and cancer (Gorain et al., 2022b).
- *Antimicrobial and antiviral activities*: Many phyto herbal constituents exhibit antimicrobial and antiviral properties, making them effective therapeutic weapons against infectious diseases. For example, garlic contains allicin, a compound with broad-spectrum antimicrobial activity. It can fight bacteria, viruses, fungi, and parasites. Echinacea, known for its immunomodulatory effects, also possesses antiviral properties and can help prevent or alleviate symptoms of viral infections such as the common cold or influenza.
- *Immunomodulatory effects*: Phyto herbal therapy can modulate the immune system, enhancing its protective functions or reducing excessive immune responses. Medicinal mushrooms contain beta-glucans that stimulate immune cells and enhance immune function. Examples include reishi, maitake, and shiitake. Astragalus, an herb used in traditional Chinese medicine, also boosts immune activity. These immunomodulatory effects make phyto herbal therapy valuable in supporting immune health and managing immune-related conditions (Kumar et al., 2023).
- *Neuroprotective properties*: Several phyto herbal constituents have demonstrated neuroprotective effects and may be beneficial in managing neurological disorders. For example, ginkgo biloba extract has been studied for its neuroprotective properties, which may help in diseases like Alzheimer's disease and stroke. Additionally, herbs like bacopa, ashwagandha, and Gotu kola have been traditionally used to support brain health and cognitive function.
- *Gastrointestinal support*: Phyto herbal therapy is commonly used to support gastrointestinal health and manage digestive disorders. Herbs like peppermint, ginger, and chamomile have carminative properties and can help alleviate symptoms such as bloating, indigestion, and nausea. Aloe vera has been used for centuries for its soothing effects on the digestive tract and is often used to manage conditions like irritable bowel syndrome and gastric ulcers (Siafaka et al., 2016).
- *Cardiovascular benefits*: Certain phyto herbal constituents offer cardiovascular benefits and can be used to support heart health. For instance, hawthorn extract has been used traditionally to support cardiovascular function and manage conditions like hypertension, angina, and heart failure. Garlic, known for its cardiovascular benefits, helps reduce blood pressure and cholesterol levels. Resveratrol from red grapes has also shown cardioprotective effects.

- *Stress management*: Phyto herbal therapy can serve as a therapeutic weapon against stress and anxiety. Herbs such as ashwagandha, holy basil, and chamomile possess adaptogenic properties, helping the body adjust to stress and restore balance. They can reduce stress hormone levels, promote relaxation, and improve overall well-being (Singh Bakshi et al., 2022).

Nanocarriers: Tailored Delivery Vehicles

Phytochemicals, despite their therapeutic potential, often face limitations such as poor bioavailability, instability, and off-target effects. This is where nanocarriers come into play. These nanoscale vehicles, typically made from biocompatible materials like polymers, lipids, or natural carbohydrates, act as miniature Trojan horses, encapsulating and delivering phytochemicals effectively.

- *Enhanced solubility and stability*: Many phyto herbal constituents have limited solubility and stability, which can affect their bioavailability and therapeutic efficacy. Nanocarriers can overcome these challenges by encapsulating the phytochemicals, protecting them from degradation, and improving their solubility. This ensures that an adequate concentration of the active compounds reaches the wound site, enhancing their therapeutic effects.
- *Controlled release*: Nanocarriers can be engineered to provide controlled and sustained release of phyto herbal constituents. This controlled release profile can prolong the presence of the active compounds at the wound site, ensuring a continuous therapeutic effect. By modulating the properties of nanocarriers such as size, surface charge, and composition, the release kinetics of the phytochemicals can be tailored to match the wound healing process (Hajialyani et al., 2018).
- *Targeted delivery*: Nanocarriers can be designed to selectively target the wound site, improving the localization and accumulation of phyto herbal agents. Surface modifications of nanocarriers with ligands or antibodies that recognize specific receptors or markers on the wound site can enhance their binding and uptake by the cells in the wound area. This targeted delivery approach increases the concentration of the active compounds at the site of action, improving their therapeutic efficacy while minimizing off-target effects.
- *Penetration enhancement*: Wound healing often requires the delivery of phyto herbal agents to deeper layers of the skin. However, the stratum corneum can pose a significant barrier to drug penetration. Nanocarriers can be engineered to overcome this obstacle by incorporating penetration enhancers or utilizing their small size and unique physicochemical properties to penetrate the skin barrier. This allows the phytochemicals to reach the deeper layers of the wound, where they can exert their therapeutic effects more effectively (Monika & Chandraprabha, 2020).
- *Combination therapy*: Nanocarriers allow the co-delivery of multiple phyto herbal constituents or the combination of phytochemicals with other therapeutic agents such as antibiotics or growth factors. This approach facilitates synergistic effects, where the combined agents work together to enhance wound healing outcomes. For example,

nanocarriers can be loaded with both curcumin and a growth factor to promote collagen synthesis and tissue regeneration simultaneously.

- *Imaging and diagnostics:* Nanocarriers can be engineered to incorporate imaging agents or diagnostic probes, enabling real-time monitoring of wound healing progress. By incorporating contrast agents or fluorescent dyes, nanocarriers can provide information about the distribution and retention of the phytochemicals at the wound site (Solati et al., 2021). This imaging capability allows healthcare professionals to assess the efficacy of the therapy and make informed decisions regarding the treatment plan.

Mechanisms of Action: A Synergistic Symphony

The therapeutic action of nanophytoherbals stems from a synergistic interplay between the encapsulated phytochemicals and the nanocarriers:

- *Direct action*: Phytochemicals directly interact with cellular targets, exerting their antimicrobial, anti-inflammatory, and other therapeutic effects.
- *Indirect action*: Nanocarriers themselves may possess intrinsic antibacterial or anti-inflammatory properties, further enhancing the overall therapeutic impact.
- *Synergistic effects*: The combined action of the phytochemicals and the nanocarrier can produce synergistic effects, amplifying their individual therapeutic potential.

Applications Across the Wound Healing Spectrum

The application of nanophytoherbal therapy using nanocarriers offers diverse benefits across the wound healing spectrum. From acute to chronic wounds, these innovative approaches have shown potential in improving healing outcomes. Here are some applications of nanophytoherbal therapy in wound care:

- *Acute wound healing*: Nanophytoherbal therapy can enhance the healing of acute wounds, such as surgical incisions, abrasions, and lacerations. Nanocarriers loaded with phytochemical constituents can be applied topically to the wound site, providing a controlled release of active compounds that promote inflammation resolution, tissue regeneration, and accelerated wound closure.
- *Chronic wound management*: Chronic wounds, including diabetic ulcers, pressure ulcers, and venous ulcers, often face impaired healing processes. Nanophytoherbal therapy offers potential solutions for managing these wounds. Nanocarriers can deliver bioactive phytochemical compounds with antimicrobial, anti-inflammatory, and regenerative properties directly to the chronic wound site, promoting healing, reducing infection risk, and stimulating tissue repair.
- *Biofilm eradication*: Biofilms are commonly associated with chronic wounds and can impede the healing process. Nanophytoherbal therapy can effectively target biofilms using phytochemicals with antimicrobial properties (Safta et al., 2022). Nanocarriers

loaded with these agents can penetrate the biofilm matrix, disrupting its structure and eradicating microbial colonies. This approach helps create a favorable environment for healing by reducing infection and promoting tissue regeneration.

- *Scar management*: Nanophytoherbal therapy shows promise in managing scars resulting from wounds. Phytochemical compounds with anti-inflammatory and collagen-modulating properties can be encapsulated in nanocarriers and applied topically to the affected area (Ganesan & Choi, 2016). These compounds may help minimize scar formation, promote scar remodeling, and improve the cosmetic appearance of scars.
- *Pain management*: Wound-associated pain is a common concern, particularly in chronic wounds. Nanophytoherbal therapy can aid in pain management by delivering phytochemical constituents with analgesic properties to the wound site. Nanocarriers can provide sustained release of these agents, offering prolonged pain relief, reducing reliance on systemic analgesics, and improving patient comfort during the healing process (Xu et al., 2023).
- *Diagnostic and monitoring tools*: Nanocarriers can be functionalized with diagnostic agents or probes to enable real-time monitoring of wound healing progress. These nanophytoherbal systems can provide information on wound status, such as inflammation levels, microbial presence, or tissue regeneration (Nagoba & Davane, 2019).

Medicinal Plants and Bioactive Compounds

The natural world possesses immense healing potential, with medicinal plants having been used for centuries to treat various ailments. This rich history of herbal medicine is now converging with cutting-edge nanotechnology, resulting in nanophytoherbals, a revolutionary approach to wound care therapy (Table 1).

From ancient times, humans have turned to nature for healing, and wound care is a prime example. The bark of willow trees eased ancient pains, while honey's antimicrobial properties were valued in Egyptian medicine. Modern science is now uncovering the secrets behind these traditional remedies, highlighting the powerful phytoherbal constituents that serve as nature's arsenal for wound healing.

- *Antibacterial Guardians:* Wounds are battlegrounds against invisible foes—bacteria. Here, potent plant warriors rise to the defense. Curcumin, the golden warrior from turmeric, wields its sharp turmericinoids, puncturing bacterial membranes and sending them reeling. Thyme, with its mighty thymol, disrupts bacterial communication, leaving them disoriented and vulnerable (Johnson et al., 2018). The powerful berberine, found in barberry, locks bacterial DNA in a tight grip, preventing replication and ensuring their defeat.

Table 1. Summary of the various nanophytoherbals use in wound healing along with their therapeutic properties and geographical distribution

Nanophytoherbal Therapy	Medicinal Plant (Biological Name)	Bioactive Compound (Biological Name)	Properties	Global Distribution	References
Curcumin Nanoparticles	Turmeric (Curcuma longa)	Curcumin	Anti-inflammatory, antioxidant, antimicrobial	Widely cultivated in tropical and subtropical regions, including India, Southeast Asia, China, and Central America.	(Gorain et al., 2022a)
Honey-based Nanogels	Honey (Apis mellifera)	Manuka honey contains unique UMF factor	Antimicrobial, wound healing, anti-inflammatory	Produced by honeybees around the world, with particularly potent Manuka honey found in New Zealand, Australia, and Chile.	(Gorain et al., 2022b)
Aloe Vera Hydrogels	Aloe vera (Aloe barbadensis miller)	Acemannan, aloesin	Wound healing, anti-inflammatory, analgesic	Grows in warm, arid climates, found in Africa, the Mediterranean, the Caribbean, and India.	(Mirrezaei et al., 2020a)
Neem Leaf Emulsions	Neem (Azadirachta indica)	Azadirachtin, nimbolide	Antibacterial, antifungal, anti-inflammatory	Native to India and Burma, but widely cultivated in tropical and subtropical regions.	(Singh Bakshi et al., 2022)
Green Tea Extract Nanoparticles	Green Tea (Camellia sinensis)	Epigallocatechin gallate (EGCG)	Antioxidant, anti-inflammatory, antibacterial	Primarily grown in East Asia, including China, Japan, Taiwan, and Vietnam.	(Hajialyani et al., 2018)
Centella Asiatica Creams	Gotu Kola (Centella asiatica)	Madecassoside, asiaticoside	Wound healing, collagen synthesis, anti-inflammatory	Native to Southeast Asia and the Indian subcontinent but naturalized in tropical and subtropical regions worldwide.	(Xu et al., 2023)
Mangosteen Extract Nanocarriers	Mangosteen (Garcinia mangostana)	Xanthones, alpha-mangostin	Anti-inflammatory, antimicrobial, antioxidant	Native to Southeast Asia, particularly Indonesia, Malaysia, and Thailand.	(Singh et al., 2019)
Lavender Oil Emulsions	Lavender (Lavandula angustifolia)	Linalool, 1,8-cineole	Antibacterial, antifungal, analgesic	Primarily grown in the Mediterranean region, but cultivated in temperate climates worldwide	(Khogta et al., 2020)

- *Inflammation's Taming Hand:* Inflammation, while a crucial first responder, can sometimes overstay its welcome, hindering repair. Enter the anti-inflammatory brigade of phytochemicals. Boswellic acid, the champion from Boswellia, blocks inflammatory messengers, keeping the battlefield calm. Resveratrol, the purple champion from grapes, quenches the flames of oxidative stress, protecting tissues from collateral damage (Pandey et al., 2023).
- *Antioxidant Shields*: During the healing frenzy, free radicals, the rogue elements of the battlefield, can wreak havoc on tissues. However, the antioxidant brigade stands guard. Flavonoids, with their vibrant pigments found in berries and flowers, scavenge these radicals, shielding tissues from their destructive effects. Phenolic acids, nature's tannic guardians, bind to free radicals, rendering them harmless.
- *Regeneration Champions*: Scars whisper tales of battles won, but sometimes the stories etched are deeper than desired. This is where the tissue regeneration brigade intervenes. Madecassoside, the star player from Centella asiatica, stimulates collagen production, the building blocks of new tissue. Allantoin, found in comfrey, encourages cell proliferation, filling the gaps left by the battle. These tireless builders bridge the divide, weaving new skin where once there was a wound (Singh et al., 2019).
- *Nature's Gentle Touch*: Healing isn't just about mending tissues; it's about soothing the warrior's spirit. Here, pain-relieving phytochemicals like hypericin from St. John's wort come to the rescue. They calm inflamed nerves, dulling the sharp edges of pain and allowing the warrior to rest and recover.
- *Harnessing Nature's Wisdom*: The potential of phytochemicals in wound therapy is vast and brimming with promise. Their natural origins often translate to fewer side effects compared to some synthetic drugs, making them appealing alternatives. Traditional knowledge, passed down through generations, is now being combined with scientific rigor to develop effective and affordable herbal remedies for diverse communities (Pandey et al., 2023).
- *Beyond the Battlefield*: The utilization of phytochemicals in wound healing extends beyond typical cuts and scrapes. They can aid in diabetic wound healing, where impaired circulation poses a unique challenge. Their anti-inflammatory properties can offer relief for burns and chronic wounds. Even oral health benefits from nature's bounty, with some constituents promoting gum healing and combating mouth ulcers.
- *Nature's Harmony:* However, we must tread respectfully on this path. While powerful, herbs can interact with medications or cause sensitivities in certain individuals. Consulting a healthcare professional familiar with herbal remedies is crucial for safe and effective wound care (Oliveira da Silva et al., 2023).

Synthesis and Characterization of Nanophytoherbals

The burgeoning field of nanophytoherbals necessitates sophisticated techniques for their synthesis and characterization to ensure both effectiveness and safety. This section delves into the crucial steps involved in developing these novel wound care therapeutics:

Synthesis Methods

The synthesis and application of nanophytoherbal formulations in wound therapy involve the preparation of nanoparticles using plant-based materials, which are then incorporated into wound dressings or topical formulations. This approach combines the therapeutic properties of medicinal plants with the advantages of nanotechnology for enhanced wound healing. Below is a detailed explanation of the synthesis methods specifically for wound therapy:

- *Selection of plant material*: The first step is to select plant material with known wound healing properties. Common examples include *Aloe vera, Calendula officinalis, Centella asiatica*, and *Curcuma longa*. The selected plant should contain active compounds such as flavonoids, terpenoids, phenolic compounds, or polysaccharides that promote wound healing.
- *Extraction of active compounds*: The active compounds responsible for wound healing are extracted from the selected plant material. Various extraction methods can be used, including maceration, Soxhlet extraction, or ultrasound-assisted extraction, using suitable solvents like ethanol, methanol, or water (Lim et al., 2022).
- *Characterization of the extract*: The extract obtained from the plant material is characterized to determine its phytochemical composition, which helps identify and quantify the active compounds present. Analytical techniques such as HPLC, GC-MS, or spectrophotometry are commonly employed for this purpose.
- *Synthesis of nanoparticles*: The synthesized plant extract is then used as a reducing and stabilizing agent for preparing nanoparticles. Several methods for nanoparticle synthesis include:
  - *Chemical synthesis*: In this method, the plant extract is mixed with metal salts (e.g., silver nitrate) and a reducing agent (e.g., sodium borohydride). The reduction reaction leads to the formation of metal nanoparticles with wound healing properties (Ovais et al., 2018).
  - *Green synthesis*: Green synthesis methods utilize the reducing and capping properties of the plant extract itself. The extract is mixed with metal salts, and the reduction reaction occurs under specific conditions, such as heating or ultrasonic irradiation. This method avoids the use of toxic chemicals and is more environmentally friendly.
  - *Electrochemical synthesis*: Electrochemical methods involve the application of an electric current to generate nanoparticles. The plant extract serves as a reducing agent, and the electric current facilitates the reduction reaction at the electrode surface, leading to nanoparticle formation.
- *Characterization of nanoparticles:* The synthesized nanoparticles are characterized to determine their size, shape, stability, and surface charge. Techniques such as DLS, TEM, or SEM are commonly employed for nanoparticle characterization. The physicochemical properties of nanoparticles significantly influence their therapeutic effects and interactions with the wound microenvironment (Amjad et al., 2019).
- *Characterization techniques:* Thorough characterization of the synthesized nanophytoherbals is essential for quality control and therapeutic efficacy:

- *Particle size and size distribution*: Techniques like dynamic light scattering (DLS) and transmission electron microscopy (TEM) are used to evaluate the size and uniformity of the nanoparticles, which are crucial for targeting and drug delivery.
- *Zeta potential*: Measuring the surface charge of the nanoparticles using electrophoretic techniques helps predict their stability and interaction with cell membranes.
- *Encapsulation efficiency*: Determining the number of phytochemicals successfully encapsulated within the nanocarriers ensures optimal therapeutic delivery.
- *Surface morphology*: Scanning electron microscopy (SEM) and atomic force microscopy (AFM) provide detailed information about the surface characteristics of the nanoparticles, influencing their interaction with biological systems.
- *Drug release studies*: *In vitro* release studies simulate physiological conditions to assess the release profile of the phytochemicals from the nanocarriers, optimizing drug delivery and therapeutic action.
- *Cytotoxicity assays*: Evaluating the potential toxicity of the nanophytoherbals on healthy cells is important for ensuring their safety for wound healing applications.

- *Formulation development:* The synthesized nanoparticles are incorporated into wound dressings or topical formulations to optimize their application in wound therapy. The choice of formulation depends on factors such as the desired release profile, ease of application, and compatibility with the wound environment. Common formulation approaches include hydrogels, films, nanofibers, or creams.
- *Evaluation of wound healing properties:* The formulated nanophytoherbal product is evaluated for its wound healing properties. *In vitro* studies using cell culture models can assess cell viability, proliferation, migration, and extracellular matrix synthesis. *In vivo* studies using animal models can evaluate wound closure rates, histological analysis, and inflammatory response. These evaluations help determine the efficacy and safety of the nanophytoherbal formulation for wound therapy.
- *Optimization and scale-up:* The formulation and synthesis process may undergo optimization to enhance the desired properties and therapeutic effects of the nanophytoherbal product. Once optimized, the process can be scaled up for larger production (Pereira & Bártolo, 2016).

Considerations for Optimal Synthesis and Characterization

Optimal synthesis and characterization of nanophytoherbal systems in wound care therapy are crucial to ensure their safety, efficacy, and successful translation into clinical practice. Here are some considerations to take into account:

- *Selection of nanocarrier materials*: The choice of nanocarrier materials should be guided by factors such as biocompatibility, stability, and controlled release properties. Biocompatible materials, such as lipids, polymers, or inorganic materials, should be selected to minimize potential toxicity or adverse reactions when in contact with the wound. The materials should also be stable under physiological conditions to ensure the integrity and controlled release of phytoherbal constituents (Mishra et al., 2022).

- *Phyto herbal compound selection*: Careful consideration should be given to selecting phytoherbal compounds based on their wound healing properties, stability, and compatibility with the nanocarrier system. The phytochemicals should possess therapeutic activities relevant to wound healing, such as anti-inflammatory, antimicrobial, antioxidant, or regenerative properties. Additionally, their stability and compatibility with the nanocarrier system should be evaluated to ensure their efficacy is maintained throughout the synthesis, storage, and application processes.
- *Synthesis methods*: Various synthesis methods can be employed to fabricate nanophytoherbal systems, including emulsion techniques, nanoprecipitation, or electrospinning. The choice of synthesis method should be based on factors such as scalability, reproducibility, and the desired characteristics of the nanophytoherbal system (Maheshwari et al., 2021). Optimization of the synthesis parameters, such as solvent choice, surfactant concentration, and processing conditions, is essential to achieve the desired physicochemical properties, drug loading efficiency, and controlled release profiles.
- *Characterization techniques*: Thorough characterization of nanophytoherbal systems is necessary to understand their physicochemical properties and ensure their quality and consistency. Characterization techniques can provide information about particle size, morphology, drug loading, stability, and release kinetics. These techniques facilitate the assessment of critical parameters that affect the performance and therapeutic efficacy of the nanophytoherbal system (Lim et al., 2022).
- *Stability and storage considerations*: Stability studies should be conducted to evaluate the physical and chemical stability of the nanophytoherbal system over time and under different storage conditions. Factors such as temperature, humidity, and exposure to light should be considered. Stability testing can include assessments of drug content, particle size distribution, drug release profile, and physical integrity. Understanding the stability of the nanophytoherbal system is essential to ensure its long-term storage and effectiveness.
- *Biocompatibility and safety evaluation*: Preclinical evaluation of the nanophytoherbal system should include biocompatibility and safety assessments. These evaluations may involve *in vitro* studies using cell cultures to assess cytotoxicity, cell viability, and inflammatory responses. Animal studies can also be conducted to evaluate the systemic and local toxicity, tissue compatibility, and immune response to the nanophytoherbal system (Pandey et al., 2023).
- *In vitro and in vivo efficacy studies:* The efficacy of the nanophytoherbal system should be evaluated through *in vitro* and *in vivo* studies. The release kinetics, antimicrobial activity, anti-inflammatory effects, and cellular responses of the nanophytoherbal system can be assessed through *in vitro* studies. *In vivo* studies, using appropriate animal models, can provide insights into wound healing outcomes, including wound closure rates, tissue regeneration, inflammation reduction, and scar formation. These studies help validate the therapeutic efficacy of the nanophytoherbal system in a relevant biological context.

Therapeutic Efficacy: Pre-Clinical and Clinical Perspectives

Nanophytoherbal refers to the application of nanotechnology in combination with phytoherbal compounds for therapeutic purposes. In the context of wound care therapy, nanophytoherbal formulations enhance the efficacy of traditional herbal remedies.

Pre-Clinical Perspectives

Pre-clinical studies involve laboratory experiments conducted on cell cultures, animal models, and occasionally ex vivo tissue samples. For nanophytoherbal wound care therapy, pre-clinical research focuses on evaluating the therapeutic efficacy of these formulations. Key perspectives include:

- *Enhanced wound healing*: Nanophytoherbal formulations may exhibit antibacterial properties, accelerate the migration and proliferation of skin cells, and promote the production of extracellular matrix components such as collagen. Pre-clinical studies aim to assess these effects using *in vitro* and animal models.
- *Controlled drug delivery*: Nanotechnology facilitates the development of targeted delivery systems. By encapsulating phytoherbal compounds within nanoparticles, controlled release kinetics can be achieved, ensuring sustained therapeutic effects at the wound site. Pre-clinical studies explore the release profiles, stability, and bioavailability of these formulations.
- *Anti-inflammatory and antioxidant effects*: Many herbal compounds possess anti-inflammatory and antioxidant properties, both of which are crucial for wound healing. Nanophytoherbal formulations may enhance these effects by improving the bioavailability and cellular uptake of phytoherbal compounds. Pre-clinical research investigates the modulation of inflammatory responses and oxidative stress markers in wound models (Khogta et al., 2020).

Clinical Perspectives

Clinical studies involve human subjects and are conducted to evaluate the safety and efficacy of nanophytoherbal wound care therapies. These studies typically progress through various phases, including Phase I (safety), Phase II (efficacy), and Phase III (large-scale efficacy and side effect monitoring). Key clinical perspectives include:

- *Wound Closure and Healing*: Clinical trials assess wound closure rates, reduction in wound size, and overall healing of patients treated with nanophytoherbal formulations. Comparative studies against standard wound care approaches may be conducted to determine the therapeutic superiority of nanophytoherbal therapy (Dewi et al., 2022).
- *Safety and Tolerability:* Evaluating the safety profile and tolerability of nanophytoherbal formulations is essential. Clinical trials monitor adverse events, assess local and systemic toxicity, and determine the optimal dosage regimen. These studies provide insights into potential side effects or risks associated with the therapy.
- *Patient Satisfaction and Quality of Life*: In addition to assessing wound healing efficacy, clinical studies consider patient-reported outcomes, such as pain relief, improvement in mobility, and overall quality of life. Patient satisfaction surveys and

quality-of-life assessments help gauge the holistic impact of nanophytoherbal wound care therapy.

In summary, both pre-clinical and clinical perspectives are vital in evaluating the therapeutic efficacy of nanophytoherbal wound care therapy. Pre-clinical studies provide insights into mechanisms of action, while clinical studies assess safety, efficacy, and patient-centered outcomes. Together, these perspectives contribute to establishing the therapeutic potential of nanophytoherbal formulations in wound care.

Safety Considerations and Challenges

The use of nanophytoherbal formulations for wound care therapy introduces specific safety considerations and challenges that must be addressed. Here are some critical points to consider:

- *Nanomaterial Toxicity*: Nanoparticles utilized in nanophytoherbal formulations may possess unique physicochemical properties that influence their toxicity profiles. It is essential to thoroughly investigate the potential toxicity of these nanoparticles, assessing their effects on cellular function, tissue compatibility, and systemic distribution. Pre-clinical studies should evaluate the long-term effects and potential accumulation of nanoparticles within the body.
- *Drug-Drug Interactions*: Nanophytoherbal formulations often contain multiple active components from herbal extracts along with nanoparticles. It is vital to examine the interactions between these components and traditional drugs to ensure there are no adverse effects or compromised therapeutic outcomes. Drug-drug interaction studies should be conducted to identify any potential interactions that could affect the safety or efficacy of the therapy.
- *Allergic Reactions*: Both phytoherbal compounds and nanoparticles have the potential to elicit allergic reactions in susceptible individuals. Identifying and assessing potential allergens present in nanophytoherbal formulations is crucial. Clinical trials should include thorough screening for allergies and monitor for any signs of allergic reactions during therapy (Boomi et al., 2020).
- *Skin Irritation and Sensitization*: Some nanoparticles or phytoherbal compounds may cause skin irritation or sensitization, particularly when applied topically. Evaluating the irritant potential of nanophytoherbal formulations using appropriate pre-clinical models is essential. Clinical trials should include careful monitoring of skin reactions and assessments of local tolerance.
- *Regulatory Considerations*: The application of nanophytoherbal formulations in wound care therapy may require specific regulatory approvals. Regulatory agencies often have specific guidelines and requirements for the safety assessment of nanomaterials and herbal products. Compliance with these regulatory standards is necessary to ensure the safe and ethical use of nanophytoherbal therapies in clinical practice (Singh et al., 2019).
- *Manufacturing Consistency and Quality Control*: To ensure safety and efficacy, nanophytoherbal formulations must be produced consistently. Manufacturing

processes should be meticulously controlled to minimize batch-to-batch variations. Implementing quality control measures to assess the stability, purity, and uniformity of these formulations is critical.

- *Ethical Considerations*: Ethical considerations must be addressed in the development and use of nanophytoherbal wound care therapies. This includes obtaining informed consent from study participants, ensuring transparency in reporting potential risks and benefits, and adhering to ethical guidelines governing research involving human subjects.

Future Prospects and Emerging Trends

The field of nanophytoherbal wound care therapy holds significant promise for the future, with emerging trends and advancements poised to enhance its efficacy and applicability. Here are some key prospects and trends, along with illustrative examples:

- *Targeted delivery systems*: By incorporating targeting ligands or stimuli-responsive components, researchers aim to deliver therapeutically active agents directly to the wound site. This approach can improve treatment efficacy while minimizing off-target effects. For example, nanoparticles functionalized with specific peptides or antibodies can selectively bind to receptors that are overexpressed in wound tissues, enabling site-specific delivery of therapeutic agents.
- *Combination therapies*: Combining nanophytoherbal formulations with other therapeutic modalities is an emerging trend in wound care. For instance, the incorporation of growth factors or antimicrobial agents into nanophytoherbal formulations can create synergistic effects that enhance wound healing. By integrating different therapeutic agents, researchers can address multiple aspects of wound healing, including inflammation, infection, and tissue regeneration, simultaneously.
- *Smart dressings and bandages*: The development of intelligent dressings and bandages represents another significant trend. These advanced wound dressings incorporate nanophytoherbal formulations alongside materials that offer functionalities such as sensing, controlled drug release, and moisture management. Smart dressings can provide real-time monitoring of wound parameters, allow for controlled delivery of therapeutic agents, and create an optimal environment for wound healing.
- *Bioactive scaffolds*: Integrating nanophytoherbal formulations into bioactive scaffolds can create three-dimensional structures that mimic the extracellular matrix. These scaffolds provide mechanical support, enhance cell adhesion and migration, and facilitate tissue regeneration. By combining nanophytoherbal formulations with scaffold technologies, researchers aim to develop advanced wound healing solutions that possess enhanced regenerative potential.
- *Personalized medicine approaches*: Personalized medicine is an emerging trend across various therapeutic areas, including wound care. By considering individual patient characteristics, such as genetic variations and wound-specific factors, researchers can tailor nanophytoherbal therapies to optimize treatment outcomes. Personalized

approaches may involve the use of patient-derived cells, genetic profiling, and individualized dosage regimens.

- *Advanced characterization techniques*: The development of sophisticated characterization techniques enables a deeper understanding of nanophytoherbal formulations and their interactions with wound tissues. Techniques such as high-resolution imaging, spectroscopy, and microfluidics provide valuable insights into the behavior of nanoparticles, release kinetics, and cellular responses. These techniques play a crucial role in the design and optimization of nanophytoherbal formulations for wound care therapy.

Examples of future prospects and emerging trends can be observed in research exploring the integration of nanophytoherbal formulations with stem cells, phototherapy, 3D printing, and bioengineering approaches. These advancements have the potential to revolutionize wound care by offering safer, more effective, and personalized treatment options.

Conclusion

The application of nanophytoherbal formulations for wound care therapy holds significant promise for improving wound treatment outcomes. By integrating nanotechnology with herbal medicine, these formulations offer unique advantages. Pre-clinical studies have demonstrated their efficacy in promoting wound closure, reducing inflammation, enhancing tissue regeneration, and combating infections. However, it is essential to address the safety considerations and challenges associated with nanophytoherbal therapies. Key aspects, including toxicity assessments, drug-drug interactions, allergic reactions, skin sensitization, and adherence to regulatory standards, must be thoroughly evaluated and monitored. Additionally, developing consistent manufacturing processes, implementing robust quality control measures, and considering ethical implications are vital for successfully translating nanophytoherbal therapies into clinical practice. Future prospects and emerging trends, such as targeted delivery systems, combination therapies, smart dressings, bioactive scaffolds, personalized medicine approaches, and advanced characterization techniques, further enhance the potential of nanophytoherbal wound care therapy. These advancements pave the way for safer, more effective, and personalized treatments that can revolutionize wound care management. Overall, the application of nanophytoherbal formulations in wound care therapy represents a promising avenue for improving healing outcomes. Continued research, robust clinical trials, interdisciplinary collaborations, and advancements in nanotechnology will be crucial in harnessing the full potential of nanophytoherbal therapies, ultimately benefiting patients with innovative and effective solutions for wound care management.

References

Amjad, S., Jafri, A., Sharma, A. K., & Serajuddin, M. (2019). A novel strategy of nanotized herbal drugs and their delivery in the treatment of diabetes: Present status and future prospects. *Journal of Herbal Medicine*, *17–18*, 100279.

Boomi, P., Ganesan, R., Prabu Poorani, G., Jegatheeswaran, S., Balakumar, C., Gurumallesh Prabu, H., Anand, K., Marimuthu Prabhu, N., Jeyakanthan, J., & Saravanan, M. (2020). Phyto-Engineered Gold Nanoparticles (AuNPs) with Potential Antibacterial, Antioxidant, and Wound Healing Activities Under *in vitro* and *in vivo* Conditions. *International Journal of Nanomedicine*, *15*, 7553–7568.

Dewi, M. K., Chaerunisaa, A. Y., Muhaimin, M., & Joni, I. M. (2022). Improved Activity of Herbal Medicines through Nanotechnology. *Nanomaterials*, *12*(22), 4073.

Ganesan, P., & Choi, D. K. (2016). Current application of phytocompound-based nanocosmeceuticals for beauty and skin therapy. *International Journal of Nanomedicine*, 1987, 11, 1987–2007.

Gorain, B., Pandey, M., Leng, N. H., Yan, C. W., Nie, K. W., Kaur, S. J., Marshall, V., Sisinthy, S. P., Panneerselvam, J., Molugulu, N., Kesharwani, P., & Choudhury, H. (2022a). Advanced drug delivery systems containing herbal components for wound healing. *International Journal of Pharmaceutics*, *617*, 121617.

Gorain, B., Pandey, M., Leng, N. H., Yan, C. W., Nie, K. W., Kaur, S. J., Marshall, V., Sisinthy, S. P., Panneerselvam, J., Molugulu, N., Kesharwani, P., & Choudhury, H. (2022b). Advanced drug delivery systems containing herbal components for wound healing. *International Journal of Pharmaceutics*, *617*, 121617.

Hajialyani, M., Tewari, D., Sobarzo-Sánchez, E., Nabavi, S. M., Farzaei, M. H., & Abdollahi, M. (2018). Natural product-based nanomedicines for wound healing purposes: therapeutic targets and drug delivery systems. *International Journal of Nanomedicine*, *Volume 13*, 5023–5043.

Johnson, T., Gómez, B., McIntyre, M., Dubick, M., Christy, R., Nicholson, S., & Burmeister, D. (2018). The Cutaneous Microbiome and Wounds: New Molecular Targets to Promote Wound Healing. *International Journal of Molecular Sciences*, *19*(9), 2699.

Khogta, S., Patel, J., Barve, K., & Londhe, V. (2020). Herbal nano-formulations for topical delivery. *Journal of Herbal Medicine*, *20*, 100300.

Kumar, M., Keshwania, P., Chopra, S., Mahmood, S., & Bhatia, A. (2023). Correction: Therapeutic Potential of Nanocarrier-Mediated Delivery of Phytoconstituents for Wound Healing: Their Current Status and Future Perspective. *AAPS PharmSciTech*, *24*(7), 206.

Lim, C. L., Raju, C. S., Mahboob, T., Kayesth, S., Gupta, K. K., Jain, G. K., Dhobi, M., Nawaz, M., Wilairatana, P., de Lourdes Pereira, M., Patra, J. K., Paul, A. K., Rahmatullah, M., & Nissapatorn, V. (2022). Precision and Advanced Nano-Phytopharmaceuticals for Therapeutic Applications. *Nanomaterials*, *12*(2), 238.

Maheshwari, S., Tiwari, R. K., & Singh, L. (2021). Green expertise: Synthesis of Silver nanoparticles for wound healing application an overview. *Research Journal of Pharmacy and Technology*, *14*(2), 1149–1154.

Mirrezaei, N., Yazdian-Robati, R., Oroojalian, F., Sahebkar, A., & Hashemi, M. (2020a). Recent Developments in Nano-Drug Delivery Systems Loaded by Phytochemicals for Wound Healing. *Mini-Reviews in Medicinal Chemistry*, *20*(18), 1867–1878.

Mirrezaei, N., Yazdian-Robati, R., Oroojalian, F., Sahebkar, A., & Hashemi, M. (2020b). Recent Developments in Nano-Drug Delivery Systems Loaded by Phytochemicals for Wound Healing. *Mini-Reviews in Medicinal Chemistry*, *20*(18), 1867–1878.

Mishra, Y., Amin, H. I. M., Mishra, V., Vyas, M., Prabhakar, P. K., Gupta, M., Kanday, R., Sudhakar, K., Saini, S., Hromić-Jahjefendić, A., Aljabali, A. A. A., El-Tanani, M., Serrano-Aroca, Ã., Bakshi, H., & Tambuwala, M. M. (2022). Application of nanotechnology to herbal antioxidants as improved phytomedicine: An expanding horizon. *Biomedicine & Pharmacotherapy*, *153*, 113413.

Monika, P., & Chandraprabha, M. N. (2020). *Phytonanotechnology for Enhanced Wound Healing Activity* (pp. 111–128).

Nagoba, B., & Davane, M. (2019). Studies on wound healing potential of topical herbal formulations- do we need to strengthen study protocol? *Journal of Ayurveda and Integrative Medicine*, *10*(4), 316–318.

Oliveira da Silva, L., Assunção Ferreira, M. R., & Lira Soares, L. A. (2023). Nanotechnology Formulations Designed with Herbal Extracts and Their Therapeutic Applications – A Review. *Chemistry & Biodiversity*, *20*(8), e202201241.

Ovais, M., Ahmad, I., Khalil, A. T., Mukherjee, S., Javed, R., Ayaz, M., Raza, A., & Shinwari, Z. K. (2018). Wound healing applications of biogenic colloidal silver and gold nanoparticles: recent trends and future prospects. *Applied Microbiology and Biotechnology*, *102*(10), 4305–4318.

Pandey, V., Barve, K., & Londhe, V. (2023). Synthesis and characterization of nanoherbal formulations for topical wound healing applications. In *Nanotechnology in Herbal Medicine* (pp. 255–278). Elsevier.

Pereira, R. F., & Bártolo, P. J. (2016). Traditional Therapies for Skin Wound Healing. *Advances in Wound Care*, *5*(5), 208–229.

Qadir, A., Jahan, S., Aqil, M., Warsi, M. H., Alhakamy, N. A., Alfaleh, M. A., Khan, N., & Ali, A. (2021a). Phytochemical-Based Nano-Pharmacotherapeutics for Management of Burn Wound Healing. *Gels*, *7*(4), 209.

Qadir, A., Jahan, S., Aqil, M., Warsi, M. H., Alhakamy, N. A., Alfaleh, M. A., Khan, N., & Ali, A. (2021b). Phytochemical-Based Nano-Pharmacotherapeutics for Management of Burn Wound Healing. *Gels*, *7*(4), 209.

Safta, D. A., Bogdan, C., & Moldovan, M. L. (2022). Vesicular Nanocarriers for Phytocompounds in Wound Care: Preparation and Characterization. *Pharmaceutics*, *14*(5), 991.

Siafaka, P. I., Zisi, A. P., Exindari, M. K., Karantas, I. D., & Bikiaris, D. N. (2016). Porous dressings of modified chitosan with poly(2-hydroxyethyl acrylate) for topical wound delivery of levofloxacin. *Carbohydrate Polymers*, *143*, 90–99.

Singh Bakshi, I., Chopra, H., Sharma, M., Kaushik, D., Pahwa, R., & Haryanto. (2022). Herbal bioactives for wound healing application. In *Herbal Bioactive-Based Drug Delivery Systems* (pp. 259–282). Elsevier.

Singh, S., Jangde, R., & Daharwal, S. J. (2019). An Updated Review on Herbal Drug in Wound Healing. *Research Journal of Pharmacy and Technology*, *12*(6), 3089.

Solati, K., Karimi, M., Rafieian-Kopaei, M., Abbasi, N., Abbaszadeh, S., & Bahmani, M. (2021). Phytotherapy for Wound Healing: The Most Important Herbal Plants in Wound Healing Based on Iranian Ethnobotanical Documents. *Mini-Reviews in Medicinal Chemistry*, *21*(4), 500–519.

Xu, Z., Dong, M., Yin, S., Dong, J., Zhang, M., Tian, R., Min, W., Zeng, L., Qiao, H., & Chen, J. (2023). Why traditional herbal medicine promotes wound healing: Research from immune response, wound microbiome to controlled delivery. *Advanced Drug Delivery Reviews*, *195*, 114764.

Chapter 13

Applications of Nanophytoherbals in Skin Care Therapy

Shiwali Sharma[1]
Narinderpal Kaur[1,*]
Parul Sood[1]
Gagandeep Kaur[1]
and Pallavi Bassi[2]
[1]Chitkara University School of Pharmacy, Chitkara University, Himachal Pradesh, India
[2]Chitkara College of Pharmacy, Chitkara University, Punjab, India

Abstract

Phytocompounds are chemical compounds derived from plants and their metabolism. In modern medicine, these compounds play a vital role in the development of numerous medications. The utilization and exploration of phytocompounds contribute significantly to traditional medicine practices. In the cosmeceutical sector, however, several challenges are associated with the use of phyto-based products, including poor penetration, instability of compounds, and the need for enhanced and sustained delivery for beauty-based skin therapies. Nanosized delivery technologies are currently being employed to address these drawbacks. These technologies aim to overcome the limitations of traditional formulations by facilitating the sustained release of bioactive compounds derived from plants in cosmeceutical products. By minimizing particle size and adopting advanced delivery systems, nanotechnology enhances the penetration of bioactive compounds into the skin, potentially improving the efficacy of cosmeceutical formulations for beauty and skincare. This chapter broadly explores the applications of nanophytocompounds in various cosmeceutical products, highlighting the incorporation of nanodelivery technologies for the effective delivery of these phytocompounds in skin therapy.

Keywords: nanodelivery technologies, nanophyto-herbals, nanophytocompound, skincare, nanotherapy, phytoconstituents, health, research, age

---

* Corresponding Author's Email: narinderpal.kaur@chitkarauniversity.edu.in.

In: Phyto-Nanomedicine
Editors: Hitesh Chopra, Vinod Kumar Gauttam, Ajmer Singh Grewal et al.
ISBN: 979-8-89530-317-7

Introduction

Recently, many cosmeceutical products have been introduced to the market. The term "cosmeceuticals" was coined by Albert Kligman to describe cosmetics that incorporate pharmaceutical compounds in topical formulations that influence the skin's biological functions (Rathod et al., 2020). In other words, cosmeceuticals represent the amalgamation of pharmaceuticals and cosmetics (Goyal et al., 2022). The exploration of cosmeceuticals is rapidly expanding within the personal care industry, encompassing a wide range of products from facial treatments to skin and body care. For centuries, bioactive compounds derived from plants have been integrated into cosmeceutical formulations, resulting in a diverse array of treatments aimed at enhancing beauty across various applications, including facial, skin, lip, nail, and hair care. These compounds provide beneficial effects for numerous concerns such as hair loss, inflammation, psoriasis, photo-aging, and the harmful effects of ultraviolet (UV) rays (Hwang et al., 2013). However, commercially available phyto-based cosmeceuticals remain limited in number, including products like acne lotions containing vitamin E, tea extract in nano-shampoos, and anti-aging skincare kits, as well as aloe vera and vitamin E in UV-protecting moisturizers.

Nanocosmeceuticals Derived from Phytoconstituents for Skin Therapy

Nanoantiaging

Aging is a continuous progression from birth to death, commencing at conception and concluding at the end of life. Products available in the market aim to moisturize, firm, and brighten the skin, providing advanced skincare solutions. Lohani et al. (2014) examined nanoproducts designed to enhance beauty, including formulations such as Skin Caviar Ampoules, Hydra Zen Cream, and Revitalift. These products incorporate phytocompounds delivered through various nanotechnology methods. They are specifically formulated to address skin aging factors associated with oxidative stress, potentially preventing premature aging. The antioxidant properties of compounds like resveratrol and curcumin have been shown to delay the effects of aging while enhancing the delivery of phytocompounds for treating various skin conditions (Friedrich et al., 2015).

Nanomoisturizer

Maintaining a perfectly functioning stratum corneum is essential for healthy skin. The use of moisturizers helps prevent skin dehydration while enhancing its beauty and flexibility by retaining moisture (Shim et al., 2016). Formulations such as nanoemulsions, nanoliposomes, and solid lipid nanocarriers can significantly improve skin appearance. Various ongoing studies are exploring nanoemulsions containing vegetable oils for their potential application as moisturizing agents in skincare products. Looking ahead, vegetable oils are poised to become significant substitutes for traditional moisturizers, providing effective hydration for managing conditions associated with dry skin (Bernardi et al., 2011).

Nanoskin Cleanser

Cleansers and soaps often contain surfactants that can disrupt the integrity of the hydrolipidic film, leading to lipid-depleted areas on the epidermis's surface. The importance of the skin barrier function is widely recognized as crucial for maintaining skin hydration and homeostasis. Ongoing research is exploring various phyto-based nano-compounds to enhance skin cleansing efficacy. The effectiveness of compounds containing phyto-constituents in cleansing the skin and their correlation with skin conditions like acne has been extensively investigated (Yang et al., 2009). For example, nanosized liposomal lauric acid, measuring approximately 113 nm, demonstrated enhanced antimicrobial properties against acne. Additionally, one study utilizing niosomes, which combined curcumin and lauric acid, showed increased antimicrobial effectiveness in combating skin infections associated with acne (Pornpattananangkul et al., 2013).

Nanosunscreens

Sunscreens are topical cosmetic products classified as cosmeceuticals, designed to shield the skin from UV exposure. The primary aim of these topical sunscreens is to protect the skin from the harmful effects of sunlight, whether by absorbing or reflecting radiation. However, they often do not provide complete sun protection for sensitive areas such as the eyes and lips. A recent study by Bulla et al. investigated the use of bioactive and phyto-based compounds derived from Schinus terebinthifolius Raddi in sunscreens. The study revealed that these compounds possess antioxidant properties and sun-blocking activities (Bulla et al., 2015). The development of poly(lactic-co-glycolic) acid nanoparticles, measuring 90–100 nm, encapsulating phytoflavonoids, demonstrated improved sunscreen efficacy along with enhanced antioxidant effects.

Nanolip Care

A rapidly expanding sector in nanotechnology is nano-lip care cosmetics. Currently, a variety of nanoscale synthetic and metal particles are employed for efficient lip protection and color enhancement. These products provide longer-lasting effects and ensure uniform distribution across the lips (Lohani et al., 2014). Lip care products containing phyto-constituents are available at both macro and micro levels. Substances such as coconut oil, curcumin, and other bioactive compounds are recognized for their enhanced lubricating properties (Kamairudin et al., 2014). Recently, pigments derived from plant betalains, extracted from indole, have been introduced as innovative dietary colorants. The extraction and encapsulation of these compounds not only enhance storage stability but also expand their utility. For example, Bixa orellana is used as a colorant in lip jelly, offering superior organoleptic properties for lipsticks. Similarly, propolis is utilized in novel lipstick formulations. Despite these advancements, the application of nanotechnology in the development of phyto-based lipsticks remains in its early stages (Khan, 2015).

Nano-Delivery System in Cosmeceuticals for Healthcare and Beauty

The demand for nano-sized ingredients, particularly bioactive and phyto-based compounds, has increased in cosmeceuticals due to the limitations of synthetic bioactive ingredients. These compounds can be effectively administered via nano delivery systems (Ahmad et al., 2014). Nanodelivery systems facilitate the penetration of phyto-bioactive compounds and improve their solubility. Appropriate nanodelivery techniques enhance the penetration of these active phyto-based ingredients, thereby increasing the effectiveness of cosmeceuticals (Islamian and Mehrali, 2015). The efficacy of these phyto-based compounds within nanotechnology systems depends on factors such as the bioactive ingredient's hydrophilicity or hydrophobicity, formulation type (emulsion or gel), degradability, toxicity, and size. This section explores various nanotechnology delivery systems that are useful in developing phyto-bioactive compound-based nano-cosmeceuticals (Scalia et al., 2013).

Solid Lipid Nanoparticles

Cosmeceutical companies utilize this technology for both beauty and therapeutic purposes. Products developed using this method exhibit enhanced stability, scalability, and storage compared to traditional formulations. For instance, curcumin-loaded solid lipid nanoparticles measuring 210 nm demonstrated improved anti-inflammatory activity in hydrogels designed for porcine skin treatment. However, certain solid lipid nanoparticles combined with quercetin exhibited larger particle sizes, averaging 574 nm (Zamarioli et al., 2015). Previous investigations have indicated that solid lipid nanoparticles incorporating plant-based bioactive ingredients have shown promising effects in enhancing both efficacy and health benefits.

Lipoid Incorporated Nano-Capsules

Lipoid-incorporated nanocapsules exhibit significant potential in the cosmeceutical and healthcare sectors (Weiss-Angeli et al., 2012). These delivery systems have demonstrated enhanced efficacy in delivering bioactive, plant-based ingredients for oral therapy, fostering advancements in cosmeceutical development through topical applications. While synthetic compounds widely utilize this technique, the application of phytocompounds in cosmeceuticals remains limited. Recent studies have shown that lipid-core nanocapsules encapsulating resveratrol and curcumin, measuring 201 nm, result in increased polyphenol retention in the skin, thereby enhancing skin protection (Friedrich et al., 2015). Additionally, lipid-derived nanocapsules containing resveratrol, prepared at 207 nm, have been found to promote skin protection and enhance the bioactivity of these compounds under UV radiation (Detoni et al., 2012). Furthermore, chitosan hydrogels combined with nanocapsules carrying capsaicinoids improve skin protection by regulating the release of these active compounds (Contri et al., 2014).

Nanophytosomes

Phytosomes represent an innovative technology, particularly for enhancing the bioavailability of plant polyphenolics in skincare and various therapeutic applications (Allam et al., 2015). This technique offers significant advantages through the chemical bonding that occurs between lipid bilayers and polyphenolics, ensuring increased physical stability and prolonged effectiveness of these compounds (Shakeri & Sahebkar, 2015). Recent studies utilizing extracts from Citrus aurantium and Glycyrrhiza glabra in phytosomes have demonstrated improvements in skin aging by boosting bioavailability. Additionally, gold nanoparticles combined with quercetin-rich extracts, measuring 100 nm, have been shown to enhance efficacy.

Fullerene

The presence of a spherical π-electron moiety in materials enhances intermolecular interactions. Buckminsterfullerene, or C60, is a notable example of a spherical π-electron carbon cluster (Dombi et al., 2015). However, C60 has limited solubility in common solvents, necessitating its functionalization for integration into various solid forms for material science applications. Fullerene-based photodynamic therapy has been utilized for the treatment of skin-related diseases, often in combination with bioactive compounds like curcumin (Zhang et al., 2015). Future research may advance cosmeceutical therapies, improving protective mechanisms and enhancing efficacy through synergistic effects.

Carbon Nanotubes

Carbon nanotubes are cylindrical structures formed by rolling up graphene sheets, typically with a diameter of around one nanometer. Recent research worldwide has unveiled the remarkable electrical and mechanical properties of these molecular-scale wires. Advances in nanotube growth have significantly contributed to both the fundamental understanding and practical applications of nanotubes (Ilbasmis-Tamerc et al., 2012). Current studies have explored the conjugation of single-walled carbon nanotubes with curcumin to enhance its delivery system (Li et al., 2014). Additionally, the incorporation of hyaluronic acid into carbon nanotubes for drug delivery has been examined, highlighting the need for further evaluation of their biosafety in clinical trials (Tripodo et al., 2015). However, there remains a gap in research regarding the use of plant-based bioactive compounds in carbon nanotubes within the context of cosmeceuticals and skin care.

Nanoscale Phytoconstituents in Cosmeceuticals and Their Role in Skin Therapy

Nanoscopic phytoconstituents are increasingly gaining popularity as essential components in cosmeceuticals for addressing skin-related conditions such as anti-aging and UV protection, enhancing both beauty and therapeutic benefits. The enhanced effects of bioactive compounds as skin protectors can be attributed to their polyphenol content and reduced particle size

(Suwannateep et al., 2013). To improve skin protection and elevate bioavailability, refining bioactive compounds in conjunction with nanodelivery technologies is an effective strategy (Detoni et al., 2012). For instance, the encapsulation of quercetin within a solid lipid nanoparticle system demonstrated improved skin retention and enhanced antioxidant activity (Han et al., 2014). Additionally, co-encapsulating curcumin and resveratrol within lipoid core nanocapsules significantly increased the availability of resveratrol to the skin (Friedrich et al., 2015). Numerous other phytobioactive compounds have also been effectively encapsulated in various nanodelivery systems to amplify beauty and therapeutic applications. Table 1 provides a list of some plant-based nanocompounds and their roles in skin and beauty care.

Table 1. Provides a list of some nano plant-based compounds and their roles in skin and beauty care

Phytocompounds	Nanodelivery Methods	Size (nm)	Applications	References
Rice bran oil	Nanoemulsion	69	Moisturizers Antiaging Skin care	Bernardi et al., 2011
Lavender extract	Polymeric poly(lactic-co-glycolic) acid (PLGA) nanoparticle	301-303	Antiaging	Pereira et al., 2015
Rosemary extract	Solid lipid nanocarriers Nanostructured lipid carriers	57 and 68	Antioxidant (skin) & Antioxidant	Lacatusu et al., 2010
Lutein	Nanostructured lipid carriers and nanoemulsion	150-350	Skin care	Mitri et al., 2011
Hinokitiol	Poly(epsilon-caprolacton) nanocapsules	223	Hair care	Hwang & Kim, 2013
Curcumin	Nanoencapsulation	190 and 276	Skin care	Suwannateep et al., 2012
Tocopherol	Nanostructured lipid carriers and nanoemulsion	67 and 576	Skin care	Abla & Banga, 2014
Resveratrol	Solid lipid nanoparticles versus nanostructured lipid carriers	287.2 and 110.5	Skin care	Gokce et al., 2012
Lycopene	Transfersomes Ethosomes	124 154	Skin care	Ascenso et al., 2015

Nanocurcumin

Chemically, curcumin is a polyphenol, specifically a diarylheptanoid, that belongs to the curcuminoid group, which are the phenolic pigments responsible for the yellow color of turmeric (Sindhu et al., 2021). It plays a regulatory role in intracellular signaling pathways governing the invasion, inflammation, apoptosis, and progression of cancerous cells. The unique intrinsic features of curcumin molecules enable them to target intracellular enzymes, DNA, and RNA. Numerous studies have explored the physical and chemical characteristics as well as the therapeutic potential of curcumin for various ailments, including Alzheimer's disease, cancer, diabetes, cardiovascular diseases, inflammatory bowel disease, wound healing, and rheumatoid arthritis. However, the bioavailability of curcumin, particularly when taken orally, is notably low, posing limitations to its therapeutic utilization (Oskuee et al., 2016). Nanotechnology, a revolutionary scientific field, has made significant advancements since its inception, particularly in agriculture and food production systems. The exploration of unique material characteristics at the nanoscale (10^-9 m) has resulted in widespread applications across various industries. The evolution of nanotechnology can be traced through different polymer generations. The first generation, prevalent between 2000 and 2005, included ceramics and coatings. The second generation, spanning from 2005 to 2010, featured active nanostructures with applications in slow-releasing medicines. The third generation, from 2010 onwards, involved nanostructures, such as evolutionary and robotic systems, forming an ensemble with similar performance but partial intelligence. Notably, the fourth generation focuses on molecular nanosystems, consisting of atomic design molecular devices with novel functions, with nanomems showing promise for the future of nanosystems. The construction of nano devices can be achieved through top-down (etching/molding) or bottom-up (atom/molecule assembly) processes (Tavano et al., 2014).

Nano *Aloe vera*

Aloe vera is rich in a variety of bioactive constituents, including carbohydrates, proteins, vitamins, and minerals, extracted from the inner parts of its leaves. These components find considerable applications in both skincare and medicine (Manca et al., 2014). Aloe vera gel significantly boosts moisturizing activity and exhibits anti-aging effects by promoting the synthesis of fibers such as elastin and collagen. Additionally, it aids in wound healing (Tabandeh et al., 2014). The elevated levels of moisture, bioactive compounds, and minerals in Aloe vera gel enhance its moisturizing effects and provide protection for the skin. Consequently, Aloe vera is frequently used in beautifying products, including gels, lotions, and creams (Yamauchi et al., 2015). Furthermore, liposomes have demonstrated improved collagen synthesis and enhanced growth of skin cell lines, suggesting their potential use in improving the quality of skincare products. Researchers have patented technologies related to nanoemulsions incorporating nanosized extracts of Aloe vera. These resultant products exhibit rejuvenating effects on the skin and show protective benefits against wrinkles. Moreover, co-encapsulation of curcumin with Aloe vera has been shown to enhance the bioavailability of phyto-compounds to the skin, providing an effective antioxidant protection system (Kitture et al., 2015). Previous studies indicate that the nano-compounds derived from Aloe vera significantly enhance its efficacy in beauty applications.

Nano-Vitamin C

Vitamin C, which is predominantly found in plants, plays a crucial role in healthcare and significantly contributes to skin and beauty care, particularly in collagen synthesis (Crisan et al., 2015). However, vitamin C is prone to degradation when exposed to ultraviolet radiation or harsh environmental conditions, making a consistent supply essential for maintaining skin health and beauty. Nanodelivery techniques provide a solution by sustaining vitamin C supplementation without compromising its therapeutic potential upon application to the skin. Recent research in nanotechnology has explored various approaches for utilizing vitamin C in beauty, skin, and health applications, including solid lipid nanoparticles and nano-structured lipoid carriers. A solid lipid nanoparticle encapsulating vitamin C, with a particle size ranging from 200 to 225 nm, was developed as an effective carrier that protects vitamin C against apoptotic effects (Guney et al., 2014). Another approach involves the use of nano-liposomes containing vitamin C, which were shown to enhance skin permeation with a particle size ranging from 66 to 130 nm. Furthermore, nano-liposomes demonstrated improved stability and increased antioxidant activity compared to conventional liposomes, even after a storage period of 60 days (Yang et al., 2013).

Nano-Vitamin E

Vitamin E, a fat-soluble and heat-stable compound, is widely utilized in various cosmetic formulations due to its skin protective properties, including anti-wrinkle effects, enhanced skin moisturization, and prevention of skin diseases (Korać and Khambholja, 2011). However, many cosmetic preparations contain precursors of the active form of tocopherol, limiting the conversion to its active form within the skin and, consequently, reducing skin protection. Additionally, the natural presence of vitamin E in human skin can be rendered inactive due to the interference of solar radiation. Nanodelivery techniques offer a solution by ensuring adequate delivery, prolonged release, and sustained availability of vitamin E, thereby enhancing its beauty-related benefits. For example, a vitamin E nanoemulsion has been developed that demonstrates improved bioavailability compared to micro-sized emulsions (Kotyla et al., 2008). This innovative approach addresses the challenges associated with vitamin E delivery and contributes to improved beauty outcomes. Furthermore, solid lipid nanoparticles containing vitamin E, with a size of approximately 292 nm, have been developed to enhance skin protection activity (Teo et al., 2010). As nanotechnology continues to evolve, it is expected to optimize vitamin E delivery in cosmetic preparations, leading to improved beauty care and stability.

Nano-Green Tea

Natural extracts of green tea are rich in bioactive compounds such as epicatechin, epigallocatechin, catechin, and epigallocatechin-3-gallate, making them a potent source of antioxidants widely utilized in beauty and skincare management. These compounds, each with unique potential, play crucial roles in the formulation of cosmetic products. The components of green tea contribute to various skincare functions, including anti-aging effects and the prevention of UV-induced photoaging (Ikeda et al., 2013). Nanotechnology enhances the bioavailability of these compounds, expanding the potential of green tea cosmeceuticals. Montenegro et al., (2014) highlighted recent research efforts that focus on utilizing green tea catechins in the preparation of anti-aging creams and as delivery agents for fullerene. Similarly, Fang et al., developed liposomes containing catechins from green tea, with nanoparticle sizes ranging from 130 to 268 nm, which demonstrated improved antioxidant activity in the skin. Another study found that green tea liposomes with a size of 138 nm enhanced catechin delivery via ethanol, facilitating transdermal absorption (Fang et al., 2006). Furthermore, nano-liposomes of green tea polyphenols were formulated using fat globule membranes from milk and soy lipids, aiming to enhance antioxidant activity in cellular models (Gülseren & Corredig, 2013).

Nano-Lycopene

Lycopene, a bioactive and plant-based natural compound, has numerous applications in skincare, including antioxidant and anti-aging activities (Stahl et al., 2012). However, its lipophilic nature and limited penetration through the skin pose challenges for its effective use in skincare products. Recent advancements have focused on the development of lycopene ethosomes and transfersomes with nanoparticle sizes of 153 nm and 124 nm, respectively. These formulations enhance the bioavailability of lycopene to the skin, demonstrating significant potential for antioxidant activity.

Nanotoxicity

The use of nanocosmeceuticals raises concerns about toxicity due to their small size, which facilitates easy penetration through membranes and interactions with proteins and cells. Although several studies indicate that polymers used in cosmetic preparations do not exhibit deleterious effects, and natural products are generally regarded as having fewer side effects, it is crucial to conduct extensive clinical screening before these products are applied. Despite their potential benefits, the widespread use of nanocosmeceuticals may still lead to adverse effects. Therefore, before the commercial progression and development of these products, further clinical research and support are essential to ensure their safety and efficacy.

Conclusion

The increasing demand for the utilization of nano-sized bioactive compounds derived from plants has driven the expansion of nano-cosmeceuticals, particularly for skin care therapies. These therapies encompass various aspects such as moisturization, whitening effects, sunblock, anti-aging, and overall skin health. Researchers are pursuing nanocosmeceuticals as high-demand solutions due to their ability to enhance skin appeal, offering improved retention, stability, and prolonged efficacy. The size of nanosized compounds varies, contributing to their versatility and suitability for diverse skincare applications. Identifying and evaluating bioactive compounds from a wide range of plant species requires a standardized and integrated approach. More research is needed on the targeted release of nanosized compounds to understand the mechanisms behind safe and effective formulations. Ongoing exploration in this field is crucial for advancing nanocosmeceutical research, which enhances the therapeutic effects of cosmeceuticals, leading to improved formulations that address various skincare concerns with greater precision and effectiveness.

References

Abla, M. J., & Banga, A. K. (2014). Formulation of tocopherol nanocarriers and *in vitro* delivery into human skin. *International Journal of Cosmetic Science*, 36(3), 239–246.

Ahmad, I., Akhter, S., Ahmad, M. Z., Shamim, M., Rizvi, M. A., Khar, R. K., & Ahmad, F. J. (2014). Collagen loaded nano-sized surfactant based dispersion for topical application: formulation development, characterization and safety study. *Pharmaceutical Development and Technology*, 19(4), 460–467.

Allam, A. N., Komeil, I. A., & Abdallah, O. Y. (2015). Curcumin phytosomal softgel formulation: Development, optimization, and physicochemical characterization. *Acta Pharmaceutica*, 65(3), 285–297.

Ascenso, A., Raposo, S., Batista, C., Cardoso, P., Mendes, T., Praça, F. G., Bentley, M. V., & Simões, S. (2015). Development, characterization, and skin delivery studies of related ultradeformable vesicles: transfersomes, ethosomes, and transethosomes. *International Journal of Nanomedicine*, 10, 5837–5851.

Bernardi, D. S., Pereira, T. A., Maciel, N. R., Bortoloto, J., Viera, G. S., Oliveira, G. C., & Rocha-Filho, P. A. (2011). Formation and stability of oil-in-water nanoemulsions containing rice bran oil: *in vitro* and *in vivo* assessments. *Journal of Nanobiotechnology*, 9, 44.

Bulla, M. K., Hernandes, L., Baesso, M. L., Nogueira, A. C., Bento, A. C., Bortoluzzi, B. B., Serra, L. Z., & Cortez, D. A. (2015). Evaluation of Photoprotective Potential and Percutaneous Penetration by Photoacoustic Spectroscopy of the Schinus terebinthifolius Raddi Extract. *Photochemistry and Photobiology*, 91(3), 558–566.

Chen-yu, G., Chun-fen, Y., Qi-lu, L., Qi, T., Yan-wei, X., Wei-na, L., & Guang-xi, Z. (2012). Development of a quercetin-loaded nanostructured lipid carrier formulation for topical delivery. *International Journal of Pharmaceutics*, 430(1-2), 292–298.

Contri, R. V., Katzer, T., Ourique, A. F., da Silva, A. L., Beck, R. C., Pohlmann, A. R., & Guterres, S. S. (2014). Combined effect of polymeric nanocapsules and chitosan hydrogel on the increase of capsaicinoids adhesion to the skin surface. *Journal of Biomedical Nanotechnology*, 10(5), 820–830.

Crisan, D., Roman, I., Crisan, M., Scharffetter-Kochanek, K., & Badea, R. (2015). The role of vitamin C in pushing back the boundaries of skin aging: An ultrasonographic approach. *Clinical, Cosmetic and Investigational Dermatology*, 8, 463–470.

Detoni, C. B., Souto, G. D., da Silva, A. L., Pohlmann, A. R., & Guterres, S. S. (2012). Photostability and skin penetration of different E-resveratrol-loaded supramolecular structures. *Photochemistry and Photobiology*, 88(4), 913–921.

Dombi, G. W., Purohit, K., Martin, L. M., & Yang, S. C. (2015). Collagen gel formation in the presence of a carbon nanobrush. *Journal of Materials Science: Materials in Medicine*, 26(1), 5356.

Fang, J. Y., Lee, W. R., Shen, S. C., & Huang, Y. L. (2006). Effect of liposome encapsulation of tea catechins on their accumulation in basal cell carcinomas. *Journal of Dermatological Science*, 42(2), 101–109.

Friedrich, R. B., Kann, B., Coradini, K., Offerhaus, H. L., Beck, R. C., & Windbergs, M. (2015). Skin penetration behavior of lipid-core nanocapsules for simultaneous delivery of resveratrol and curcumin. *European Journal of Pharmaceutical Sciences*, 78, 204–213.

Gokce, E. H., Korkmaz, E., Dellera, E., Sandri, G., Bonferoni, M. C., & Ozer, O. (2012). Resveratrol-loaded solid lipid nanoparticles versus nanostructured lipid carriers: Evaluation of antioxidant potential for dermal applications. *International Journal of Nanomedicine*, 7, 1841–1850.

Goyal, A., Sharma, A., Kaur, J., Kumari, S., Garg, M., Sindhu, R. K., Rahman, M. H., Akhtar, M. F., Tagde, P., Najda, A., Banach-Albińska, B., Masternak, K., Alanazi, I. S., Mohamed, H. R. H., El-Kott, A. F., Shah, M., Germoush, M. O., Al-Malky, H. S., Abukhuwayjah, S. H., Altyar, A. E., Bungau, S. G., & Abdel-Daim, M. M. (2022). Bioactive-based cosmeceuticals: An update on emerging trends. *Molecules*, 27(3), 828.

Gülseren, I., & Corredig, M. (2013). Storage stability and physical characteristics of tea-polyphenol-bearing nanoliposomes prepared with milk fat globule membrane phospholipids. *Journal of Agricultural and Food Chemistry*, 61(13), 3242–3251.

Guney, G., Kutlu, H. M., & Genç, L. (2014). Preparation and characterization of ascorbic acid loaded solid lipid nanoparticles and investigation of their apoptotic effects. *Colloids and Surfaces B: Biointerfaces*, 121, 270–280.

Han, S. B., Kwon, S. S., Jeong, Y. M., Yu, E. R., & Park, S. N. (2014). Physical characterization and permeation of solid lipid nanoparticles for transdermal delivery of quercetin. *International Journal of Cosmetic Science*, 36(6), 588–597.

Hwang, B., Noh, E., Kim, J., Kim, J., You, Y., Hwang, J., Kwon, K., & Lee, Y. (2013). Curcumin inhibits UVB-induced matrix metalloproteinase-1/3 expression by suppressing the MAPK-p38/JNK pathways in human dermal fibroblasts. *Experimental Dermatology*, 22(5), 371–374.

Hwang, S. L., & Kim, J. C. (2008). *In vivo* hair growth promotion effects of cosmetic preparations containing hinokitiol-loaded poly(epsilon-caprolactone) nanocapsules. *Journal of Microencapsulation*, 25(5), 351–356.

Ikeda, S., Kanoya, Y., & Nagata, S. (2013). Effects of a foot bath containing green tea polyphenols on interdigital tinea pedis. *Foot*, 23(2–3), 58–62.

Ilbasmis-Tamerc, S., & Degim, I. T. (2012). A feasible way to use carbon nanotubes to deliver drug molecules: Transdermal application. *Expert Opinion on Drug Delivery*, 9(8), 991–999.

Kamairudin, N., Gani, S. S., Masoumi, H. R., & Hashim, P. (2014). Optimization of natural lipstick formulation based on pitaya (Hylocereus polyrhizus) seed oil using D-optimal mixture experimental design. *Molecules*, 19(10), 16672–16683.

Khameneh, B., Halimi, V., Jaafari, M. R., & Golmohammadzadeh, S. (2015). Safranal-loaded solid lipid nanoparticles: Evaluation of sunscreen and moisturizing potential for topical applications. *Iranian Journal of Basic Medical Sciences*, 18(1), 58–63.

Khan, M. I., & Giridhar, P. (2015). Plant betalains: Chemistry and biochemistry. *Phytochemistry*, 117, 267–295.

Kitture, R., Ghosh, S., More, P. A., Date, K., Gaware, S., Datar, S., Chopade, B. A., & Kale, S. N. (2015). Curcumin-loaded, self-assembled aloe vera template for superior antioxidant activity and trans-membrane drug release. *Journal of Nanoscience and Nanotechnology*, 15(6), 4039–4045.

Korać, R. R., & Khambholja, K. M. (2011). Potential of herbs in skin protection from ultraviolet radiation. *Pharmacognosy Reviews*, 5(10), 164–173.

Kotyla, T., Kuo, F., Moolchandani, V., Wilson, T., & Nicolosi, R. (2008). Increased bioavailability of a transdermal application of a nano-sized emulsion preparation. *International Journal of Pharmaceutics*, 347(1–2), 144–148.

Lacatusu, I., Badea, N., Murariu, A., Nichita, C., Bojin, D., & Meghea, A. (2010). Antioxidant capacity of lipid nanoparticles loaded with rosemary extract. *Molecular Crystals and Liquid Crystals*, 523 (1), 260–272.

Li, H., Zhang, N., Hao, Y., Wang, Y., Jia, S., Zhang, H., Zhang, Y., & Zhang, Z. (2014). Formulation of curcumin delivery with functionalized single-walled carbon nanotubes: Characteristics and anticancer effects *in vitro. Drug Delivery*, 21(5), 379–387.

Lohani, A., Verma, A., Joshi, H., Yadav, N., & Karki, N. (2014). Nanotechnology-based cosmeceuticals. *ISRN Dermatology*, 2014, 843687.

Lu, W. C., Chiang, B. H., Huang, D. W., & Li, P. H. (2014). Skin permeation of D-limonene-based nanoemulsions as a transdermal carrier prepared by ultrasonic emulsification. *Ultrasonics Sonochemistry*, 21(2), 826–832.

Manca, M. L., Castangia, I., Caddeo, C., Pando, D., Escribano, E., Valenti, D., Lampis, S., Zaru, M., Fadda, A. M., & Manconi, M. (2014). Improvement of quercetin protective effect against oxidative stress skin damages by incorporation in nanovesicles. *Colloids and Surfaces. B, Biointerfaces*, 123, 566–574.

Mitri, K., Shegokar, R., Gohla, S., Anselmi, C., & Müller, R. H. (2011). Lipid nanocarriers for dermal delivery of lutein: Preparation, characterization, stability, and performance. *International Journal of Pharmaceutics*, 414(1–2), 267–275.

Montenegro, L. (2014). Nanocarriers for skin delivery of cosmetic antioxidants. *Journal of Pharmaceutical Research*, 2(4), 73–92.

Pereira, F., Baptista, R., Ladeiras, D., Madureira, A. M., Teixeira, G., Rosado, C., Fernandes, A. S., Ascensão, L., Oliveira Silva, C., Pinto Reis, C., & Rijo, P. (2015). Production and characterization of nanoparticles containing methanol extracts of Portuguese lavenders. Measurement, 74, 170–177.

Islamian, J. P., & Mehrali, H. (2015). Lycopene as a carotenoid provides radioprotectant and antioxidant effects by quenching radiation-induced free radical singlet oxygen: An overview. *Cell Journal*, 16(4), 386–391.

Pornpattananangkul, D., Fu, V., Thamphiwatana, S., Zhang, L., Chen, M., Vecchio, J., Gao, W., Huang, C. M., & Zhang, L. (2013). *In vivo* treatment of Propionibacterium acnes infection with liposomal lauric acids. *Advanced Healthcare Materials*, 2(10), 1322–1328.

Rahimi, H. R., Nedaeinia, R., Shamloo, A. S., Nikdoust, S., & Oskuee, R. K. (2016). Novel delivery system for natural products: Nano-curcumin formulations. *Avicenna Journal of Phytomedicine*, 6(4), 383.

Raj, S., Jose, S., Sumod, U. S., & Sabitha, M. (2012). Nanotechnology in cosmetics: Opportunities and challenges. *Journal of Pharmacy & Bioallied Sciences*, 4(3), 186–193.

Rathod, S., Mali, S., Shinde, N., & Aloorkar, N. (2020). Cosmeceuticals and beauty care products: Current trends with future prospects. *Research Journal of Topical and Cosmetic Science*, 11(1), 45–51.

Scalia, S., Franceschinis, E., Bertelli, D., & Iannuccelli, V. (2013). Comparative evaluation of the effect of permeation enhancers, lipid nanoparticles, and colloidal silica on *in vivo* human skin penetration of quercetin. Skin Pharmacology and Physiology, 26(2), 57–67.

Shakeri, A., & Sahebkar, A. (2015). Phytosome: A fatty solution for efficient formulation of phytopharmaceuticals. *Recent Patents on Drug Delivery & Formulation*, 10(1), 7–10.

Shim, J. H., Park, J. H., Lee, J. H., Lee, D. Y., Lee, J. H., & Yang, J. M. (2016). Moisturizers are effective in the treatment of xerosis irrespectively from their particular formulation: Results from a prospective, randomized, double-blind controlled trial. *Journal of the European Academy of Dermatology and Venereology*, 30(2), 276–281.

Sindhu, R. K., Verma, R., Salgotra, T., Rahman, M. H., Shah, M., Akter, R., Murad, W., Mubin, S., Bibi, P., Qusti, S., Alshammari, E. M., Batiha, G. E., Tomczyk, M., & Al-Kuraishy, H. M. (2021). Impacting the remedial potential of nano delivery-based flavonoids for breast cancer treatment. *Molecules*, 26(17), 5163.

Stahl, W., & Sies, H. (2012). Photoprotection by dietary carotenoids: Concept, mechanisms, evidence, and future development. *Molecular Nutrition & Food Research*, 56(2), 287–295.

Suwannateep, N., Wanichwecharungruang, S., Fluhr, J., Patzelt, A., Lademann, J., & Meinke, M. C. (2013). Comparison of two encapsulated curcumin particulate systems contained in different formulations with regard to *in vitro* skin penetration. *Skin Research and Technology*, 19(1), 1–9.

Suwannateep, N., Wanichwecharungruang, S., Haag, S. F., Devahastin, S., Groth, N., Fluhr, J. W., Lademann, J., & Meinke, M. C. (2012). Encapsulated curcumin results in prolonged curcumin activity *in vitro* and radical scavenging activity ex vivo on skin after UVB-irradiation. *European Journal of Pharmaceutics and Biopharmaceutics*, 82(3), 485–490.

Tabandeh, M. R., Oryan, A., & Mohammadalipour, A. (2014). Polysaccharides of Aloe vera induce MMP-3 and TIMP-2 gene expression during the skin wound repair of rat. *International Journal of Biological Macromolecules*, 65, 424–430.

Tanaka, M., Misawa, E., Yamauchi, K., Abe, F., & Ishizaki, C. (2015). Effects of plant sterols derived from Aloe vera gel on human dermal fibroblasts *in vitro* and on skin condition in Japanese women. *Clinical, Cosmetic and Investigational Dermatology*, 8, 95–104.

Tavano, L., Muzzalupo, R., Picci, N., & de Cindio, B. (2014). Co-encapsulation of lipophilic antioxidants into niosomal carriers: Percutaneous permeation studies for cosmeceutical applications. *Colloids and Surfaces B: Biointerfaces*, 114, 144–149.

Teo, B. S., Basri, M., Zakaria, M. R., Salleh, A. B., Rahman, R. N., & Rahman, M. B. (2010). A potential tocopherol acetate loaded palm oil esters-in-water nanoemulsions for nanocosmeceuticals. *Journal of Nanobiotechnology*, 8, 4.

Tripodo, G., Trapani, A., Torre, M. L., Giammona, G., Trapani, G., & Mandracchia, D. (2015). Hyaluronic acid and its derivatives in drug delivery and imaging: Recent advances and challenges. *European Journal of Pharmaceutics and Biopharmaceutics*, 97(Pt B), 400–416.

Weiss-Angeli, V., Poletto, F. S., de Marco, S. L., Salvador, M., da Silveira, N. P., Guterres, S. S., & Pohlmann, A. R. (2012). Sustained antioxidant activity of quercetin-loaded lipid-core nanocapsules. *Journal of Nanoscience and Nanotechnology*, 12(3), 2874–2880.

Yang, D., Pornpattananangkul, D., Nakatsuji, T., Chan, M., Carson, D., Huang, C. M., & Zhang, L. (2009). The antimicrobial activity of liposomal lauric acids against Propionibacterium acnes. *Biomaterials*, 30(30), 6035–6040.

Yang, S., Liu, C., Liu, W., Yu, H., Zheng, H., Zhou, W., & Hu, Y. (2013). Preparation and characterization of nanoliposomes entrapping medium-chain fatty acids and vitamin C by lyophilization. *International Journal of Molecular Sciences*, 14(10), 19763–19773.

Zamarioli, C. M., Martinsh, R. M., Carvalho, E. C., & Freitas, L. A. P. (2015). Nanoparticles containing curcuminoids (Curcuma longa): Development of topical delivery formulation. *Revista Brasileira de Farmacognosia*, 25(1), 53–60.

Zhang, Z., Chen, X., Rao, W., Long, F., Yan, L., & Yin, Y. (2015). Preparation of novel curcumin-imprinted polymers based on magnetic multi-walled carbon nanotubes for the rapid extraction of curcumin from ginger powder and kiwi fruit root. *Journal of Separation Science*, 38(1), 108–114.

Chapter 14

Applications of Nanophytoherbals in Obesity Therapy

Karan Goel
Abhishek Marwari
Kirti Goel
Jasmine Chaudhary
and Akash Jain*
M.M. College of Pharmacy, Maharishi Markandeshwar (Deemed to be University), Mullana, Ambala, Haryana, India

Abstract

Nanophytoherbals represent a fusion of nanotechnology and phytotherapy aimed at optimizing the efficacy of bioactive phytochemicals for treating obesity. These innovative formulations utilize nanocarriers to encapsulate plant extracts, thereby enhancing their bioavailability and enabling precise delivery to targeted sites. Existing obesity treatments often face limitations due to insufficient long-term effectiveness. In contrast, nanomedicine provides novel nanoscale platforms to address these challenges through tailored and targeted therapeutic strategies. Nanophytoherbals exhibit anti-obesity properties through various pathways, including appetite regulation, metabolic modulation, inflammation reduction, microbiota modification, and inhibition of adipogenesis. Conducting safety evaluations is essential due to the potential toxicity of nanoparticles. Green nanotechnology supports the environmentally friendly and efficient production of these products on a large scale while adhering to rigorous quality assurance measures. Emerging applications involve precise medication delivery techniques and combinations with gene therapy. Although nanophytoherbals hold promise for addressing obesity through personalized therapy, challenges remain concerning ethical considerations, cost-efficiency, and regulatory frameworks that require resolution.

Keywords: nanophytoherbs, green nanotechnology, weight management, obesity, targeted delivery system

* Corresponding Author Email: akash.jain@mmumullana@org.

In: Phyto-Nanomedicine
Editors: Hitesh Chopra, Vinod Kumar Gauttam, Ajmer Singh Grewal et al.
ISBN: 979-8-89530-317-7

Abbreviations

BMI	Body Mass Index BMI
WHO	World Health Organization
CDCP	Centers for Disease Control and Prevention
AOMs	Anti-Obesity Medications
GMP	Good Manufacturing Practices
DLS	Dynamic Light Scattering
NTA	Nanoparticle Tracking Analysis

Introduction

Nanophytoherbals result from the fusion of two influential disciplines: nanotechnology and phytotherapy. These novel formulations leverage the therapeutic properties of plant-derived compounds while capitalizing on the advantages of nanoscale technology. By reducing medicinal plant extracts into nano-sized particles, nanophytoherbals achieve higher bioavailability, precise targeted distribution, and enhanced effectiveness of bioactive compounds (Bhattacharya et al., 2022). Phytotherapy, often referred to as herbal medicine, has been used for centuries to address various health conditions due to the wide range of beneficial substances found in plants. However, the effectiveness of traditional herbal treatments may be limited by inadequate solubility, restricted bioavailability, and a lack of precise delivery to specific tissues or cells in the body. In contrast, nanotechnology focuses on the manipulation and study of materials and structures at the nanoscale, typically ranging from 1 to 100 nanometers (Babazadeh et al., 2018; Bhattacharya et al., 2022). At this scale, materials exhibit distinct characteristics that are often not observed in larger quantities, such as increased surface area, altered chemical reactivity, and improved permeability. Nanophytoherbals effectively address the drawbacks of traditional herbal formulations by encapsulating plant-derived compounds in nanoscale carriers such as liposomes, nanoparticles, or nanoemulsions. The application of nanotechnology to phytotherapy holds promising prospects for enhancing the management of various health conditions, including obesity, cancer, diabetes, and cardiovascular disorders (Chavda et al., 2023; Koklesova et al., 2023). These formulations can selectively target specific cells or tissues, deliver therapeutic agents in a controlled manner, and minimize the risk of systemic side effects. Furthermore, nanophytoherbals have the potential to revolutionize personalized medicine by enabling customized therapies tailored to the unique characteristics of each patient, including their genetic makeup, metabolic processes, and health conditions. The ongoing advancements in nanotechnology and plant science create significant opportunities for the future of healthcare through the development and commercialization of nanophytoherbals (WAHI et al., 2024). Obesity is a chronic condition characterized by an excessive accumulation of body fat, leading to various health issues. It is typically diagnosed when an individual's body mass index (BMI) is 30 or higher. From 1975 to 2022, the prevalence of obesity among children and adolescents (ages 5 to 19) increased from 4% to 18%, resulting in more than a fourfold rise in global obesity rates. As of March 2023, the prevalence of obesity in the US reached 41.9% and continues to rise. Excess weight or obesity is associated with numerous health problems, including cardiovascular disease, stroke, type 2 diabetes, and various forms of cancer (Müller et al., 2022). Several factors can influence the development of these conditions, including genetic predisposition, metabolic processes, environmental conditions, individual behaviors, and cultural influences. Successfully managing obesity often requires a holistic approach that includes dietary changes, lifestyle modifications, and, if necessary, medical intervention. According to the World Health Organization (WHO), obesity largely results from an imbalance between calorie intake and calorie expenditure (Kim, 2020; Müller et al., 2022). The WHO emphasizes the importance of community and environmental factors in reducing the burden of obesity and enhancing access to nutritious food options. The Centers for Disease Control and Prevention (CDC) note that obesity is influenced by several variables, including dietary choices, physical activity, sleep patterns, genetic susceptibility, and environmental factors. They highlight the need to address these issues at the individual, community, and societal levels to effectively combat the obesity epidemic (Kim, 2020; Mauro et al., 2008; Müller et al., 2022).

Current Challenges in Obesity Therapy

The treatment of obesity faces numerous obstacles and constraints. A significant challenge is the development of effective anti-obesity medications (AOMs) that can substantially and consistently reduce excessive weight while minimizing the risks of cardiovascular disease, abuse potential, tachyphylaxis, and other adverse effects that have historically plagued this area of research (Müller et al., 2022). Another constraint is the limited long-term effectiveness of current therapies. Although interventions such as lifestyle modifications, medication administration, and bariatric surgery often lead to initial weight loss, sustaining these results over the long term proves challenging, as many individuals experience weight regain. Additionally, the high costs associated with maintaining a nutritious diet and the inability to finance enrollment in commercial weight loss programs create significant barriers to effective obesity management (Kim, 2020). The complexity of obesity is further compounded by individual variability. Given its multifaceted nature, the effectiveness of treatments can vary widely among individuals, making it difficult to devise universally applicable strategies. Psychological factors, including stress, depression, and emotional eating, can also hinder treatment outcomes, necessitating a comprehensive approach that addresses both physical and mental health. Social determinants of health, such as socioeconomic status and access to healthcare services, play a crucial role in the prevalence of obesity and the accessibility of treatment. The existence of unequal access to evidence-based obesity care highlights the urgent need for improved healthcare infrastructure and policies that promote health equity (Kim, 2020; Mauro et al., 2008; Müller et al., 2022). Additional challenges include competing health issues, short appointment durations that do not allow adequate time for discussions about weight management, and insufficient training in obesity medicine among primary care practitioners. Weight stigma and discrimination exacerbate the difficulties associated with obesity treatment, negatively affecting individuals' self-esteem, treatment adherence, and willingness to seek help. Addressing cultural biases and fostering inclusivity in healthcare settings are essential for delivering effective and compassionate obesity treatment (Oshman et al., 2023). Moreover, obesity is a complex, chronic condition characterized by multiple factors leading to excessive fat accumulation and, in some cases, reduced well-being. Addressing this issue requires a comprehensive strategy that includes adopting a healthy diet, engaging in regular physical activity, and implementing environmental and policy changes to support healthier choices. To effectively tackle the existing obstacles in obesity treatment, a holistic approach is necessary. This approach should consider the diverse needs of individuals affected by obesity and recognize the social, economic, and environmental factors that contribute to the condition. Allocating resources toward research, education, policy initiatives, and community-based interventions is crucial for advancing obesity prevention and treatment and improving health outcomes for individuals and communities affected by obesity (Heymsfield et al., 2018; Oshman et al., 2023).

Nanomedicine and Nanophytoherbals: A Potential Alternative Therapy

Nanomedicine, an emerging discipline that integrates nanotechnology with healthcare, holds significant promise for addressing obesity, a disorder characterized by its complexity and diversity. By utilizing nanoscale materials and technologies, nanomedicine offers innovative approaches for the prevention, diagnosis, and treatment of obesity. Specifically designed nanoparticles for drug delivery can target adipose tissue or metabolic pathways associated with obesity, enhancing treatment effectiveness while minimizing systemic adverse effects. Additionally, nanosensors and imaging agents enable continuous monitoring of metabolic processes and disease progression, facilitating early detection and tailored treatment strategies. Moreover, nanotechnology-based platforms can create novel solutions for metabolic health and weight management within the realms of tissue engineering and regenerative medicine. Overall, nanomedicine has considerable potential to combat obesity through personalized and targeted therapies (Sanders, 2018; Sharma et al., 2021). The combination of nanotechnology with phytotherapy, referred to as nanophytoherbals, presents a promising alternative for obesity treatment. These formulations leverage the medicinal properties of plant-derived substances, known as phytochemicals, while capitalizing on the advantages of nanoscale delivery systems. By encapsulating bioactive phytochemicals within nanoparticles, nanophytoherbals enhance their bioavailability, stability, and targeted delivery to adipose tissue or metabolic pathways related to obesity (Malik et al., 2023; Saini et al., 2010). This targeted approach not only improves the efficacy of phytochemicals in promoting weight loss and metabolic health but also reduces the risk of systemic adverse effects. Furthermore, nanophytoherbals can be tailored to address specific metabolic dysfunctions or comorbidities associated with obesity, offering personalized and comprehensive therapeutic options. By influencing appetite, metabolism, inflammation, and other obesity-related factors, nanophytoherbals provide a natural and sustainable strategy for weight management (Malik et al., 2023; Saini et al., 2010; Sharma et al., 2021).

Mechanisms of Action of Nanophytoherbals in Obesity Treatment

Nanophytoherbals, derived from plants and formulated at the nanoscale, have attracted considerable interest in the field of obesity therapy due to their potential therapeutic properties. These formulations synergistically combine nanotechnology and phytotherapy to enhance the bioavailability, targeted delivery, and effectiveness of bioactive compounds found in medicinal plants (Heymsfield et al., 2018). Nanophytoherbals exert their effects in obesity therapy through multiple pathways.

- *Appetite Regulation:* Certain phytochemicals found in plants have been shown to influence appetite regulation by modulating the secretion of hormones such as leptin, ghrelin, and adiponectin. Nanoformulations can enhance the bioavailability of these phytochemicals, thereby facilitating better regulation of appetite control mechanisms (Sanders, 2018; Sim & Wong, 2021).
- *Metabolic Modulation:* Nanophytoherbals can target metabolic pathways involved in lipid metabolism, glucose homeostasis, and energy expenditure. For example, they may inhibit key enzymes responsible for lipid synthesis or promote the activation of enzymes involved in lipid breakdown, thus helping to reduce fat accumulation (Malik et al., 2023).
- *Inflammation Reduction:* Chronic low-grade inflammation is often associated with obesity and contributes to metabolic dysfunction. Phytochemicals with anti-inflammatory properties, such as polyphenols and flavonoids, can mitigate inflammation by inhibiting pro-inflammatory cytokines and signaling pathways. Nanotechnology facilitates the targeted delivery of these compounds, enhancing their anti-inflammatory effects (Sanders, 2018, Munjal et al., 2020).
- *Enhanced Thermogenesis:* Some phytochemicals have been found to promote thermogenesis, the process by which the body generates heat and burns calories. By activating thermogenic pathways, nanophytoherbals may increase energy expenditure and aid in weight loss (Oshman et al., 2023).
- *Gut Microbiota Modulation:* The gut microbiota plays a crucial role in energy metabolism and adiposity. Certain plant-derived compounds can modulate the composition and function of the gut microbiota in ways that favor metabolic health. Nanoformulations can protect these compounds from degradation in the gastrointestinal tract, improving their delivery to the gut and enhancing their probiotic or prebiotic effects (Kim, 2020).
- *Adipogenesis Inhibition:* Adipogenesis, the process of fat cell formation, is a key target in obesity treatment. Phytochemicals in nanophytoherbals may interfere with adipocyte differentiation and proliferation, thus reducing fat accumulation in adipose tissue (Müller et al., 2022; WAHI et al., 2024).
- *Antioxidant Activity:* Oxidative stress is closely linked to obesity-related complications such as insulin resistance and cardiovascular diseases. Phytochemicals with antioxidant properties, when delivered in nanoformulations, can scavenge free radicals and attenuate oxidative stress, thereby improving overall metabolic health (Kim, 2020; Müller et al., 2022).
- *Blood Glucose Regulation:* Some plant-derived compounds exhibit hypoglycemic effects by enhancing insulin sensitivity, promoting glucose uptake by cells, or inhibiting carbohydrate digestion and absorption. Nanoencapsulation enhances the stability and solubility of these compounds, improving their efficacy in regulating blood glucose levels (Malik et al., 2023; Sharma et al., 2021).

Table 2. Evidence-based studies on the use of nanophytoherbs as obesity treatment and management tools

Study	Constituents	Methods/Model	Outcomes	Reference
Nanocurcumin for Obesity Management	Curcumin	*In vivo* study using obese mice	Reduced adipose tissue inflammation, improved insulin sensitivity, lowered serum lipid levels	(Sim & Wong, 2021)
Nanoresveratrol for Weight Control	Resveratrol	Clinical trial with obese individuals	Significant reductions in body weight, waist circumference, and adiposity index	(Ranjit & Klabunde, 2007; Yusuf et al., 2023)
Nanogreen Tea Extract for Metabolic Health	Green tea extract	Animal study using obese mice	Improved glucose tolerance, insulin sensitivity, and lipid metabolism	(Malik et al., 2023; Sharma et al., 2021)
Nanocapsaicin for Appetite Regulation	Capsaicin	Randomized controlled trial with overweight subjects	Reduced appetite, energy intake, and body weight	(Malik et al., 2023; Patra et al., 2018; Sharma et al., 2021)
Nanoemulsified Omega-3 Fatty Acids for Weight Loss	Omega-3 fatty acids	Animal study with obese rats	Decreased body weight, adiposity, and serum lipid levels	(Patra et al., 2018; Ranjit & Klabunde, 2007; Yusuf et al., 2023)

Evidence-Based Studies on the Use of Nanophytoherbs as Obesity Treatment and Management Tools

Evidence-based investigations are essential for assessing the efficacy of nanophytoherbals in obesity treatment and management, as discussed in Table 1. Such research plays a pivotal role in determining the therapeutic potential of nanophytoherbals and guiding their integration into clinical practice for effective obesity management.

Safety and Tolerability of Nanophytoherbals

Ensuring the safety and tolerability of nanophytoherbals for obesity management necessitates thorough preclinical and clinical studies. Due to their small size and increased surface area, nanoparticles may exhibit unique toxicological properties that could lead to adverse effects on cells, tissues, or organs if they accumulate in the body or interact unpredictably with biological systems (Müller et al., 2022). Biocompatibility studies, including cell viability assays, immunotoxicity assessments, and histopathological analyses, are essential for evaluating compatibility with biological systems (Khogta et al., 2020). Additionally, pharmacokinetic studies are crucial for understanding the absorption, distribution, metabolism, and excretion of these formulations, providing insights into their biodistribution and potential systemic exposure (Khogta et al., 2020). Nanophytoherbals may also interact with proteins, nucleic acids, or other biomolecules, potentially causing unintended biological effects or adverse reactions (Raman et al., 2022). Concerns regarding organ toxicity arise from the potential accumulation of nanoparticles in organs such as the liver, kidneys, or spleen, which could lead to dysfunction or damage over time (Khogta et al., 2020; Raman et al., 2022). Clinical trials are essential for monitoring adverse events, vital signs, and laboratory parameters to assess the safety profile in obese individuals (Patra et al., 2018). Long-term follow-up studies are also necessary to track patients treated with nanophytoherbals over extended periods, evaluating their safety, tolerability, and potential adverse effects in the context of obesity management (Yusuf et al., 2023).

Formulation and Delivery of Nanophytoherbals for Obesity Therapy

Nanophytoherbals for obesity treatment leverage nanotechnology to enhance the therapeutic properties of herbal medications and improve their bioavailability. The creation of these formulations follows a systematic approach that integrates concepts from nanotechnology and pharmacological sciences. The initial stages involve the production of nanoparticles using various materials, such as lipids, polymers, or metals, while maintaining precise control over their size and surface characteristics. These nanoparticles serve as carriers for bioactive phytochemicals derived from medicinal plants recognized for their anti-obesity properties (Ranjit & Klabunde, 2007; Sanders, 2018; Yusuf et al., 2023). Nanophytoherbals, including nanodrugs and nanocarrier systems based on phytochemicals, demonstrate potential in addressing obesity. The encapsulation process employs techniques like solvent evaporation or nanoprecipitation to entrap the phytochemicals within the nanoparticle matrix, ensuring their protection and enabling controlled release. Additionally, nanoparticles may undergo surface modification to enhance their stability, biocompatibility, and targeting capabilities. Functionalization using ligands or polymers allows for precise targeting of adipose tissue or metabolic pathways implicated in obesity (Ranjit & Klabunde, 2007; Sanders, 2018; Sim & Wong, 2021). The method of delivering nanophytoherbals may vary based on the desired therapeutic outcome and the specific tissue targeted. Oral administration is often preferred for systemic effects, while localized delivery can be achieved through topical application or direct injection. Ensuring the safe elimination of nanophytoherbals from the body after their therapeutic effects requires careful investigation of their biodegradability and biocompatibility. Rigorous quality control measures are implemented at every stage of the formulation process to ensure reproducibility and uniformity. Stability testing assesses the physical and chemical stability of the product under varying conditions to confirm its effectiveness and shelf life (Müller et al., 2022; Patra et al., 2018; Yusuf et al., 2023). The development of scalable manufacturing procedures aims to produce nanophytoherbals in large quantities for clinical applications, adhering to GMP standards to ensure product quality, safety, and regulatory compliance. However, the pharmaceutical industry continues to face challenges in scaling operations and managing the costs associated with developing nanotechnology products. These issues may impact the thorough assessment of the safety and tolerability of advanced drug delivery systems based on nanotechnology (Heymsfield et al., 2018; Sanders, 2018; Sim & Wong, 2021).

Potential Applications of Nanophytoherbals in Obesity Therapy

Drug Doses Specifications

Nanophytoherbals offer precise medication dosage specifications due to their controlled release characteristics and enhanced bioavailability. This accuracy enables healthcare professionals to administer the exact dosage of phytochemicals needed to elicit therapeutic effects on the metabolic pathways associated with obesity. Furthermore, nanophytoherbals can be formulated with specific dose potencies, ranging from minimal to substantial concentrations, to accommodate varying degrees of obesity and individual patient characteristics (Ansari et al., 2012).

Green Nanotechnology-Based Assemblies

Green nanotechnology-based assemblies involve the use of eco-friendly and sustainable methods for the creation and production of nanomaterials. These assemblies are characterized by their environmentally conscious design, aiming to minimize ecological footprints and promote sustainability throughout the manufacturing process (Raman et al., 2022). Green nanotechnology-based assemblies for nanophytoherbals in obesity treatment encompass:

- *Plant-derived nanomaterials*: Utilizing renewable plant-derived materials such as cellulose, chitosan, or lignin as building blocks for nanoparticle synthesis. These materials are biocompatible and readily available, making them ideal candidates for green nanotechnology-based assemblies (Khogta et al., 2020).

- *Solvent-free fabrication*: Employing solvent-free or aqueous-based fabrication techniques minimizes the use of organic solvents and reduces environmental pollution. Techniques such as nanoprecipitation, emulsification, and electrospinning can be adapted to align with green synthesis approaches (Ranjit & Klabunde, 2007).
- *Bioinspired design:* Drawing inspiration from nature to design nanomaterials with specific properties and functionalities. Mimicking natural processes such as self-assembly and biomineralization allows for the creation of complex nanostructures using sustainable and biocompatible building blocks (Malik et al., 2023).
- *Energy-efficient processing*: Implementing energy-efficient manufacturing processes, such as microwave-assisted synthesis or green synthesis using solar energy, helps minimize energy consumption and reduce carbon footprints (Raman et al., 2022).

Gene Therapy and Polyplex Micelles-Based Delivery

The objective of gene therapy in obesity treatment is to target the fundamental genetic mechanisms contributing to metabolic dysfunction and weight gain. By administering therapeutic genes that encode proteins involved in energy metabolism, adipogenesis regulation, or appetite control, gene therapy aims to rectify genetic abnormalities or dysfunctions related to obesity. Nanophytoherbals can be designed to encapsulate gene vectors, such as plasmid DNA or viral vectors, facilitating their targeted delivery to adipose tissue or metabolic organs (Ansari et al., 2012; Yao et al., 2020). Polyplex micelles are nanoscale delivery systems composed of biocompatible polymers that spontaneously form micelle-like structures, capable of enclosing and protecting nucleic acids. These polyplex micelles offer several advantages for gene delivery, including enhanced stability, increased cellular uptake, and controlled release of genetic payloads. Additionally, they can be modified with targeting ligands or surface alterations to ensure precise distribution to adipocytes or metabolic organs (Afzal et al., 2022; Patra et al., 2018; Yao et al., 2020). The integration of gene therapy with polyplex micelle-based delivery methods enables the development of customized treatment approaches for obesity. Nanophytoherbals serve as versatile platforms for encapsulating both phytochemicals and genetic payloads, allowing for a synergistic effect and precise control over metabolic pathways associated with obesity. Furthermore, the use of natural and biocompatible materials in nanophytoherbals ensures safety and compatibility with living organisms, thereby reducing the likelihood of adverse effects typically associated with gene therapy (Khogta et al., 2020; Saini et al., 2010; Sanders, 2018).

Drug Delivery Technologies and Machinery

Drug delivery technologies are essential for enabling precise control over drug release, targeting specific tissues, and enhancing therapeutic efficacy while minimizing side effects. Key technologies and machinery used in the development of nanophytoherbals include:

- *Nanoparticle synthesis equipment*: Various types of equipment, such as reactors, mixers, and sonicators, are employed for the synthesis of nanoparticles. These machines provide precise control over particle size, shape, and surface properties, which are critical for optimizing the performance of nanophytoherbals in obesity therapy (Ansari et al., 2012).
- *Encapsulation techniques*: Drug encapsulation within nanoparticles is achieved through methods such as nanoprecipitation, emulsification, or solvent evaporation. Equipment like homogenizers, microfluidic devices, and spray dryers is utilized to ensure uniform drug distribution and efficient encapsulation of phytochemicals within nanophytoherbals (Yao et al., 2020).
- *Surface modification systems*: Surface modification of nanoparticles with targeting ligands, polymers, or protective coatings is crucial for enhancing stability, biocompatibility, and targeted delivery. Equipment such as coaters, plasma reactors, and functionalization reactors enable precise control over surface chemistry and functionality (Malik et al., 2023).
- *Particle size analysis instruments*: Accurate characterization of nanoparticle size distribution is vital for ensuring product consistency and performance. Particle size analyzers, including dynamic light scattering and nanoparticle tracking analysis systems, provide valuable insights into the size distribution and stability of nanophytoherbals formulations (Ranjit & Klabunde, 2007).
- *Drug release testing devices: In vitro* dissolution testers or dialysis systems are used to evaluate drug release kinetics from nanophytoherbals. These devices enable researchers to assess the release profile of phytochemicals from nanoparticles under simulated physiological conditions, guiding formulation optimization and dosage regimen design (Oshman et al., 2023).
- *Targeted delivery systems*: Equipment such as microfluidic devices or electrospray systems facilitates the precise engineering of nanoparticles for targeted delivery to specific tissues or cells involved in obesity. These systems enable the incorporation of targeting ligands or surface modifications to enhance nanoparticle accumulation and uptake at the desired site of action (WAHI et al., 2024).
- *Scale-up manufacturing equipment*: Scalable manufacturing equipment, including high-pressure homogenizers, spray dryers, and fluidized bed reactors, is utilized to produce nanophytoherbals in large quantities for clinical translation. These machines ensure consistent product quality, reproducibility, and compliance with Good Manufacturing Practices (GMP) regulations (Ansari et al., 2012; Koklesova et al., 2023).

Antiviral and Antibacterial Applications

Nanophytoherbals leverage the inherent antimicrobial properties of phytochemicals encapsulated within nanoparticles, enhancing targeted delivery and bioavailability through nanotechnology (Patra et al., 2018). Key aspects of their applications in antiviral and antibacterial treatments include:

- *Phytochemical antimicrobial activity:* Many phytochemicals derived from medicinal plants exhibit inherent antiviral and antibacterial properties. Compounds such as flavonoids, alkaloids, and terpenoids demonstrate broad-spectrum antimicrobial activity against various viruses, bacteria, and fungi. By encapsulating these phytochemicals within nanoparticles, their antimicrobial efficacy can be enhanced and directed toward specific pathogens (Afzal et al., 2022).
- *Nanoparticle delivery systems*: Nanophytoherbals function as effective delivery systems for phytochemicals with antimicrobial activity. The nanoparticles protect the encapsulated compounds from degradation, prolong their circulation time in the body, and facilitate their uptake by target cells or microorganisms. This targeted delivery minimizes off-target effects and enhances the therapeutic efficacy of nanophytoherbals in combating viral and bacterial infections (Yao et al., 2020).
- *Viral inhibition*: Nanophytoherbals have shown potential in inhibiting viral replication and infectivity. Phytochemicals encapsulated within nanoparticles can target mechanisms involved in viral entry, replication, or release, disrupting the viral life cycle and reducing viral load. Furthermore, nanophytoherbals may modulate host immune responses, enhancing antiviral defenses and reducing viral pathogenicity (Yusuf et al., 2023).
- *Bacterial eradication*: These formulations exhibit antibacterial activity against various bacterial pathogens, including drug-resistant strains. Phytochemicals encapsulated within nanoparticles can disrupt bacterial cell membranes, inhibit essential enzymes, or interfere with bacterial signaling pathways, leading to bacterial growth inhibition and eradication. Additionally, nanophytoherbals may enhance the action of conventional antibiotics, overcoming antibiotic resistance and improving treatment outcomes (Sanders, 2018; Sim & Wong, 2021).
- *Biofilm disruption*: Nanophytoherbals have been studied for their ability to disrupt bacterial biofilms, which are complex microbial communities that resist conventional antibiotics. Phytochemicals encapsulated within nanoparticles can penetrate biofilm matrices, inhibit biofilm formation, and disperse pre-formed biofilms, thus enhancing the efficacy of antimicrobial treatments and preventing recurrent infections (Ansari et al., 2012; Sanders, 2018).
- *Topical and systemic applications*: Nanophytoherbals can be administered both topically and systemically to treat viral and bacterial infections. Topical formulations, such as creams or ointments, deliver nanophytoherbals directly to infected skin or mucous membranes. In contrast, systemic formulations, such as oral or intravenous preparations, enable widespread distribution and targeted action against systemic infections.

Clinical Practice, Future Perspectives, and Complications Facing Nanophytoherbs as Obesity Therapy (Table 3)

Table 3. Clinical practice, future perspectives, and complications facing nanophytoherbs as obesity therapy

Aspect	Clinical Practice	Future Perspectives	Complications Facing Nanophytoherbs	Reference
Patient Assessment	Perform thorough evaluations, considering the degree of obesity, accompanying medical conditions, and individual preferences for therapy.	Incorporation into personalized medicine for customized treatment strategies based on individual criteria.	Potential safety risks related to nanoparticle toxicity, immunogenicity, and off-target effects.	(Patra et al., 2018)
Treatment Planning	Design customized treatment programs by integrating nanophytoherbs with other therapeutic approaches.	Progress in nanotechnology enables the development of innovative formulations that have improved effectiveness and precise delivery to specific targets.	Obstacles related to regulations, such as rigorous approval procedures and restricted rules for nanophytoherbs.	(Yao et al., 2020)
Monitoring and Follow-up	Consistently observe and evaluate the advancement, gauging the reduction in weight, metabolic indicators, and any negative consequences.	Incorporation into multimodal treatments, including combining nanophytoherbs with gene therapy and digital inputs.	Issues related to cost-effectiveness and accessibility, especially in situations with low resources.	(Afzal et al., 2022)
Patient Education	Offer explicit details on treatment objectives, anticipated outcomes, potential advantages, and any drawbacks.	Progress in the field of personalized medicine has enabled the development of customized treatment approaches that take into account individual genetic characteristics.	Key ethical issues include ensuring informed consent, respecting patient autonomy, and promoting fair access to treatment.	(Ansari et al., 2012)

Conclusion

Nanophytoherbals merge nanotechnology and herbal therapy, showing significant promise in effectively targeting obesity. These formulations may address the limitations of traditional phytotherapy by enhancing the bioavailability, stability, and targeted delivery of bioactive phytochemicals derived from medicinal plants. Nano-enhanced herbal formulations combat obesity through various mechanisms, including appetite control, metabolic regulation, inflammation reduction, microbiota modulation, and inhibition of fat cell growth. Preclinical and clinical research increasingly supports the effectiveness and safety of these treatments. However, thorough evaluations of nanoparticle toxicity, their interactions with biological systems, pharmacokinetics, organ accumulation, and potential adverse effects in clinical settings are crucial. The application of advanced green engineering technologies and stringent production processes ensures the quality and consistency of these formulations. Emerging applications include precise medication administration, gene therapy, combinations of polyplex micelles, and the use of plant-derived nanomaterials compatible with living organisms, all integrated with eco-friendly technologies. By incorporating personalized therapeutic integration, customized dosing, and multimodal digital health platforms, treatment programs can be developed to prioritize individual patient needs and preferences. Despite these advancements, challenges remain, including regulatory policies, ethical concerns, scaling-up processes, and cost-effectiveness issues that require proactive solutions. Overall, nanophytoherbals represent a new generation of innovative phytopharmaceuticals, potentially paving the way for effective approaches to combat the global obesity epidemic through natural and personalized medicine strategies.

References

Afzal, O., Altamimi, A. S. A., Nadeem, M. S., Alzarea, S. I., Almalki, W. H., Tariq, A., Mubeen, B., Murtaza, B. N., Iftikhar, S., Riaz, N., & Kazmi, I. (2022). Nanoparticles in Drug Delivery: From History to Therapeutic Applications. *Nanomaterials*, 12(24), 4494.

Ansari, S., Sameem, Mohd., & Islam, F. (2012). Influence of nanotechnology on herbal drugs: A Review. *Journal of Advanced Pharmaceutical Technology & Research*, 3(3), 142.

Babazadeh, A., Zeinali, M., & Hamishehkar, H. (2018). Nano-Phytosome: A Developing Platform for Herbal Anti-Cancer Agents in Cancer Therapy. *Current Drug Targets*, 19(2), 170–180.

Bhattacharya, T., Soares, G. A. B. e, Chopra, H., Rahman, Md. M., Hasan, Z., Swain, S. S., & Cavalu, S. (2022). Applications of Phyto-Nanotechnology for the Treatment of Neurodegenerative Disorders. *Materials*, 15(3), 804.

Chavda, V. P., Nalla, L. V., Balar, P., Bezbaruah, R., Apostolopoulos, V., Singla, R. K., Khadela, A., Vora, L., & Uversky, V. N. (2023). Advanced Phytochemical-Based Nanocarrier Systems for the Treatment of Breast Cancer. *Cancers*, 15(4), 1023.

Heymsfield, S., Aronne, L. J., Eneli, I., Kumar, R., Michalsky, M., Walker, E., Wolfe, B. M., Woolford, S. J., & Yanovski, S. (2018). Clinical Perspectives on Obesity Treatment: Challenges, Gaps, and Promising Opportunities. *NAM Perspectives,* Discussion Paper, National Academy of Medicine, Washington, DC.

Khogta, S., Patel, J., Barve, K., & Londhe, V. (2020). Herbal nano-formulations for topical delivery. *Journal of Herbal Medicine*, 20, 100300.

Kim, T. N. (2020). Barriers to Obesity Management: Patient and Physician Factors. *Journal of Obesity & Metabolic Syndrome*, 29(4), 244–247.

Koklesova, L., Jakubikova, J., Cholujova, D., Samec, M., Mazurakova, A., Šudomová, M., Pec, M., Hassan, S. T. S., Biringer, K., Büsselberg, D., Hurtova, T., Golubnitschaja, O., & Kubatka, P. (2023). Phytochemical-based nanodrugs going beyond the state-of-the-art in cancer management—Targeting cancer stem cells in the framework of predictive, preventive, personalized medicine. *Frontiers in Pharmacology*, 14, 1121950.

Malik, S., Muhammad, K., & Waheed, Y. (2023). Emerging Applications of Nanotechnology in Healthcare and Medicine. *Molecules*, 28(18), 6624.

Mauro, M., Taylor, V., Wharton, S., & Sharma, A. M. (2008). Barriers to obesity treatment. *European Journal of Internal Medicine*, 19(3), 173–180.

Müller, T. D., Blüher, M., Tschöp, M. H., & DiMarchi, R. D. (2022). Anti-obesity drug discovery: advances and challenges. *Nature Reviews Drug Discovery*, 21(3), 201–223.

Oshman, L., Othman, A., Furst, W., Heisler, M., Kraftson, A., Zouani, Y., Hershey, C., Cho, T.-C., Guetterman, T., Piatt, G., & Griauzde, D. H. (2023). Primary care providers' perceived barriers to obesity treatment and opportunities for improvement: A mixed methods study. *PLOS ONE*, 18(4), e0284474.

Patra, J. K., Das, G., Fraceto, L. F., Campos, E. V. R., Rodriguez-Torres, M. del P., Acosta-Torres, L. S., Diaz-Torres, L. A., Grillo, R., Swamy, M. K., Sharma, S., Habtemariam, S., & Shin, H.-S. (2018). Nano based drug delivery systems: recent developments and future prospects. *Journal of Nanobiotechnology*, 16(1), 71.

Raman, S., Murugaiyah, V., & Parumasivam, T. (2022). Andrographis paniculata Dosage Forms and Advances in Nanoparticulate Delivery Systems: An Overview. *Molecules*, 27(19), 6164.

Ranjit, K. T., & Klabunde, K. J. (2007). Nanotechnology: Fundamental Principles and Applications. In *Kent and Riegel's Handbook of Industrial Chemistry and Biotechnology* (pp. 328–344). Springer US.

Saini, R., Saini, S., & Sharma, S. (2010). Nanotechnology: The future medicine. *Journal of Cutaneous and Aesthetic Surgery*, 3(1), 32.

Sanders, W. C. (2018). *Basic Principles of Nanotechnology*. CRC Press.

Sharma, A., Sabharwal, P., & Dada, R. (2021). Herbal medicine—An introduction to its history. In *Herbal Medicine in Andrology* (pp. 1–8). Elsevier.

Sim, S., & Wong, N. (2021). Nanotechnology and its use in imaging and drug delivery (Review). *Biomedical Reports,* 14(5), 42.

Wahi, A., Bishnoi, M., Raina, N., Singh, M. A., Verma, P., Gupta, P. K., Kaur, G., Tuli, H. S., & Gupta, M. (2024). Recent updates on nano-phyto-formulations based therapeutic intervention for cancer treatment. *Oncology Research*, 32(1), 19–47.

Yao, Y., Zhou, Y., Liu, L., Xu, Y., Chen, Q., Wang, Y., Wsu, S., Deng, Y., Zhang, J., & Shao, A. (2020). Nanoparticle-Based Drug Delivery in Cancer Therapy and Its Role in Overcoming Drug Resistance. *Frontiers in Molecular Biosciences*, 7, 193.

Yusuf, A., Almotairy, A. R. Z., Henidi, H., Alshehri, O. Y., & Aldughaim, M. S. (2023). Nanoparticles as Drug Delivery Systems: A Review of the Implication of Nanoparticles' Physicochemical Properties on Responses in Biological Systems. *Polymers*, 15(7), 1596.

Chapter 15

Applications of Immune-Boosting Phytoherbals with Nanoparticle Delivery

Vishnu Mittal*
and Abhinav Singhal
Guru Gobind Singh College of Pharmacy, Yamunanagar, Haryana, India

Abstract

The chapter presents a comprehensive investigation into immune-modulating phytoherbals and their potential applications when combined with nanoparticle delivery systems. It explores a diverse range of phytoherbals known for their immunomodulatory properties, evaluating their compatibility with various nanoparticle formulations. The primary objective is to assess and leverage the immunomodulatory effects of selected phytoherbals by examining their potential impact on the immune system. A critical focus is placed on integrating traditional herbal knowledge with modern nanotechnology, providing a holistic perspective on advancing immune-boosting interventions. The methodology employs a multidisciplinary approach, incorporating principles from immunology, pharmacology, and nanotechnology. Inclusion criteria encompass studies that specifically focus on the application of immune-boosting phytoherbals with nanoparticle delivery. The gathered data offer a comprehensive overview of the current state of knowledge in this emerging field, facilitating the evaluation of immune response modulation and comprehensive safety assessments. Results indicate that the enhanced bioavailability and sustained release of active compounds contribute to a heightened immune response, showcasing promising synergies between immune-boosting phytoherbals and nanoparticle delivery systems. The realization of the full therapeutic potential underscores the importance of adopting a holistic approach to harness the benefits of nanotechnology for improved healthcare outcomes. The potential synergies between traditional herbal medicine and modern nanotechnology are highlighted, emphasizing the significance of a holistic approach to immune system modulation.

Keywords: immunomodulation, phytoherbals, nanoparticle delivery, bioavailability, safety assessment, immunotherapy

* Corresponding Author's Email: vishnumittal720@gmail.com.

In: Phyto-Nanomedicine
Editors: Hitesh Chopra, Vinod Kumar Gauttam, Ajmer Singh Grewal et al.
ISBN: 979-8-89530-317-7

Abbreviations

NDDS	Novel Drug Delivery Systems
RES	Reticuloendothelial System
NPs	Nanoparticles
CNTS	Carbon Nanotubes
IV	Intravenously
PLGA	Poly(D,L-Lactide-Co-Glycolide)
PLA	Poly (Lactic Acid)
EGCG	Epigallocatechin Gallate
TAMs	Tumor-Associated Macrophages
OVA	Ovalbumin
Dex-NPs	Dextran Nanoparticles
APCs	Antigen-Presenting Cells

Introduction

A significant emphasis has been placed in the last few decades on the creation of novel drug delivery systems (NDDS) for herbal medications. Two key requirements should ideally be met by these innovative carriers. First, they should administer the medication at a pace determined by the body's needs throughout the course of therapy. Second, they should target the active ingredients of herbal medicine to the specific area of action (Bray et al., 2021). Nanodosage forms have been developed in phyto-formulation research, offering several advantages for herbal drugs (Greco, 2019). As a result, novel drug delivery methods utilizing nanosized formulations may enhance the effectiveness of plant medicines and address their limitations in the future. This can be achieved through targeting strategies and the enhanced permeability and retention effect phenomenon (Arnold et al., 2022). Traditional liposomes tend to be trapped by the reticuloendothelial system (RES), making it simple to deliver agents to this system. The effectiveness of herbal cosmetic formulations on the human body can also be improved by employing advanced techniques. Similarly, additional vesicular systems, such as nanoemulsions, ethosomes, and transferosomes, serve as highly beneficial assemblies with numerous advantages for the distribution of herbal medicines. Some of these benefits are outlined in this article. Herbal remedies have been extensively used around the world since ancient times. Both practitioners and patients have recognized the superior therapeutic benefits of herbal remedies, noting that they tend to have fewer side effects than contemporary medications (Shnoudeh et al., 2022).

Immune-Boosting Phytoherbals with Nanoparticle Delivery

Many rasayanas, or therapeutic plants known for their unique capabilities against specific microorganisms, are derived from a diverse spectrum of plants. Immunomodulatory compounds are also extracted from various medicinal plants and plant extracts. These phytochemicals possess antioxidant and anti-inflammatory properties. They can suppress the synthesis of interleukin (IL)-12/IL-18-induced IFN-γ, activate natural killer cells, inhibit the release of pro-inflammatory cytokines, or act as inhibitors by concealing the glycans on the viral envelope. This study focuses on specific phytochemicals and their potential mechanisms of action in modulating an individual's immune response to combat SARS-CoV-2 infection (Turashvili et al., 2017). In recent decades, nanoparticles have garnered significant attention due to their distinct physicochemical and physiological characteristics, which differ markedly from those of their bulk form. Many of their size-dependent physical properties—such as surface reactivity, melting points, and optical, magnetic, and catalytic capabilities—are essential for drug delivery applications, ranging from viruses to human cells. Before using a material as a drug delivery vehicle, it is crucial to investigate its immune response within the body. To prevent adverse immune reactions, nanomaterials must be designed thoughtfully and systematically, taking metabolic considerations into account (Hawkins et al., 1988). The lack of logical design has contributed to the failure of several therapeutic trials involving nanostructured materials. Thus, the aim of this study is to provide a comprehensive overview of how nanomaterials interact with the immune system, addressing one of these metabolic challenges. We will first present a brief overview of the structural and compositional diversity of nanomaterials reported in the literature and their interactions with the immune system (Dean et al., 2008). The application of immune-boosting phytoherbals combined with nanoparticle delivery represents a groundbreaking approach that integrates traditional herbal medicine with advanced nanotechnology to enhance immune support therapies. This concept can be applied in several ways:

- *Nanoparticle delivery systems*: Nanoparticles are tiny particles with dimensions on the nanometer scale. These characteristics make nanoparticles ideal carriers for delivering phytochemicals from medicinal herbs to targeted cells or tissues in the body.
- *Encapsulation of phytochemicals*: Phytochemicals are bioactive compounds found in plants that provide various health benefits, including immune-boosting properties. However, their efficacy can be limited by factors such as poor solubility, low bioavailability, and rapid metabolism in the body (Bardou et al., 2003).
- *Targeted delivery*: Nanoparticles can be engineered to selectively deliver immune-boosting phytochemicals to immune cells, such as macrophages, dendritic cells, or lymphocytes (Harvey et al., 1999).
- *Synergistic effects*: Combining multiple immune-boosting phytochemicals from different herbs into a single nanoparticle formulation can lead to synergistic effects, where the combined therapeutic effect is greater than the sum of the individual effects. This synergism can enhance immune modulation and provide broader protection against infectious agents and diseases.
- *Long-acting formulations*: Nanoparticle delivery systems can also prolong the release of phytochemicals, resulting in sustained immune modulation over an extended period.
- *Reduced toxicity*: By delivering phytochemicals directly to immune cells or tissues, nanoparticle formulations can reduce systemic exposure and minimize potential toxicity compared to conventional administration routes. This targeted delivery approach enhances the safety profile of immune-boosting therapies (Sorlie et al., 2001).

- *Potential applications*: Immune-boosting phytoherbals with nanoparticle delivery have various potential applications, including prevention & treatment of infectious diseases, autoimmune disorders, & cancer immunotherapy. Additionally, these formulations can serve as adjuvants to enhance the efficacy of vaccines by boosting the immune response.

Immune-Boosting Phytoherbals

The application of immune-boosting phytoherbals with nanoparticle delivery systems holds great promise for enhancing immune health and combating a wide range of diseases. However, further research is needed to optimize nanoparticle formulations, evaluate their safety and efficacy in preclinical and clinical studies, and translate these findings into practical therapeutic strategies for human health (Bhushan et al., 2021). Historically, plants have been utilized both in whole and extract forms for therapeutic purposes. Phytochemicals, also known as secondary metabolites, are compounds produced by plants that play significant roles in traditional medicine. The use of secondary metabolites in herbal medicine is supported by evidence of their diverse biological functions. Their pharmacological actions indicate potential for treating fungal and bacterial infections as well as degenerative conditions, including cancer and diabetes (Galmarini et al., 2012). However, several challenges hinder the clinical application of these compounds, including poor absorption and distribution, along with generally low target specificity. These factors reduce the bioavailability of phytochemicals and ultimately diminish their biological activity. Additionally, high dosages are often required to achieve the desired effects, and some phytochemicals exhibit low stability and susceptibility to acidic environments. One notable example is *Pueraria lobata* (Willd.) Ohwi, from which the principal active ingredient, puerarin, has been isolated from the roots. Puerarin exhibits a wide range of pharmacological activities but is most soluble at only 7.56 mg/mL in a pH 7.4 phosphate buffer, which limits its use. Research on enhancing the bioavailability of puerarin has rapidly expanded in recent years. Various nanotechnologies have been explored to improve puerarin's bioavailability, with some methods demonstrating faster absorption than puerarin suspension (Lall et al., 2015). Figure 1 illustrates the phytoconstituents derived nanomedicines designed for the immune system.

The Tmax is shorter, supporting the enhanced absorption of puerarin. Furthermore, SLN-puerarin exhibited a bioavailability more than three times that of puerarin suspension. The goal of numerous researchers is to create a safe and effective drug delivery system. Recent advancements in the field of nanotechnology have led to a resurgence in the popularity of herbal medicine formulations. Nanoparticles have altered and enhanced the pharmacokinetic properties of various pharmaceuticals, and their application is anticipated to boost the bioavailability and bioactivity of herbal remedies. Many well-known herbal extracts, such as ginseng, green tea, milk thistle, hawthorn, Ginkgo biloba, and grape seed, have also been processed using the phytosome method (Kesarwani et al., 2013). Medications can be adsorbed or linked to the surface of nanoparticles, as well as incorporated or dissolved within them. Encapsulating drugs in nanoparticles (NPs) can enhance their solubility and pharmacokinetics. In some cases, this can also advance the clinical development of novel chemical entities that have stalled in pharmacokinetic research.

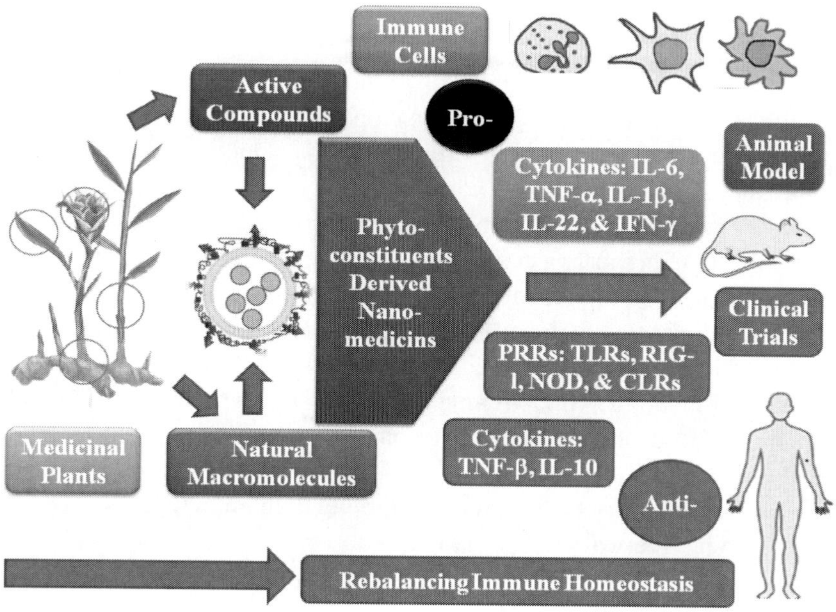

Figure 1. Phytoconstituents derived nanomedicines for immune system.

Biodegradable natural and synthetic high molecular polymers primarily serve as carriers for these nanoparticles (Goyal et al., 2011). Herbal treatments are generally considered safer and less expensive than synthetic medications. However, herbal medicines do have certain drawbacks, including poor solubility, stability, and absorption. Some may undergo chemical and physical degradation, which reduces their medicinal potency. Nanotechnology-based herbal medicinal formulations aim to address these issues (Bonifacio et al., 2014). The immune system protects the host from infections and cancers, adapting to meet the body's evolving needs in response to both internal and external environments. Various perturbations can cause the immune system to either become suppressed or overstimulated. Therefore, before any novel chemicals or biological entities can be used in industry, biology, or medicine, they must undergo thorough investigations into their interactions with the immune system. Nanoscale particles can be artificially produced or found in nature. When nanoparticles interact with the immune system, they can provide potential medical benefits, such as in vaccines or treatments for autoimmune and inflammatory diseases (Chauhan et al., 2009). The following are potential advantages of using nanoparticle-based delivery systems:

- Site-specific delivery of genes, peptides, and medications
- Increased stability both *in vivo* and *in vitro*
- Reduced side effects

Immunosuppression

Immunosuppression can occur either accidentally or voluntarily. While it has the potential to reduce the body's resistance to infections and malignant cells, immunosuppression can also enhance the therapeutic effects of treatments for autoimmune diseases and allergies, as well as minimize the rejection of transplanted organs. Traditional toxicological studies have primarily focused on the undesirable consequences of immunosuppression; however, there is limited research specifically addressing the effects of nanoparticles in this context. Most studies to date have examined how nanoparticles induce inflammation. One of the few investigations into immunosuppression found that inhaling carbon nanotubes (CNTs) inhibits B cell activity, with a crucial component of this reported immunosuppressive process being TGF-β produced by alveolar macrophages (Shrivastava et al., 2014). Further research has shown that nanoparticles can effectively deliver immunosuppressive medications and that they can prevent the immunosuppressive qualities of small-molecule drugs. For instance, in a mouse model of arthritis, glucocorticoids were delivered intravenously (IV) to the inflamed joints using poly(D,L-lactide-co-glycolide) (PLGA) nanoparticles. The targeted and regulated release of steroids from the PLGA nanoparticles led to a complete remission of the inflammatory response and increased efficacy. Another example is Abraxane, a chemotherapy agent approved by the FDA, which is a colloidal suspension of nanoparticles containing human serum albumin with paclitaxel bound to it (Agarwal et al., 2013).

Immunostimulation

Recent evidence suggests that cancer progression may be accelerated by the activation of the complement system at tumor sites, which in turn enhances tumor-associated immune cells and encourages their transformation into a tumor-supportive phenotype. This reaction could impact the effectiveness of nanoparticle formulations as treatment or diagnostic tools for cancer. Conversely, if nanoparticles are designed for subcutaneous (SC) administration, complement activation may enhance vaccine efficacy (Singh et al., 2011). The rapidly expanding field of nanomedicine has highlighted these findings, underscoring the need to clarify the relationship between complement activation and nanoparticle toxicity. Understanding this relationship is crucial for advancing nanotechnology-based formulations for medicinal applications, even though many questions remain unanswered (Nayak et al., 2010). Table 1 provides a summary of the applications of immune-boosting phytoherbals combined with nanoparticle delivery systems.

Nanotechnology

Known as a submicrometer system, a nanoscale system has a particle diameter of 0.1 μm. Researchers are increasingly investigating this nanotechnology due to its numerous advantages related to various factors, such as the route of administration and improved therapeutic effects. Because nanoscale systems can minimize negative effects, enhance activity, and reduce dosages, many studies have linked herbal medicine with nanotechnology (Chidambaram et al., 2011). Herbal medications utilizing nanotechnology-based delivery systems hold significant promise and possess unique qualities. For example, they can transform unstable, poorly absorbed, and less soluble compounds into potentially effective medications. Consequently, nanotechnology-based delivery systems provide a viable strategy to enhance the efficacy of herbal medicine and address some of its inherent challenges (Thapa et al., 2013).

Table 1. Some examples of applications of immune-boosting phytoherbals with nanoparticle delivery

Phytoherbal	Active Compound(s)	Nanoparticle Type	Application/Use
Echinacea	Echinacoside	Liposomes	Boosting immune response against infections promoting overall immune health
	Alkamides	Polymeric	
	Polysaccharides	Nanoparticles	
Turmeric	Curcumin	Polymeric	Providing antioxidant support (Hou et al., 2008)
		Nanoparticles	
Astragalus	Astragaloside IV	Liposomes	Supporting immune system function, improving resistance to infections, and enhancing overall health
	Polysaccharides	Polymeric	
Ginseng	Ginsenosides	Liposomes	Improving immune response, reducing inflammation, & increasing resistance to infections
	Polysaccharides	Polymeric	
Garlic	Allicin	Liposomes	Enhancing immune function, reducing oxidative stress & providing antimicrobial support
	Alliin	Polymeric	
Green Tea	Epigallocatechin Gallate (EGCG)	Liposomes	Boosting immune response, providing antioxidant (Yen et al., 2008)
		Polymeric	Support, and reducing inflammation
Elderberry	Anthocyanins	Liposomes	Strengthening immune function, reducing duration & severity of cold and flu symptoms
	Flavonoids	Polymeric	
Reishi Mushroom	β-glucans	Liposomes	Enhancing immune function, modulating inflammation, and supporting overall health
	Triterpenoids	Polymeric	
Andrographis	Andro-grapholides	Liposomes	Supporting immune response against infections, reducing inflammation, and promoting respiratory health
		Polymeric	
Cat's Claw	Alkaloids	Liposomes	Boosting immune system function, reducing oxidative stress, & supporting gastrointestinal health
	Quinovic Acid	Polymeric	
Licorice	Glycyrrhizin	Liposomes	Enhancing immune function, reducing inflammation, & supporting respiratory health
	Flavonoids	Polymeric	
Schisandra	Lignans	Liposomes	Improving immune response, enhancing liver function, and reducing stress
	Schisandrins	Polymeric	
Olive Leaf	Oleuropein	Liposomes	Supporting immune system function, providing antioxidant support, and promoting cardiovascular health
	Hydroxytyrosol	Polymeric	
Rhodiola	Salidroside	Liposomes	Enhancing immune function, reducing fatigue, and supporting stress adaptation
	Rosavin	Polymeric	
Ginseng (Panax ginseng)	Ginsenosides	Liposomes	Improving immune response, reducing inflammation & increasing resistance to infections
		Polymeric	

Table 1. (Continued)

Phytoherbal	Active Compound(s)	Nanoparticle Type	Application/Use
Ashwagandha (Withania somnifera)	Withanolides	Liposomes	Enhancing immune function, reducing stress, and promoting overall well-being (Ajazuddin et al., 2010)
	Withaferin A	Polymeric	
HolyBasil (Ocimum sanctum)	Eugenol	Liposomes	Boosting immune system function, reducing inflammation & providing antioxidant support
	Ursolic acid	Polymeric	
	Rosmarinic acid	nanoparticles	
Moringa (Moringa oleifera)	Quercetin	Liposomes	Enhancing immune function, providing antioxidant support & promoting overall health
	Kaempferol	Polymeric	
Aloe Vera	Acemannan	Liposomes	Supporting immune response, reducing inflammation, & promoting skin health
	Polysaccharides	Polymeric	

Nanotechnology-Based Drug Delivery System for Phytochemical Compounds

Seventy percent of the active compounds derived from plants are hydrophobic, according to the literature. One strategy to enhance the bioavailability and bioactivity of phytochemical substances is to employ innovative technologies. The ability to develop appropriate drug delivery formulations is crucial for the advancement of novel nanotechnology-based therapeutics. Effective disease prevention and treatment necessitate the administration of phytochemicals. These delivery methods, which can boost the bioactivity of phytochemical substances, include lipid- and polymer-based systems (Gupta et al., 2010). Two varieties of nanoparticle systems, solid lipid nanoparticles (SLNs) and nanostructured lipid carriers (NLCs), feature lipid cores made from either solid or liquid-lipid blends. The bioavailability of medications that undergo significant first-pass metabolism and exhibit hydrophobicity can be increased by using nanoemulsions. The components of the nanoemulsion system consist of water-soluble cosolvents, oils, lipids, surfactants, and water (Aw et al., 2012). The most prevalent and extensively researched class of nanocarriers comprises lipid-based nanostructures. Among these, the delivery of liposomes and phytosomes is considered the most effective strategy. Liposomes can enhance the solubility, effectiveness, and bioavailability of medications due to their high levels of biocompatibility and biodegradability. They can encapsulate both lipophilic and hydrophilic medications. For instance, tetrandrine and curcumin are phytochemicals with limited solubility, resulting in reduced bioavailability (Elzoghby et al., 2012). The results demonstrated that following encapsulation into liposome carriers, both tetrandrine and curcumin exhibited improved solubility and bioavailability. Additionally, *in vivo* studies have indicated that this system poses no significant risk to zebrafish. However, liposomes can present challenges, such as self-leakage and stability issues when exposed to certain medications. The addition of dioleoylphosphatidylcholine (DP) markedly increases both the loading dose and encapsulation efficiency of tetrandrine and curcumin. Furthermore, the particle size distribution is significantly enhanced (Cajot et al., 2012). Figure 2 illustrates the different types of nano-phytoconstituents.

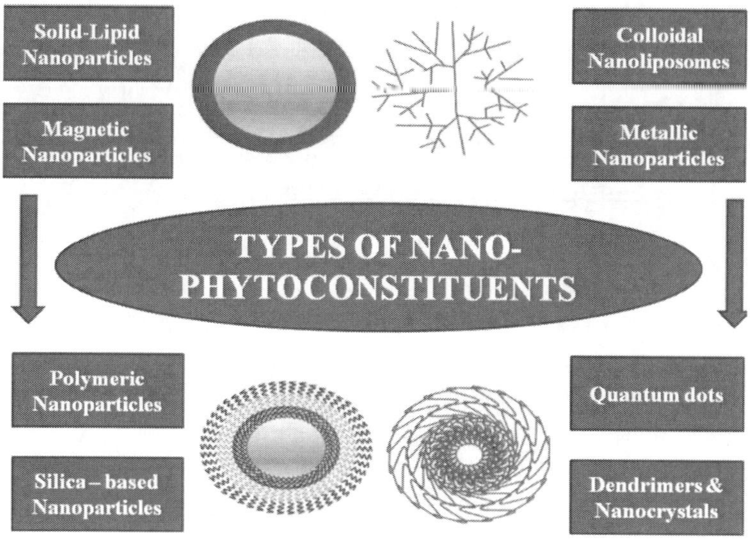

Figure 2. Types of different nano-phytocontituents.

Strategies for Specific Delivery to Immune Cells

Tumor-associated macrophages (TAMs) refer to the predominant immune cells that invade tumors, specifically macrophages. However, these receptors are also found in healthy macrophages and monocytes, playing a crucial role in the immune system's functionality (Mukerjee et al., 2009). Dendritic cells (DCs) are capable of binding to dextran nanoparticles (Dex-NPs) treated with acetal. Given that DCs function as antigen presenters, various strategies are employed in the development of vaccines utilizing these nanocarriers to enhance DC activity. These strategies may include the use of adjuvants or the incorporation of ovalbumin (OVA) protein peptides, such as OT-1. Such approaches can stimulate CD8+ T cells, with some also capable of stimulating CD4+ T cells and promoting their proliferation. This can amplify the immune response surrounding the tumor and impede its growth. Additional studies have indicated that mannose-modified nanoparticles can improve dendritic cells' uptake of antigens (Verma et al., 2013). Table 2 outlines the nanoparticles and their interactions with the immune system.

Table 2. Nanoparticles and immune system interaction

Sr. No.	Nanoparticles	Interactions
1	Neutrophils	– Modulating migration – Depleting inflammation-related neutrophils – Neutrophil-based drug delivery – Neutrophil membrane-coated techniques
2	T/B lymphocytes	– Inducing T cell-related immune tolerance – Depleting auto-reactive – T lymphocytes Inhibiting auto-reactive B lymphocytes
3	Inflammation-related molecules	– Neutralizing inflammatory cytokines – Scavenging ROS and RNS – Inhibiting activity of MPO – Eliminating cell-free DNA
4	Monocytes/ Macrophages	– Inhibiting monocyte production and egression – Modulating mobilization and recruitment – Depleting hyperactive macrophages – Modulating macrophage polarization – Macrophage biomimetic techniques
5	Dendritic cells	– Inducing tolerogenic phenotype – Regulating antigen presentation
6	NK cells	– Enhancing cytotoxicity towards unwanted cells – NK cell monitoring techniques

Nano Formulations in Immunology

Nanomaterials are classified into "soft" or "hard" categories based on their composition, size, and structure. This classification framework, introduced by Tomalia, highlights the diverse techniques used to create these materials. Hard nanostructures, which often incorporate noble metals such as silver, gold, and platinum, are noteworthy for their unique optical and electrical properties. These characteristics enable their application in various fields, including imaging, sensors, catalysis, optical filters, medical biology, and cancer treatment. Metal nanoparticles serve as theranostic agents, offering a dual platform for therapeutic and diagnostic applications, while also exhibiting bactericidal properties. Additionally, they demonstrate efficacy in cancer therapies through photothermal and radiation treatments (Hammond, 2017). The synthesis of these nanoparticles can be achieved through various chemical, photochemical, and radiolytic processes. The specific properties of the resulting nanomaterials depend on the synthesis method, which can be fine-tuned by selecting appropriate precursors and technologies. Metal nanoparticles tend to agglomerate during growth and nucleation, necessitating the use of various ligands, stabilizers, and supports to control their development. Among these, micelles and polymers have proven effective, with commercially available polymers and ligands such as calixarenes, cyclodextrins, and macrocycles serving as reliable stabilizing agents. However, concerns regarding the release of certain metals into biological media during imaging due to their toxicity have been raised (Poon et al., 2011). Quantum dots (QDs) exhibit distinct physico-optical characteristics that could significantly advance diagnostic and therapeutic applications. Nonetheless, their intrinsic toxicity limits potential translational uses, necessitating further surface passivation, which can occasionally lead to a quenching of luminescence (Richards et al., 2005). Soft nanoparticles, primarily composed of various precursors like lipids (liposomes), polymers, dendrimers, and other organic compounds, form the backbone of nanotechnology-driven medicine. These nanoparticles possess advantageous features, including significant drug loading capacity, programmed release capabilities, low toxicity, high biocompatibility, and improved photoluminescence and quantum yield. Their properties make soft nanoparticles particularly appealing for biomedical applications, especially in therapeutic contexts. Surface modifications can enhance their water solubility and facilitate conjugation with biomolecules for targeted therapeutic action (Sekaly, 2008). Moreover, their potential as theranostic agents is amplified when coupled with fluorescent dyes and/or therapeutic compounds. In summary, while nanoparticles have a wide range of applications from biofouling to electronics, this work emphasizes their interactions with the immune system in the context of cancer therapy (Tomalia, 2009).

Liposomes

Among the first members of the soft nanomaterials are liposomes. These structures are created from phospholipids, which consist of a hydrophilic head and a hydrophobic tail. When using aqueous solvents, liposomes generate vesicle-like formations that can entrap medications in their core. The hydrophobic and hydrophilic interactions between lipids and lipid-water lead to bilayered structures. Since plasma lipoproteins are naturally occurring lipid nanoparticles and phospholipids make up the foundation of cell membranes, liposomes are biocompatible and typically exhibit little to no toxicity (Jain et al., 2008). Many medications, including doxorubicin and amphotericin, have significantly increased therapeutic indices since the introduction of liposomes in medicine. This is accomplished by enhancing pharmacokinetics and biodistribution. However, liposomes often face rapid removal from circulation due to opsonization by plasma constituents and internalization by macrophages in the reticuloendothelial system (RES). A popular solution to this challenge is the use of PEGylation polymers. PEG chains enhance the concentration of hydrated groups on the surface, reducing the formulation's internalization by the RES by sterically inhibiting hydrophobic and electrostatic interactions with plasma proteins. Liposomes vary greatly in size, which influences their interaction with the immune system. Larger liposomes typically experience greater clearance than smaller ones (Andre et al., 2016).

Polymeric Nanoparticles

Numerous biodegradable polymers with low off-target toxicities have been employed as drug delivery vehicles, enhancing therapeutic efficacy. Specialized polymers, such as PLA and PLGA, have garnered significant interest due to their ability to release chemotherapeutic drugs in a controlled manner while maintaining biocompatibility. Additionally, other polymers derived from natural sources, such as chitosan and sodium alginate, have also been utilized as drug delivery agents. Another significant category of soft nanomaterials includes lipid- or protein-based nanoparticles, which offer unique properties for targeted therapy (Guerineau et al., 2019).

Nanoparticle Mediated Immunotoxicity

The immunotoxicity of nanoparticles is a crucial factor to consider in clinical settings, despite their high payload capacity, low dosage, and targeting ability, which make them desirable candidates for cancer treatment. The interaction between nanoparticles (NPs) and biological agents is vital for their effective distribution, clearance, and accumulation *in vivo*, especially for the systemic delivery of medications. The primary role of the immune system is to defend the body from foreign objects considered dangerous. The immune system can be divided into two main categories: innate and adaptive immunity. Innate immunity produces a non-specific inflammatory response when it encounters exogenous bioactive substances, such as strains of bacteria or viruses. This system utilizes various receptors to recognize pathogens, leading to the activation of the acquired immune system by antigen-presenting cells (APCs). Upon initial contact with biofluids, NPs are exposed to different proteins, resulting in the formation of a protein corona, also known as the crown effect (Clement et al., 2020).

Size and Structural Importance of Nanoparticles in Immunological Considerations

Large-sized NPs typically interact with APCs that are widely distributed throughout tissues. In contrast, NPs smaller than 200 nm tend to circulate through lymphatic and venous drainage, enhancing antigen presentation. A significant challenge for NP utilization is their retention in the liver, which is primarily influenced by size; larger NPs are retained more than smaller ones. However, smaller NPs are quickly removed by the lymphatic system, allowing local dendritic cells to absorb them. In addition to size, the shape of NPs plays a crucial role in determining an appropriate immune response. Reports indicate that macrophages are significantly more likely to absorb rod-shaped NPs with a higher surface area compared to spherical NPs. This preference is largely attributed to the vesicles formed, which facilitate easier engulfment through micropinocytosis. The aspect ratio of rod-shaped NPs has also been shown to influence the release of cytokines; a higher aspect ratio correlates with increased levels of several inflammatory markers, such as IL-6 and IFN-γ. Furthermore, studies have investigated complement activation using nanoparticles with altered shapes but the same surface area (Willis et al., 1998).

Conclusion

In conclusion, integrating immune-boosting phytoherbals with nanoparticle delivery systems represents a promising avenue for advancing immunotherapy. This comprehensive investigation highlights the potential synergies between traditional herbal medicine and modern nanotechnology, emphasizing the importance of a holistic approach to immune system modulation. The globalization of trade has facilitated the integration of diverse herbal medicines worldwide, providing a rich pool of therapeutic agents. Nanotechnology-based delivery systems address the limitations of herbal medicines, such as low solubility, bioavailability, and stability. By encapsulating phytochemical constituents in nanoparticles, their pharmacological activity can be enhanced, expanding their clinical applications. However, developing these nanotechnology-based delivery systems requires further review, particularly regarding safety and toxicity profiles, to ensure their effectiveness in treating various diseases. The rapid development of nanotechnology has equipped researchers with new tools for immune modulation, particularly in managing inflammatory diseases. Immunomodulatory nanodrugs hold significant potential to target and accumulate in inflamed tissues, addressing the pathogenic factors of inflammatory diseases more effectively than current palliative treatments.

References

Agarwal, P., Shashi, A., Amreen, F., & Verma, A. (2013). Current scenario of herbal technology worldwide: An overview. *International Journal of Pharmaceutical Sciences & Research, 4*, 4105–4117.

Ajazuddin, & Saraf, S. S. (2010). Applications of novel drug delivery system for herbal formulations. *Fitoterapia, 81*(7), 680–689.

André, E., Boutonnet, B., Charles, P., Martini, C., Aguiar-Hualde, J. M., Latil, S., Guérineau, V., Hammad, K., Ray, P., Guillot, R., & Huc, V. (2016). A new, simple and versatile strategy for the synthesis of short segments of zigzag-type carbon nanotubes. *Chemistry, 22*(9), 3105–3114.

Ansari, S. H., Islam, F., & Sameem, M. (2012). Influence of nanotechnology on herbal drugs: A review. *Journal of Advanced Pharmaceutical Technology & Research, 3*(3), 142–146.

Arnold, M., Morgan, E., Rumgay, H., Mafra, A., Singh, D., Laversanne, M., Vignat, J., Gralow, J. R., Cardoso, F., Siesling, S., & Soerjomataram, I. (2022). Current and future burden of breast cancer: Global statistics for 2020 and 2040. *Breast, 66*, 15–23.

Aw, M. S., Addai-Mensah, J., & Losic, D. (2012). A multi-drug delivery system with sequential release using titania nanotube arrays. *Chemical Communications, 48*(27), 3348–3350.

Bardou, V. J., Arpino, G., Elledge, R. M., Osborne, C. K., & Clark, G. M. (2003). Progesterone receptor status significantly improves outcome prediction over estrogen receptor status alone for adjuvant endocrine therapy in two large breast cancer databases. *Journal of Clinical Oncology, 21*(10), 1973–1979.

Bhushan, A., Gonsalves, A., & Menon, J. U. (2021). Current state of breast cancer diagnosis, treatment, and theranostics. *Pharmaceutics, 13*(5), 723.

Bonifácio, B. V., Silva, P. B., Dos Santos Ramos, M. A., Silveira Negri, K. M., Bauab, T. M., & Chorilli, M. (2014). Nanotechnology-based drug delivery systems and herbal medicines: A review. *International Journal of Nanomedicine, 9*, 1–15.

Bray, F., Ferlay, J., Soerjomataram, I., Siegel, L., Torre, A., & Ahmedin, D. (2021). GLOBOCAN estimates of incidence and mortality worldwide for 36 cancers in 185 countries. *Global Cancer Statistics, 73*, 209–249.

Cajot, S., Van Butsele, K., Paillard, A., Passirani, C., Garcion, E., Benoit, J. P., Varshney, S. K., & Jérôme, C. (2012). Smart nanocarriers for pH-triggered targeting and release of hydrophobic drugs. *Acta Biomaterialia, 8*(12), 4215–4223.

Chauhan, N. S., Rajan, G., & Gopalakrishna, B. (2009). Phytosomes: Potential phyto-phospholipid carriers for herbal drug delivery. *Journal of Pharmacy Research, 2*(7), 1267–1270.

Chidambaram, M., Manavalan, R., & Kathiresan, K. (2011). Nanotherapeutics to overcome conventional cancer chemotherapy limitations. *Journal of Pharmacy & Pharmaceutical Sciences, 14*(1), 67–77.

Clément, M., Abdellah, I., Ray, P., Martini, C., Coppel, Y., Remita, H., Lampre, I., & Huc, V. (2020). Synthesis and NMR study of trimethylphosphine gold(I)-appended calix[8]arenes as precursors of gold nanoparticles. *Inorganic Chemistry Frontiers, 7*(4), 953–960.

Dean-Colomb, W., & Esteva, F. J. (2008). Her2-positive breast cancer: Herceptin and beyond. *European Journal of Cancer, 44*(18), 2806–2812.

Elzoghby, A. O., Samy, W. M., & Elgindy, N. A. (2012). Protein-based nanocarriers as promising drug and gene delivery systems. *Journal of Controlled Release, 161*(1), 38–49.

Galmarini, D., Galmarini, C. M., & Galmarini, F. C. (2012). Cancer chemotherapy: A critical analysis of its 60 years of history. *Critical Reviews in Oncology/Hematology, 84*(2), 181–199.

Goyal, A., Kumar, S., Nagpal, M., Singh, I., & Arora, S. (2011). Potential of novel drug delivery systems for herbal drugs. *Indian Journal of Pharmaceutical Education & Research, 45*, 225–235.

Greco, S. J. (2019). Breast cancer risk in a rapidly aging population: Advances and approaches to study the aging tissue microenvironment. *Breast Cancer, 11*, 111–113.

Guérineau, V., Rollet, M., Viel, S., Lepoittevin, B., Costa, L., Saint-Aguet, P., Laurent, R., Roger, P., Gigmes, D., Martini, C., & Huc, V. (2019). The synthesis and characterization of giant calixarenes. *Nature Communications, 10*(1), 113.

Gupta, V. K., Karar, P. K., Ramesh, S., Misra, S. P., & Gupta, A. (2010). Nanoparticle formulation for hydrophilic and hydrophobic drugs. *International Journal of Research in Pharmaceutical Sciences, 1*, 163–169.

Hammond, P. T. (2017). Nano tools pave the way to new solutions in infectious disease. *ACS Infectious Diseases, 3*(8), 554–558.

Harvey, J. M., Clark, G. M., Osborne, C. K., & Allred, D. C. (1999). Estrogen receptor status by immunohistochemistry is superior to the ligand-binding assay for predicting response to adjuvant endocrine therapy in breast cancer. *Journal of Clinical Oncology, 17*(5), 1474–1481.

Hawkins, R. A., Killen, E., Tesdale, A. L., Sangster, K., Thomson, M., Steele, R. J., & Blackie, R. A. (1988). Oestrogen receptors, lactate dehydrogenase and cellularity in human breast cancer. *Clinica Chimica Acta; International Journal of Clinical Chemistry, 175*(1), 89–96.

Hou, J., & Zhou, S. W. (2008). Formulation and preparation of glycyrrhizic acid solid lipid nanoparticles. *Acta Academiae Medicinae Militaris Tertiae, 30*, 1043–1045.

Jain, P. K., & El-Sayed, M. A. (2008). Noble metal nanoparticle pairs: Effect of medium for enhanced nanosensing. *Nano Letters, 8*(12), 4347–4352.

Kesarwani, K., Gupta, R., & Mukerjee, A. (2013). Bioavailability enhancers of herbal origin: An overview. *Asian Pacific Journal of Tropical Biomedicine, 3*(4), 253–266.

Lall, R. K., Syed, D. N., Adhami, V. M., Khan, M. I., & Mukhtar, H. (2015). Dietary polyphenols in prevention and treatment of prostate cancer. *International Journal of Molecular Sciences, 16*(2), 3350–3376.

Mukerjee, A., & Vishwanatha, J. K. (2009). Formulation, characterization and evaluation of curcumin-loaded PLGA nanospheres for cancer therapy. *Anticancer Research, 29*(10), 3867–3875.

Nayak, A. P., Tiyaboonchai, W., Patankar, S., & Madhusudhan, B. (2010). Curcuminoids loaded lipid nanoparticles: Novel approach to treat malaria treatment. Amsterdam: Elsevier.

Poon, Z., Chang, D., Zhao, X., & Hammond, P. T. (2011). Layer-by-layer nanoparticles with a pH-sheddable layer for *in vivo* targeting of tumor hypoxia. *ACS Nano, 5*(6), 4284–4292.

Richards, R., & Bönnemann, H. (2005). Synthesis approaches to metallic nanomaterials, applications and impact. *Wiley-VCH Verlag, 3*.

Sekaly, R. P. (2008). The failed HIV Merck vaccine study: A step back or a launching point for future vaccine development? *Journal of Experimental Medicine, 205*(1), 7–12.

Shnoudeh, A. J., Qadumii, L., Zihlif, M., Al-Ameer, H. J., Salou, R. A., Jaber, A. Y., & Hamad, I. (2022). Green synthesis of gold, iron and selenium nanoparticles using phytoconstituents: Preliminary evaluation of antioxidant and biocompatibility potential. *Molecules, 27*(4), 1334.

Shrivastava, A. K., Srivastava, A. K., & Prakash, D. (2014). Herbal immunomodulators: A review. *International Journal of Pharmaceutical Sciences & Research, 5*, 1192–1207.

Singh, R. P., Singh, S. G., Naik, H., Jain, D., & Bisla, S. (2011). Herbal excipients in novel drug delivery system. *International Journal of Comprehensive Pharmacy, 2*, 1–7.

Sørlie, T., Perou, C. M., Tibshirani, R., Aas, T., Geisler, S., Johnsen, H., Hastie, T., Eisen, M. B., Van De Rijn, M., Jeffrey, S. S., Thorsen, T., Quist, H., Matese, J. C., Brown, P. O., Botstein, D., Lønning, P. E., & Børresen-Dale, A. L. (2001). Gene expression patterns of breast carcinomas distinguish tumor subclasses with clinical implications. *Proceedings of the National Academy of Sciences of the United States of America, 98*(19), 10869–10874.

Sørlie, T., Borgan, E., Myhre, S., Vollan, H. K., Russnes, H., Zhao, X., Nilsen, G., Lingjaerde, O. C., Børresen-Dale, A. L., & Rødland, E. (2010). The importance of gene-centering microarray data. *Lancet Oncology, 11*(8), 719–720.

Thapa, R. K., Khan, G. M., Baral, K. P., & Thapa, P. (2013). Herbal medicine incorporated nanoparticles: Advancements in herbal treatment. *Asian Journal of Biomedical & Pharmaceutical Sciences, 3*(24), 7–14.

Tomalia, D. A. (2009). In quest of a systematic framework for unifying and defining nanoscience. *Journal of Nanoparticle Research, 11*(6), 1251–1310.

Turashvili, G., & Brogi, E. (2017). Tumor heterogeneity in breast cancer. *Frontiers in Medicine, 4*, 227.

Verma, H., Prasad, S. B., Singh, Y., & Singh, H. (2013). Herbal drug delivery system: A modern era prospective. *International Journal of Current Pharmaceutical Review & Research, 4*(3), 88–101.

Willis, M., & Forssen, E. (1998). Ligand-targeted liposomes. *Advanced Drug Delivery Reviews, 29*(3), 249–271.

Yen, F. L., Wu, T. H., Lin, L. T., Cham, T. M., & Lin, C. C. (2008). Nanoparticles formulation of *Cuscuta chinensis* prevents acetaminophen-induced hepatotoxicity in rats. *Food & Chemical Toxicology, 46*(5), 1771–1777.

Chapter 16

Applications of Nanophytoherbals in Inflammation Therapy

Swati Verma[1]
Manasvi Saini[2]
Neelam Singh[3]
Chaitanya Vinayak Narayan[1,*]
[1]I.T.S. College of Pharmacy, Delhi-Meerut Road, Ghaziabad, Uttar Pradesh, India
[2]College of Pharmacy, Shivalik Campus, Dehradun, Uttrakhand, India
[3]Noida Institute of Engineering and Technology (Pharmacy Institute), Greater Noida, Uttar Pradesh, India

Abstract

Inflammation is a crucial response orchestrated by the immune system to ensure survival in the face of infection and tissue injury. This process is vital for maintaining normal tissue balance. The intricate molecular mechanisms underlying inflammation are initiated by recognizing specific patterns associated with infection or tissue damage. Key regulators control the entire inflammatory response by selectively expressing pro-inflammatory molecules. However, prolonged inflammation can have severe adverse effects on health. Nanoformulations of herbal phytoconstituents have emerged as a promising approach to manage inflammation. These nanophytoherbals provide a positive direction for addressing inflammatory conditions. Phototherapeutic strategies necessitate a scientific approach for delivering active herbal extracts in a controlled manner to enhance patient collaboration and minimize the need for recurrent doses. This is achievable through the development of novel drug delivery systems (NDDS) for herbal components. NDDS can reduce the need for repeated doses to overcome ineffectiveness while enhancing potency by decreasing toxicity and increasing drug bioavailability. Furthermore, an overview of current advancements in this field highlights characteristics that contribute to favorable outcomes. Looking ahead, the combination of nano-photothermal constituents with existing therapies presents an opportunity to manage inflammation effectively and mitigate its consequences over time.

Keywords: inflammation, nanoparticles, nanophytoherbal constituents, NDDS, bioavailability

* Corresponding Author's Email: chaitanayvinayak@gmail.com.

In: Phyto-Nanomedicine
Editors: Hitesh Chopra, Vinod Kumar Gauttam, Ajmer Singh Grewal et al.
ISBN: 979-8-89530-317-7

Abbreviations

ALA	Alpha-lipoic acid
RES	Resveratrol
SLNs	Solid lipid nanoparticles
PNPs	Polymeric Nanoparticles
PPH	Polyphenols
Eos	Essential oils
NDDS	Novel drug delivery systems
PEG2	Prostaglandin 2
NOS	Nitric oxide synthase

Introduction

In higher-living organisms, inflammation acts as a defense mechanism against harmful stimuli such as microbial infections, tissue damage, and other adverse conditions. It serves as an essential part of the immune system's response to protect the body. Foreign bodies, such as diseases, thorns, or irritants, can trigger this response. Pathogens like bacteria, viruses, parasites, and fungi are common causes of inflammation, with bacteria and viruses being the most frequent infectious agents responsible for initiating this process. Inflammation is crucial in containing infections, repairing tissue, and restoring normal function (Zeng et al., 2017). Endotoxins are toxic substances released by bacteria, particularly Gram-negative bacteria, that can trigger inflammation by activating immune cells. In addition to bacterial toxins, viruses entering the body can also provoke an inflammatory response by infecting and killing host cells. Inflammation can also arise due to inadequate blood flow to affected areas, leading to a lack of oxygen (hypoxia) and nutrients. This impaired circulation, often seen in conditions like ischemia, disrupts cellular function and can cause tissue damage. Oxygen plays a critical role in cellular functions, including wound healing, brain protection, and overall cellular metabolism. A deficiency in oxygen can hinder these vital processes, leading to adverse health outcomes (González-Muniesa et al., 2016). Injury and infection initiate inflammation, a critical immune response that helps with wound healing and controlling infections. Key to this process are pattern recognition receptors (PRRs), such as mannose-binding lectin-like receptors and nucleotide-binding oligomerisation domains (NODs). These receptors recognize molecular patterns associated with pathogens or cellular damage. Upon activation, they trigger intracellular signaling pathways, notably the nuclear factor-κB (NF-κB) pathway, which plays a pivotal role in regulating the immune response. This signaling leads to the production of adhesion molecules, which facilitate the movement of immune cells to the site of injury or infection, accelerating the inflammatory process. This cascade ensures that the immune system can respond effectively to eliminate harmful stimuli and promote tissue repair (Watkins et al., 1995). The initiation of the inflammatory response begins when cells in the affected area release chemical substances known as cytokines, which include interleukins, growth factors, and chemokines. These cytokines are essential for activating immune cells and orchestrating the body's defense mechanisms. They facilitate the movement of leukocytes (white blood cells) to the site of inflammation, where these cells work to eliminate harmful agents, such as pathogens, and clear away damaged or dead tissue. During inflammation, a key physiological response is vasodilation, which increases blood flow to the affected area. This increased blood circulation helps deliver immune cells and nutrients to the site of injury or infection, promoting the healing process. However, the enhanced blood flow can also cause a reduction in blood pressure, especially if widespread vasodilation occurs, leading to a drop in systemic vascular resistance. This complex interplay of cellular signals and blood flow changes is central to managing infections and repairing tissue damage during the inflammatory process (Serhan et al., 2010). After the inflammatory response subsides, the body activates repair mechanisms to restore the injured tissue and fill any gaps with fibrous tissue, a process critical for wound healing and tissue regeneration (Tidball, 2005). Herbal products, derived from plants and microorganisms, offer therapeutic benefits due to the natural compounds produced by these organisms. These medicines can address a wide range of health conditions, including bacterial infections, inflammation, and even cancer. Herbal remedies are often favored for their potency, accessibility, and cost-effectiveness, in addition to having minimal or no side effects. Furthermore, many people consider herbal medicines safer and more effective compared to synthetic drugs (EI-Refai et al., 2018). However, despite their benefits, herbal medications face some challenges. For example, they often have poor solubility in water, making them difficult to absorb effectively. Additionally, their therapeutic effects may be limited due to rapid metabolism in the body, and their stability can be compromised by light sensitivity (Oguntibeju, 2018). Many herbal medications are widely used today to combat inflammation due to their numerous benefits. Resveratrol (RES), a naturally occurring polyphenolic phytoalexin, is produced by over 70 plant species in response to stress, with its levels influenced primarily by fungal presence and weather conditions. Found in fruits like blueberries, blackberries, and peanuts (Chung et al., 2020). RES has been shown to possess significant anti-inflammatory properties. It helps protect against inflammation by reducing the production and release of pro-inflammatory substances, altering the synthesis of compounds involved in inflammation, and inhibiting specific immune cells or enzymes responsible for generating pro-inflammatory molecules. Resveratrol exerts these effects by acting on transcription factors like AP-1 and NF-kappa B, which play crucial roles in the production of pro-inflammatory mediators (de Sá Coutinho et al., 2018). Ginger, the root of the Zingiber officinale plant, has long been recognized as a natural remedy for inflammation. Its active compounds, gingerols and shogaols, exhibit potent anti-inflammatory effects. Ginger works by promoting heat production and inhibiting the release of pro-inflammatory substances, effectively reducing inflammation, swelling, and pain. This versatile herb has traditionally been used to address various health issues, including colds, digestive problems, and migraines (Funk et al., 2016). Garlic (Allium sativum L.) has been widely used as a remedy for inflammation due to its rich content of organic sulfur compounds, with allicin being the primary active component in its volatile oil. Allicin exhibits a range of biological properties, including anti-inflammatory, antibacterial, and antifungal effects. Although the precise mechanism of garlic's action remains unclear, studies suggest that its anti-inflammatory properties may result from its ability to inhibit the COX-2 enzyme, which blocks the production of prostaglandin (PEG2) and nitric oxide in macrophage cells (Lee et al., 2012). Chili pepper is a widely used spice worldwide, with its primary active ingredient being capsaicin (CAP), known for its inflammation-reducing properties. Capsaicin has been formulated into patches and gels for the treatment of discomfort. Its anti-inflammatory effect is attributed to its ability to inhibit the activity of the COX-2 enzyme, which subsequently reduces the activation of nitric oxide synthase (NOS) and lowers the production of prostaglandin E2 (Lu et al., 2020). Lipoic acid, a disulfide compound derived from octanoic acid, includes alpha-lipoic acid (ALA), which is a form of thioctic acid naturally produced by animals and plants. Its anti-inflammatory properties arise from its ability to suppress pro-inflammatory cytokines, inhibit NF-κB activation, and stimulate nitric oxide synthase. Research has demonstrated a close connection between its antioxidant properties and its anti-inflammatory effects (Wang and Xia, 2014). Curcumin, a hydrophobic compound found in the rhizome of Curcuma longa, comprises small polyphenols. Historically, it has been used as a paste for pain relief (Wal et al., 2019). Nanotechnology is a cutting-edge technology with diverse applications across various industries. In pharmaceuticals, it has been employed to develop formulations that specifically target diseased organs, thereby minimizing the adverse effects associated with the accumulation of medication in unintended areas. Moreover, nanotechnology enhances patient adherence compared to traditional treatments (Son et al., 2017). Nanoparticles are minuscule particles that range in size from 1 to 100 nanometers. These microscopic particles are too small to be seen by the naked eye and possess unique chemical and physical properties compared to their larger counterparts (Wang et al., 2017). Nanoparticles are constructed from biocompatible materials that can be easily degraded, such as solid lipids or polymers. These materials can be natural, like gelatin or albumin, or synthetic, such as polylactides or polyalkylcyanoacrylates. When utilized for drug delivery in the body, nanoparticles are typically released from their matrix through processes like degradation, erosion, swelling, or diffusion. The use of nanoparticles as drug carriers offers several advantages, including a long shelf life and the capacity to hold a substantial amount of medication (Son et al., 2017). Some common nanophytoherbals that are beneficial in relieving pain are listed in Table 1.

Solid Lipid Nanoparticles (SLNs)

SLNs are small carriers composed of purified lipids derived from solid fats, stabilized by suractants. These nanoparticles typically range in size from 50 to 1000 nm and can be utilized for drug delivery via various routes, including oral and parenteral administration. SLNs combine the advantages of both polymeric nanoparticles (PNPs) and liposomes, providing effective protection against drug degradation, reduced toxicity, and excellent stability. One successful formulation involved stearic acid-based SLNs coated with poloxamer 188 and loaded with resveratrol. Using the solvent diffusion-solvent evaporation method, these lipid nanoparticles achieved a remarkable 8.035-fold increase in the oral bioavailability of resveratrol compared to a standard drug suspension (Penalva et al., 2015). Additionally, lavender essential oil can be encapsulated in SLNs and transformed into a gel for treating topical inflammation. In this formulation, cocoa butter was used as the solid lipid, while Tween 80% served as the surfactant. Given lavender's limited water solubility and low bioavailability, encapsulating it in SLNs addresses these challenges. The anti-inflammatory properties of lavender-based SLNs were evaluated using the carrageenan-induced edema method, revealing a 28 ± 0.1% inhibition of edema at a 1% concentration, compared to a 33.6 ± 0.05% inhibition by diclofenac gel (Chaudhari and Bind, 2019).

Table 1. Sources, phytoconstituents, mechanisms, and potential benefits of nanophytoherbals

Nano-phytoherbal	Source	Phyto-constituent	Mechanism	Potential benefits	References
Curcumin Nanoparticles	Turmeric (*Curcuma longa*)	Curcumin	Inhibits NF-κB pathway, reduces cytokine production	Reduces pain, swelling, and inflammation	Wal et al., 2019
Quercetin Nanoparticles	Onion (*Allium cepa*), apples (*Malus domestica*)	Quercetin	Antioxidant, inhibits histamine release, reduces oxidative stress	Alleviates chronic inflammation, supports immune function	Ozdal et al., 2019
Resveratrol Nanoparticles	Grapes (*Vitis vinifera*)	Resveratrol	Modulates inflammatory pathways and enhances antioxidant defense	Reduces markers of inflammation and oxidative damage	Chung et al., 2020
Ginger Extract Nanoparticles	Ginger (*Zingiber officinale*)	Gingerol	Inhibits COX-2 enzyme, reduces prostaglandin synthesis	Eases pain and inflammation in various conditions	Funk et al., 2016
Green Tea Extract Nanoparticles	Green Tea (*Camellia sinensis*)	Catechins (e.g., EGCG)	Antioxidant modulates inflammatory cytokines	Reduces chronic inflammation and oxidative stress	Chung et al., 2020
Boswellia Serrata Extract Nanoparticles	Frankincense (*Boswellia serrata*)	Boswellic acids	Inhibits leukotriene synthesis, modulates the immune response	Provides relief in arthritis and other inflammatory conditions	Chung et al., 2020
Aloe Vera Extract Nanoparticles	Aloe Vera (*Aloe barbadensis*)	Polysaccharides, anthraquinones	Reduces cytokine levels, promotes tissue repair	Helps in wound healing, reduces local inflammation	Surjushe et al., 2008
Guggul Extract Nanoparticles	Guggul (*Commiphora wightii*)	Guggulsterones	Inhibits pro-inflammatory enzymes, modulates lipid metabolism	Assists in managing chronic inflammatory diseases	Wang and Xia, 2014

Furthermore, curcumin was incorporated into SLNs to enhance its biopharmaceutical effectiveness. The SLNs were formulated using Compritol 888 ATO, soy lecithin, and polysorbate 80. The evaluation of these SLNs was conducted in rats with incomplete Freund's adjuvant-induced arthritis, demonstrating the potential of SLNs as an innovative method for delivering curcumin to inflamed joints (Arora et al., 2016).

Liposomes

Liposomes are small, spherical vesicles composed of natural or synthetic lipid bilayers that encapsulate a watery core. These structures can enclose hydrophilic materials within the aqueous center while lipophilic substances can be absorbed into or integrated within the lipid layers. Liposomes are classified based on several factors, including size, surface charge, lipid composition, and preparation method. They can be uni-lamellar (single bilayer) or multi-lamellar (multiple bilayers). Liposomes have demonstrated significant advantages in reducing the side effects of various medications, particularly anti-cancer and anti-fungal drugs, while simultaneously enhancing their efficacy. Furthermore, liposomal drug delivery systems have shown promise in treating chronic inflammatory diseases by minimizing the adverse effects of anti-inflammatory medications on healthy tissues (Akbarzadeh et al., 2013). Curcumin, a polyphenolic compound, faces challenges such as rapid metabolism and sensitivity to light, limiting its therapeutic potential. However, encapsulating curcumin in liposomes can mitigate these issues. By incorporating curcumin into the phospholipid bilayer, its delivery in aqueous environments is significantly improved, resulting in enhanced effectiveness (Sin et al., 2019). In one study, liposomes were employed to encapsulate curcumin through a process known as lipid hydration. The resulting liposomes were carefully analyzed for their ability to combat inflammation, focusing on key inflammatory markers such as IL-6, TNFα, and IL-8. The curcumin-loaded formulations demonstrated improved encapsulation efficiency and a significant reduction in pro-inflammatory markers, outperforming a positive control group treated with salbutamol-loaded liposomes (Ng et al., 2018). Capsaicin, which has limited solubility in body fluids and reduced bioavailability, also benefits from liposomal encapsulation. This method enhances both the bioavailability and anti-inflammatory effects of capsaicin. A liposome was developed using a combination of isopropyl myristate, sodium cholate, phospholipid, and cholesterol via the film-dispersion method (Zhu et al., 2015). Additionally, epicatechin, another natural polyphenolic compound, faces solubility challenges that can be addressed through liposomal encapsulation. When liposomes loaded with epicatechin are combined with a chitosan hydrogel, the resulting formulation not only enhances the anti-inflammatory properties of epicatechin but also prolongs its effectiveness (Joraholmen et al., 2019).

Metallic Nanoparticles

Metallic nanoparticles are materials made from metals such as platinum, gold, and titanium, known for their remarkable optical and electronic properties, which make them valuable in the medical field. Their large surface area-to-volume ratio allows for the attachment of antibodies, ligands, and carriers for gene-drug delivery and diagnostic imaging (Venkatesh, 2018). Garlic can be encapsulated in silver nanoparticles, resulting in G-Ag-NPS, which enhances its anti-inflammatory properties. Inflammation can occur when proteins lose their structural integrity, leading to the production of autoantigens, as observed in rheumatoid disorders. G-Ag-NPS effectively prevents protein structure loss even at low concentrations of 10 μM. Furthermore, at a concentration of 250 μM, G-Ag-NPS demonstrated an impressive 85% inhibition of protein structure loss, surpassing the effects of the standard anti-inflammatory drug diclofenac sodium. Notably, G-Ag-NPS also alleviates the stomach irritation commonly associated with over-the-counter anti-inflammatory medications (Vijayakumar et al., 2019). Quercetin, a natural flavonoid found in fruits such as cherries and mangoes, has recently been shown to reduce the production of inflammatory cytokines and inhibit pro-inflammatory enzymes. However, due to its limited solubility and bioavailability, researchers have explored the use of gold nanoparticles to enhance its solubility and drug availability (Ozdal et al., 2019).

Polymeric Nanoparticles (PNPs)

PNPs have a matrix structure composed of eco-friendly and bio-resorbable polymers derived from either natural or synthetic sources. Common synthetic polymers include polyacrylate, polylactide-polyglycolide copolymers, polycaprolactones, and polylactide, with the lactide-glycolide copolymer being particularly well-researched. Organic polymers such as chitosan, albumin, and alginate have also been extensively studied. The characteristics of PNPs, including their size, strength, and drug release profile, are influenced by various factors, including mixing times, drug-to-polymer ratios, molecular weight, polymer composition, solvent, pH, homogenization speed, and the solubility of the drug (Sreekumar et al., 2018). One active compound found in ginger, shogaol, was successfully incorporated into PLGA/PLA-PEG-FA nanoparticles using a simple and efficient surface-functionalizing method. These nanoparticles demonstrated therapeutic effects in treating colitis in a mouse model induced by dextran sulfate sodium (DSS). When administered orally, the shogaol-loaded nanoparticles effectively alleviated symptoms of colitis and promoted the healing of colitis wounds by regulating the expression of pro-inflammatory mediators (Ribeiro et al., 2017). Licorice contains a potent compound called glycyrrhizic acid (GA), known for its anti-inflammatory effects through the inhibition of NF-κB signaling. However, GA is rapidly broken down in the intestines and liver, which reduces its effectiveness. To enhance its bioavailability, GA was loaded into PLGA nanoparticles, facilitating oral administration (Zeeshan et al., 2019). Capsaicin, another anti-inflammatory agent, has limited bioavailability, hindering its effectiveness. Encapsulating capsaicin within PLGA nanoparticles can provide sustained release and enhance its therapeutic impact (Baskaran et al., 2017).

Polyphenols

Plant polyphenols (PPH) are a diverse collection of molecules found in many plants, ranging from simple to complex structures, all characterized by the presence of benzene rings with hydroxyl groups. In plants, these compounds play crucial roles in growth, reproduction, and defense against pathogens and diseases. PPH also significantly impact human health by interacting with proteins, enzymes, and receptors, influencing various biological processes. One of their well-studied properties is their ability to scavenge free radicals, which contributes to their anti-inflammatory effects. Notably, quercetin, resveratrol, and tannins are recognized for their pain-relieving properties. PPH can enhance the immune system's response to chronic diseases; however, their effectiveness relies on their metabolism and bioavailability—the amount of the compound that enters the bloodstream after administration (Gonzalez et al., 2011). Generally, PPH have low bioavailability due to factors such as their chemical structure, molecular weight, and limited solubility in water. Additionally, they are unstable in the gastrointestinal tract, undergo extensive phase II metabolism, and are rapidly eliminated from the body, which limits their clinical applications. To overcome these challenges, researchers have developed nano-delivery systems that can preserve the structure of these bioactive molecules. For instance, nanosized carriers containing QC, a semi-lipophilic flavonol found in plants, have been created. These carriers, called SLNs, are composed of polyethylene glycol, Tween 80, and soya lecithin, with a size of 155 nm. The encapsulation efficiency of QC in these SLNs is 91%, and these nanoparticles remain stable for over ten weeks without producing any degradation products (Barras et al., 2009).

Phytocannabinoids

Phytocannabinoids refer to the lipid-based substances derived from the hemp plant, Cannabis sativa L. The extract of cannabis contains over 460 compounds, with approximately 70 being phytocannabinoids (Esposito et al., 2016). Phytocannabinoids have been found to offer numerous therapeutic benefits, including pain relief, seizure control, sleep aid, calming effects, anesthesia, reducing inflammation, fighting infections, preventing parasites, relieving nausea, increasing appetite, promoting urination, suppressing coughs, and aiding in expectoration. However, cannabis extract is increasingly viewed as a potential substance for abuse. To address this concern, medicine has turned to nanotechnology to target the active ingredients while avoiding the psychotropic effects and other unwanted consequences. One example of this is the development of a method to enclose phytocannabinoids in nanostructured lipid carriers. These carriers are created using a specialized process of melting and ultrasonication to optimize the recovery of nanoparticles and the efficiency of drug encapsulation. Additionally, lipid nanoparticle formulations have been proposed as effective carriers for the oral delivery of cannabinoid derivatives to combat chronic pain (Duran Lobato et al., 2016).

Phytosterols

Plant sterols and stanols, collectively known as phytosterols, are naturally occurring substances found in a wide range of foods, including plant-based oils, grains, nuts, legumes, fruits, and vegetables. Among the more than 200 compounds classified as phytosterols, the most common include sitosterol, campesterol, sitostanol, and campestanol. These phytosterols possess several beneficial properties, such as reducing blood cholesterol levels by partially blocking cholesterol absorption in the intestines. They also exhibit anti-atherogenic effects, and β-sitosterol can stimulate the immune system and exhibit anti-inflammatory properties. Moreover, various studies suggest that plant sterols may have a protective effect against certain types of cancer, including colorectal, breast, and prostate cancer (Trautwein and Demonty, 2010). Despite their structural similarities to cholesterol, phytosterols have limited absorption, with less than 2% being absorbed compared to 30-60% for cholesterol. To address this challenge, nanotechnology can significantly enhance the pharmacokinetics of phytosterols (Leong et al., 2011).

Carbohydrates

Plants rely on carbohydrates for their growth and development. These carbohydrates, which constitute a significant portion of the cell wall, are crucial for its proper functioning. The structure of plants is largely influenced by three types of high molecular weight carbohydrates: pectin, hemicelluloses, and cellulose. Certain plant polysaccharides, such as those found in Echinacea purpurea and Echinacea angustifolia, exhibit anti-inflammatory properties and promote skin repair. Extracts derived from the roots of these plants contain echinacin, a polysaccharide that has shown promising anti-inflammatory effects on the skin. Additionally, pectin derived from Comarum palustre has demonstrated immune-modulating and anti-inflammatory properties (Tragni et al., 1988). The anti-inflammatory effects of sulfated polysaccharides found in Artemisia tripartita (a member of the Asteraceae family) are attributed to their ability to modify macrophage function, as well as their impact on neutrophil count and complement fixation function. Recent research has increasingly focused on utilizing nanotechnology to deliver anti-inflammatory carbohydrates (Surjushe et al., 2008).

Essential Oils (EOs)

Hydrophobic, volatile, and complex, EOs are natural compounds known for their potent aroma. These oils are produced as secondary metabolites by aromatic plants. The extraction methods for EOs date back to the Middle Ages, with origins in Arabic Spain. Techniques such as steam or hydro-distillation are renowned for their ability to preserve the antibacterial and fungicidal properties of the oils. Additionally, EOs are highly valued for their fragrance and flavor, finding applications in food preservation and medicine. In the medical field, they are utilized as remedies for pain relief, sedation, inflammation reduction, muscle relaxation, and local anesthesia (Bakkali et al., 2008).

Terpenoids

Terpenoids, found in a variety of natural sources, play a crucial role in combating inflammation. They are present in a broad range of species, including plants, lichens, insects, mosses, algae, microbes, and marine creatures. Scientists have been actively investigating the molecular mechanisms underlying the anti-inflammatory properties of terpenoids derived from plants. Numerous studies have shown that these compounds can effectively inhibit the signaling of

NF-κB, a key player in the development of cancer and inflammatory diseases (Salminen et al., 2008).

Conclusion

In recent years, there has been a growing belief in the tremendous potential of phytochemicals for the prevention and treatment of inflammatory diseases. However, their practical application has been hindered by issues such as poor bioavailability, stability, and water solubility. Furthermore, reports of side effects associated with these compounds in therapeutic use have raised concerns. To overcome these limitations, the use of nanosized drug delivery systems has been proposed. These systems can enhance the absorption of phytochemicals in the body, prolong their circulation time, protect them from early enzymatic degradation or metabolic processes, and improve their solubility and persistence. By doing so, the side effects associated with their use can be minimized. Nanotechnology holds great promise and has already made significant strides in bringing anti-inflammatory phytochemicals closer to clinical application. The increasing body of research on nanotoxicology reflects a growing understanding of and concern for the ethical implications of nanotechnology. Further studies are needed to improve the affordability and long-term safety of these drug delivery technologies at the nanoscale. This can be achieved by using biocompatible materials and ensuring that the release mechanisms are safe. By establishing a strong connection between intelligent nanoparticle design and comprehensive safety evaluations, we can pave the way for future applications of nanotechnology in biomedicine.

References

Akbarzadeh, A., Rezaei-Sadabady, R., Davaran, S., Joo, S. W., Zarghami, N., Hanifehpour, Y., Samiei, M., Kouhi, M., & Nejati-Koshki, K. (2013). Liposome: Classification, preparation, and applications. *Nanoscale Research Letters*, *8*(1), 102.

Arora, R., Kuhad, A., Kaur, I. P., & Chopra, K. (2015). Curcumin loaded solid lipid nanoparticles ameliorate adjuvant-induced arthritis in rats. *European Journal of Pain*, *19*(7), 940–952.

Bakkali, F., Averbeck, S., Averbeck, D., & Idaomar, M. (2008). Biological effects of essential oils – A review. *Food and Chemical Toxicology*, *46*(2), 446–475.

Barras, A., Mezzetti, A., Richard, A., Lazzaroni, S., Roux, S., Melnyk, P., Betbeder, D., & Monfilliette-Dupont, N. (2009). Formulation and characterization of polyphenol-loaded lipid nanocapsules. *International Journal of Pharmaceutics*, *379*(2), 270–277.

Baskaran, M., Baskaran, P., Arulsamy, N., & Thyagarajan, B. (2017). Preparation and Evaluation of PLGA-Coated Capsaicin Magnetic Nanoparticles. *Pharmaceutical Research*, *34*(6), 1255–1263.

Chaudhari, P. M., & Bind, V. M. (2019). Topical solid lipid nanoparticles based gel of lavender essential oil for anti-inflammatory activity. *Asian Journal of Pharmaceutical and Clinical Research*, 12(11), 175-182.

Chung, I. M., Subramanian, U., Thirupathi, P., Venkidasamy, B., Samynathan, R., Gangadhar, B. H., Rajakumar, G., & Thiruvengadam, M. (2020). Resveratrol Nanoparticles: A Promising Therapeutic Advancement over Native Resveratrol. *Processes*, *8*(4), 458.

De Sá Coutinho, D., Pacheco, M. T., Frozza, R. L., & Bernardi, A. (2018). Anti-Inflammatory Effects of Resveratrol: Mechanistic Insights. *International Journal of Molecular Sciences*, *19*(6), 1812.

Durán-Lobato, M., Martín-Banderas, L., Lopes, R., Gonçalves, L. M. D., Fernández-Arévalo, M., & Almeida, A. J. (2016). Lipid nanoparticles as an emerging platform for cannabinoid delivery: Physicochemical optimization and biocompatibility. *Drug Development and Industrial Pharmacy*, *42*(2), 190–198.

El-Refai, A. A., Ghoniem, G. A., El-Khateeb, A. Y., & Hassaan, M. M. (2018). Eco-friendly synthesis of metal nanoparticles using ginger and garlic extracts as biocompatible novel antioxidant and antimicrobial agents. *Journal of Nanostructure in Chemistry*, *8*(1), 71–81.

Esposito, E., Drechsler, M., Cortesi, R., & Nastruzzi, C. (2016). Encapsulation of cannabinoid drugs in nanostructured lipid carriers. *European Journal of Pharmaceutics and Biopharmaceutics*, *102*, 87–91.

Funk, J. L., Frye, J. B., Oyarzo, J. N., Chen, J., Zhang, H., & Timmermann, B. N. (2016). Anti-inflammatory effects of the essential oils of ginger (Zingiber officinale Roscoe) in experimental rheumatoid arthritis. *Pharma Nutrition*, *4*(3), 123–131.

González, R., Ballester, I., López-Posadas, R., Suárez, M. D., Zarzuelo, A., Martínez-Augustin, O., & Medina, F. S. D. (2011). Effects of flavonoids and other polyphenols on inflammation. *Critical Reviews in Food Science and Nutrition*, *51*(4), 331–362.

González-Muniesa, P., Garcia-Gerique, L., Quintero, P., Arriaza, S., Lopez-Pascual, A., & Martinez, J. A. (2016). Effects of hyperoxia on oxygen-related inflammation with a focus on obesity. *Oxidative Medicine and Cellular Longevity*, *2016*, 1–11.

Jøraholmen, M. W., Basnet, P., Tostrup, M. J., Moueffaq, S., & Škalko-Basnet, N. (2019). Localized therapy of vaginal infections and inflammation: liposomes-in-hydrogel delivery system for polyphenols. *Pharmaceutics*, *11*(2), 53.

Lee, D. Y., Li, H., Lim, H. J., Lee, H. J., Jeon, R., & Ryu, J. H. (2012). Anti-Inflammatory Activity of Sulfur-Containing Compounds from Garlic. *Journal of Medicinal Food*, *15*(11), 992–999.

Leong, W. F., Lai, O. M., Long, K., Che Man, Y. B., Misran, M., & Tan, C. P. (2011). Preparation and characterisation of water-soluble phytosterol nanodispersions. *Food Chemistry*, *129*(1), 77–83.

Lu, M., Chen, C., Lan, Y., Xiao, J., Li, R., Huang, J., Huang, Q., Cao, Y., & Ho, C. T. (2020). Capsaicin—the major bioactive ingredient of chili peppers: Bio-efficacy and delivery systems. *Food & Function*, *11*(4), 2848–2860.

Ng, Z. Y., Wong, J.-Y., Panneerselvam, J., Madheswaran, T., Kumar, P., Pillay, V., Hsu, A., Hansbro, N., Bebawy, M., Wark, P., Hansbro, P., Dua, K., & Chellappan, D. K. (2018). Assessing the potential of liposomes loaded with curcumin as a therapeutic intervention in asthma. *Colloids and Surfaces B: Biointerfaces*, *172*, 51–59.

Oguntibeju, O. (2018). Medicinal plants with anti-inflammatory activities from selected countries and regions of Africa. *Journal of Inflammation Research*, 11, 307–317.

Ozdal, Z. D., Sahmetlioglu, E., Narin, I., & Cumaoglu, A. (2019). Synthesis of gold and silver nanoparticles using flavonoid quercetin and their effects on lipopolysaccharide induced inflammatory response in microglial cells. *3 Biotech*, *9*(6), 212.

Penalva, R., Esparza, I., Larraneta, E., González Navarro, C. J., Gamazo, C., & Irache, J. M. (2015). Zein-Based Nanoparticles Improve the Oral Bioavailability of Resveratrol and Its Anti-inflammatory Effects in a Mouse Model of Endotoxic Shock. *Journal of Agricultural and Food Chemistry*, *63*(23), 5603–5611.

Ribeiro, L. N. M., Alcântara, A. C. S., Rodrigues Da Silva, G. H., Franz-Montan, M., Nista, S. V. G., Castro, S. R., Couto, V. M., Guilherme, V. A., & De Paula, E. (2017). Advances in Hybrid Polymer-Based Materials for Sustained Drug Release. *International Journal of Polymer Science*, *2017*, 1–16.

Salminen, A., Lehtonen, M., Suuronen, T., Kaarniranta, K., & Huuskonen, J. (2008). Terpenoids: Natural inhibitors of NF-κB signaling with anti-inflammatory and anticancer potential. *Cellular and Molecular Life Sciences*, *65*(19), 2979–2999.

Serhan, C. N., Ward, P. A., & Gilroy, D. W. (2010). *Fundamentals of Inflammation.* Cambridge University Press.

Sinjari, B., Pizzicannella, J., D'Aurora, M., Zappacosta, R., Gatta, V., Fontana, A., Trubiani, O., & Diomede, F. (2019). Curcumin/Liposome Nanotechnology as Delivery Platform for Anti-inflammatory Activities via NFkB/ERK/pERK Pathway in Human Dental Pulp Treated With 2-HydroxyEthyl MethAcrylate (HEMA). *Frontiers in Physiology*, *10*, 633.

Son, G. H., Lee, B. J., & Cho, C. W. (2017). Mechanisms of drug release from advanced drug formulations such as polymeric-based drug-delivery systems and lipid nanoparticles. *Journal of Pharmaceutical Investigation*, *47*(4), 287–296.

Sreekumar, S., Goycoolea, F. M., Moerschbacher, B. M., & Rivera-Rodriguez, G. R. (2018). Parameters influencing the size of chitosan-TPP nano- and microparticles. *Scientific Reports*, *8*(1), 4695.

Surjushe, A., Vasani, R., & Saple, D. (2008). Aloe vera: A short review. *Indian Journal of Dermatology*, *53*(4), 163.

Tidball, J. G. (2005). Inflammatory processes in muscle injury and repair. *American Journal of Physiology-Regulatory, Integrative and Comparative Physiology*, *288*(2), R345–R353.

Tragni, E., Galli, C. L., Tubaro, A., Del Negro, P., & Della Loggia, R. (1988). Anti-inflammatory activity of Echinacea angustifolia fractions separated on the basis of molecular weight. *Pharmacological Research Communications*, *20*, 87–90.

Trautwein, E. A., & Demonty, I. (2007). Phytosterols: Natural compounds with established and emerging health benefits. *Oléagineux, Corps Gras, Lipides*, *14*(5), 259–266.

Venkatesh, N. (2018). Metallic Nanoparticle: A Review. *Biomedical Journal of Scientific & Technical Research*, *4*(2), 3765-3775.

Vijayakumar, S., Malaikozhundan, B., Saravanakumar, K., Durán-Lara, E. F., Wang, M. H., & Vaseeharan, B. (2019). Garlic clove extract assisted silver nanoparticle – Antibacterial, antibiofilm, antihelminthic, anti-inflammatory, anticancer and ecotoxicity assessment. *Journal of Photochemistry and Photobiology B: Biology*, *198*, 111558.

Wal, P., Saraswat, N., Pal, R. S., Wal, A., & Chaubey, M. (2019). A detailed insight of the anti-inflammatory effects of curcumin with the assessment of parameters, sources of ROS and associated mechanisms. *Open Medicine Journal*, *6*(1), 64–76.

Wang, J., & Xia, Q. (2014). Alpha-lipoic acid-loaded nanostructured lipid carrier: Sustained release and biocompatibility to HaCaT cells *in vitro*. *Drug Delivery*, *21*(5), 328–341.

Wang, W., Zhang, L., Chen, T., Guo, W., Bao, X., Wang, D., Ren, B., Wang, H., Li, Y., Wang, Y., Chen, S., Tang, B., Yang, Q., & Chen, C. (2017). Anticancer effects of resveratrol-loaded solid lipid nanoparticles on human breast cancer cells. *Molecules*, *22*(11), 1814.

Watkins, L. R., Maier, S. F., & Goehler, L. E. (1995). Immune activation: The role of pro-inflammatory cytokines in inflammation, illness responses and pathological pain states. *Pain*, *63*(3), 289–302.

Zeeshan, M., Ali, H., Khan, S., Mukhtar, M., Khan, M. I., & Arshad, M. (2019). Glycyrrhizic acid-loaded pH-sensitive Poly-(Lactic-Co-Glycolic Acid) Nanoparticles for the Amelioration of Inflammatory Bowel Disease. *Nanomedicine*, *14*(15), 1945–1969.

Zeng, M. Y., Inohara, N., & Nuñez, G. (2017). Mechanisms of inflammation-driven bacterial dysbiosis in the gut. *Mucosal Immunology*, *10*(1), 18–26.

Zhu, Y., Wang, M., Zhang, J., Peng, W., Firempong, C. K., Deng, W., Wang, Q., Wang, S., Shi, F., Yu, J., Xu, X., & Zhang, W. (2015). Improved oral bioavailability of capsaicin via liposomal nanoformulation: Preparation, *in vitro* drug release and pharmacokinetics in rats. *Archives of Pharmacal Research*, *38*(4), 512–521.

Chapter 17

Nanophytochemicals as Possible Cancer-Fighting Substances

Shuchi Dave[1,*]
Priyanka Rathore[2]
Uttam Singh Baghel[3]
and Umesh Patil[4]
[1]Guru Ramdas Khalsa Institute of Science and Technology (Pharmacy), Jabalpur, Madhya Pradesh, India
[2]Sagar Institute of Research Technology and Science, Pharmacy, Bhopal, Madhya Pradesh, India
[3]Gurukul Pharmacy College, Ranpur, Kota, Rajasthan, India
[4]Department of Pharmaceutical Sciences, Dr. Harisingh Gour Vishwavidyalaya, Sagar, Madhya Pradesh, India

Abstract

Phytochemical products and remedies have been utilized for medical conditions since ancient times. The discipline of nanotechnology aims to develop devices and dosage forms within the 1-100 nm range. Safe materials such as lipids, synthetic biodegradable polymers, and polysaccharides are employed to create nanocarriers. Cancer continues to be one of the deadliest diseases, affecting a significant portion of the global population. A wealth of scientific literature identifies numerous potent plant-based anticancer agents that have been integrated into modern cancer treatment practices, including vincristine, vinblastine, paclitaxel, curcumin, podophyllotoxin, and camptothecin. Various techniques have been employed to prepare nanoherbal formulations for cancer treatment, including the emulsion-solvent evaporation method, double emulsion and evaporation method, salting out method, emulsions diffusion method, and solvent displacement method. Important challenges in this field include addressing multidrug resistance and mitigating adverse drug reactions. Due to their unique structural and functional characteristics, nanomedicines offer the potential for improved translational outcomes. This chapter outlines the potential and challenges of a drug delivery strategy based on nanotechnology for administering plant-based anticancer agents.

Keywords: nanoherbal formulation, anticancer, drug delivery, therapeutic outcomes

* Corresponding Author's Email: shuchi1801@gmail.com.

In: Phyto-Nanomedicine
Editors: Hitesh Chopra, Vinod Kumar Gauttam, Ajmer Singh Grewal et al.
ISBN: 979-8-89530-317-7

Abbreviations

ARB	Antibiotic-resistant bacteria
EGCG	Epigallocatechin gallate
PAMAM	Polyamidoamine
PTX	Paclitaxel
CUR	Curcumin
NPs	Nanoparticles
QDs	quantum dots

Introduction

Phytochemicals are relatively small molecular species found in plants, exhibiting a wide array of techno- and bifunctional properties. Recent attention has been drawn to the identification, isolation, and application of dietary phytochemicals, which have potential uses as natural pigments, antioxidants, and antimicrobials. These compounds may also enhance human health and wellness by preventing chronic illnesses such as cancer, diabetes, obesity, and cardiovascular disease. The focus on phytochemicals in food and plants has intensified as more individuals pursue healthier lifestyles grounded in nature. Scientific research increasingly demonstrates the efficacy of phytochemicals in treating various ailments and promoting better lifestyle choices. Historically utilized in medications, dietary supplements, and cosmetics, these substances are now being integrated with modern research to provide significant health benefits, especially given their lower risk profile compared to synthetic chemicals. Phytochemicals are applied in various health-enhancing practices, including gemmotherapy, aromatherapy, and phytotherapy. However, challenges such as poor solubility, low bioavailability, and the necessity of consuming them as whole foods or in combination can hinder their effective formulation for diverse applications. To fully realize the benefits of these phytochemicals, effective delivery systems, such as nano-engineered formulations, are essential. These nano-delivery methods not only enhance the solubility and stability of phytochemicals but also have the potential to prolong their average circulation time in the bloodstream, thereby improving their overall efficacy (Kim et al., 2021; Julian et al., 2022).

Nanotechnology

In nanotechnology, matter is manipulated at the nanoscale, typically at sizes smaller than 100 nanometers. This field of study holds promise across various scientific and industrial sectors, including electronics, materials science, and medicine. The term "nanophytochemical" specifically refers to the application of nanotechnology in the investigation, extraction, or utilization of phytochemicals derived from plants. Techniques such as nanoscale drug delivery systems and nanoparticle (NP) formulations aim to enhance the efficiency and bioavailability of these phytochemicals. Nanotechnology represents an innovative approach focused on handling materials at the nanoscale, which is one billionth of a meter. It encompasses the development and application of chemical, physical, and biological systems from individual molecules or atoms to submicron dimensions and the integration of the resulting nanomaterials into larger systems. Numerous NPs measuring less than 100 nm have emerged as potent drug delivery methods. These NPs provide advantages such as improved drug delivery, enhanced bioavailability, and optimized pharmacokinetics, alongside high drug loading efficiency. Inorganic NPs possess distinct nanostructural morphologies and sizes, including carbon nanotubes, ceramic NPs, quantum dots, magnetic NPs, and gold/silver NPs. Conversely, organic NPs comprise polymeric conjugates, polymeric NPs, lipid-based carriers (such as liposomes and micelles), dendrimers, and ferritin. Over the past decade, these NPs have been extensively utilized in biomedical sciences for cancer treatment through targeted drug delivery and diagnostic applications. Various nanocarriers, including polymeric NPs, mesoporous NPs, carbon nanotubes, dendrimers, liposomes, metallic NPs, and synthetic nanomaterials, serve as delivery systems for targeted therapies aimed at specific affected areas within the body.

Cancer

The progression of cancer is characterized by tumor development and subsequent metastasis, leading to increased tumor cell invasiveness and growth rates. Treatment options for cancer include chemotherapy, radiation therapy, and tumor resection, with the choice of therapy determined by the tumor's stage and location. Chemotherapy has proven highly effective, especially when combined with other medications, and utilizes both cytotoxic and cytostatic agents. Key classes of chemotherapeutics include alkylating agents, which damage DNA by covalently binding to it (e.g., carboplatin, cisplatin, oxaliplatin, cyclophosphamide, and melphalan); topoisomerase inhibitors, which inhibit DNA replication (e.g., irinotecan and doxorubicin); and tubulin-targeting agents, which disrupt mitosis by preventing the formation of mitotic spindles (e.g., vinblastine, vincristine, docetaxel, and paclitaxel). Additionally, various phytochemicals, including gums, resins, oils, alkaloids, flavonoids, phenolics, tannins, and glycosides, exhibit strong anticancer activity, with notable examples being vinblastine, vincristine, taxol, elliptinium, etoposide, colchicinamide, 10-hydroxycamptothecin, curcumol, gossypol, ipomeanol, lycobetaine, tetrandrine, homoharringtonine, monocrotaline, curdione, and indirubin. Despite advancements in cancer therapies, challenges such as poor solubility, low stability, limited biodistribution, metabolism, chemoresistance, and toxicity remain. To address these issues, nanobiotechnologies, including nanoparticles (NPs), have been employed for efficient drug delivery, enhancing the bioavailability of anticancer agents, including natural compounds. Recently, phytochemicals, such as resveratrol, ginsenosides, curcumin, and epigallocatechin gallate (EGCG), have emerged as effective anticancer agents with fewer adverse effects than traditional treatments. Specific plants with phytochemicals that exhibit anticancer properties include Artemisia annua (Artesunate) for leukemia, melanoma, lung cancer, colon cancer, renal cancer, ovarian cancer, and central nervous system tumors; Rhizoma coptidis for berberine alkaloids; Curcuma longa (curcumin) for human breast and colon cancer; Fagonia indica for MCF-7 estrogen-dependent breast cancer and MDA-MB-468 estrogen-independent breast cancer; Garcinia oblongifolia for MCF-7 breast cancer and cervical cancer (HeLa); Garcinia indica for HT-29 and HCT-116 colon cancer; Hedyotis diffusa for colorectal cancer; Morus alba for pulmonary carcinoma, colon carcinoma, and breast adenocarcinoma; and Paris polyphylla for esophageal cancer. Specifically, curcumin, derived from Curcuma longa, demonstrates anticancer properties against various malignancies, including liver, brain, and colon tumors, though its rapid metabolism, systemic clearance, low absorption, and poor bioavailability limit its therapeutic efficacy (Wang et al., 2014; Manickam et al., 2021; Yang et al., 2014).

Intersection of Phytochemicals, Nanotechnology, and Anticancer Applications

Research on the integration of phytochemicals with nanotechnology for anticancer applications is advancing steadily. Phytochemicals, naturally occurring compounds found in plants, have been extensively studied for their potential health benefits, particularly their anticancer properties. In the realm of cancer treatment, nanotechnology offers a promising platform for enhancing the delivery, stability, safety, and targeted release of these phytochemicals. Here are some key aspects of the synergy between nanotechnology, phytochemicals, and anticancer applications:

Phytochemicals in Cancer Prevention

Preclinical research has highlighted the anticancer potential of various phytochemicals, including flavonoids, alkaloids, steroids, terpenoids, and polyphenols. These compounds exert their effects through multiple mechanisms, such as inducing apoptosis, exhibiting antioxidant activity, and demonstrating anti-inflammatory properties. The potential advantages of phytochemicals in cancer therapy include boosting the immune system, minimizing inflammation, preventing DNA damage, promoting DNA repair, reducing the proliferation of cancer cells, and inhibiting the growth of damaged cells. Different phytochemicals offer unique benefits: carotenoids, found in foods like broccoli, carrots, and leafy greens, support vision, enhance immunity, prevent cancer, and maintain healthy skin. Flavonoids, present in citrus fruits, soybeans, and tea, strengthen immunity, reduce inflammation, and inhibit tumor growth. Indoles and glucosinolates, found in cruciferous vegetables, help lower cancer risk and prevent tumor growth. Inositols, such as phytic acid in bran and soybeans, prevent cell damage. Isoflavones, typically found in soy products, inhibit tumor growth and limit hormone production related to cancer. Polyphenols, including resveratrol and ellagic acid present in green tea, grapes, and berries, may prevent inflammation and the development of cancer. These diverse phytochemicals contribute to a multifaceted approach to cancer prevention and treatment.

Barriers in Phytochemical Delivery

Although phytochemicals offer numerous potential benefits, delivering them effectively to cancer cells poses significant challenges. Their therapeutic efficacy can be limited by issues such as poor solubility, low bioavailability, and off-target effects. First, the presence of various distinct bioactive components leads to a high degree of heterogeneity in phytochemical extracts, meaning that a desired biological response may arise from a combination of multiple bioactive substances rather than from a single component. Additionally, despite the development of several innovative delivery techniques, many of these methods remain costly, labor-intensive, and technologically complex. A major drawback is the reliance on live organisms, particularly mice and rats, for testing, which is often impractical due to ethical concerns surrounding the frequent need for euthanasia. Lastly, employing biological assays for the isolation, screening, and quantification of specific bioactive molecules presents further challenges.

Targeted Drug Delivery Systems

A novel approach to drug delivery, known as “drug targeting,” aims to deliver medication precisely to the intended site of action or absorption while preventing its release at non-target locations. In this method, the drug remains intact within the delivery system until it reaches the target site, where it is subsequently released without any alterations. Compared to conventional drug administration methods, tailored drug delivery systems offer several advantages, including enhanced pharmacological activity, reduced adverse effects, and lower required doses. These targeted drug delivery systems are specifically designed to deliver therapeutic agents exclusively to diseased organs, sparing healthy tissues from side effects, which is particularly crucial in cancer treatment with chemotherapeutic agents. This approach often involves functionalizing nanoparticles (NPs) with antibodies or ligands that specifically target cancer cells. By maximizing the delivery of therapeutic compounds to the tumor site, this targeted method improves treatment efficacy while minimizing damage to normal tissues.

Enhancement of Bioavailability

NPs enhance the effectiveness and longevity of phytochemical delivery by protecting these compounds from degradation and improving their absorption into the body. This enhanced delivery ensures that phytochemicals can more effectively reach and persist at tumor sites. Despite their origins in traditional phytomedicine, many contemporary pharmaceutical compounds face challenges such as instability, rapid first-pass metabolism, limited systemic availability, poor water solubility, and inadequate tissue penetration. Nanoparticle-based delivery systems address these issues by stabilizing phytochemicals and enhancing their bioavailability, thereby facilitating better therapeutic outcomes (Gunasekaran et al., 2014).

Nanotechnology for Drug Delivery

Nanotechnology offers innovative solutions to overcome the obstacles associated with the delivery of phytochemicals. By incorporating phytochemicals into NPs, their solubility and stability can be significantly enhanced. Additionally, nanocarriers can specifically target cancer cells, reducing adverse effects on healthy organs. Various types of nanoformulations, such as dendrimers, liposomes, nanosensors, nanoshells, nanorobots, and quantum dots, have been developed to address issues related to limited water solubility and inadequate bioavailability of drugs. This highlights the increasing need for pharmaceutical carriers capable of overcoming these challenges. The newly designed systems should be non-toxic, have a high drug-loading capacity, possess surface modification capabilities, offer controlled release properties, and ensure drug stability against potential chemical and physical degradation. Furthermore, these carriers should be cost-effective and viable for production. Recent advancements in drug delivery methods aim for targeted delivery with minimal drug particle sizes, which helps to minimize side effects and enhance efficacy. NPs based on lipids or polymers are specifically designed to improve the pharmacokinetics and biodistribution of therapeutic agents.

Dendrimers

The term “dendrimer” originates from the Greek word “dendron,” meaning “tree,” combined with the suffix “mer,” indicating a segment, which reflects the structure of these artificial, three-dimensional molecules with branching components. Dendrimers were first discovered in the early 1980s by Tomalia, Donald, and their colleagues. These man-made macromolecules are hyperbranched, monodisperse, and possess distinct molecular weights, allowing them to encapsulate bioactive substances effectively. Constructed step-by-step from branched monomer units, dendrimers can be tailored in shape, size, molecular weight, flexibility, density, and solubility by selecting appropriate surface functional groups and building units. Their tree-like structure provides a significant surface area for the entrapment of desired phytochemical bioactive constituents, making them valuable in pharmaceutical, medical, and nutraceutical sciences. The efficiency of nanoencapsulation using dendrimers is influenced by several factors, including the type of end groups, surface charge, pH, environmental conditions, and particle formation (Yousefi et al., 2020). For instance, camptothecin-loaded polyethylene glycol (PEG)-modified polyamidoamine (PAMAM) G5 dendrimers have been functionalized with AS1411 antinucleolin aptamers to enhance specific targeting to tumor cells and improve endocytosis. Additionally, N-acetyl-D-glucosamine has been utilized to further increase the targeting of camptothecin-loaded PAMAM dendrimers. In another example, paclitaxel (PTX)-loaded PAMAM dendrimers have demonstrated improved targeting capabilities, leading to enhanced cell uptake, cytotoxicity, and apoptosis, as well as increased solubility and bioavailability for cancer treatment (An et al., 2023).

Liposomes

Liposomes are small, artificial vesicles composed of natural, non-toxic phospholipids and cholesterol, characterized by their spherical shape. They are particularly promising drug delivery systems due to their unique hydrophobic and hydrophilic properties, along with their biocompatibility. Liposomes have a wide range of pharmacological applications and are especially effective for delivering anti-sense oligonucleotides, ribosomes, proteins/peptides, and DNA into cells. Recent research has focused on using liposomal nanovesicles to deliver phytonutrients, leveraging their ability to enhance transport across cellular barriers and provide targeted delivery to cancer cells (Chavda et al., 2022). These biocompatible and biodegradable nanoparticles are frequently employed as carriers for phytochemicals, with nanotechnology significantly improving the solubility, stability, and bioavailability of compounds such as curcumin, quercetin, resveratrol, and berberine (Yunus et al., 2017).

Quantum Dots (QDs)

QDs are nanometer-scale semiconductor crystals composed of groups II–VI or III–V elements, defined as particles whose physical dimensions are smaller than the exciton Bohr radius. When visible light strikes a semiconductor, some electrons are excited to higher energy states, and as they return to their ground state, they emit a photon of a frequency characteristic of that material. QDs, particularly those in the 2–6 nm size range, are of significant interest due to their dimensional similarities with biological macromolecules. These emerging artificial nanomaterials, such as CdSe, ZnS, and CdS, exhibit unique optical and chemical properties, making them promising platforms for cancer diagnostics and detection. Recent studies have shown that curcumin-based quantum dots enhance the degradation of bacterial biofilms. Other QD nanoparticle candidates, such as folic acid and chlorophyllin, also demonstrate potential for imaging diagnosis (Fang et al., 2017; Kim et al., 2021).

Nanoshells

One significant advancement in nanotechnology is the development of nanoshells, which consist of dielectric core components made of silica and are coated with thin layers of metals, particularly gold. Gold nanoshells have demonstrated considerable promise in various biomedical applications, including imaging, targeted therapy, gene delivery, tissue welding, and drug delivery systems. Their potential is especially notable in cancer imaging and treatment due to several advantageous properties. Gold nanoshells possess optically tunable characteristics, excellent biocompatibility, and stability, which enhances their bioavailability. They also have a high capacity for attaching to various therapeutic agents and exhibit photoluminescent properties. These features make them increasingly utilized in medical applications, particularly for cancer therapy. Cancer cells are known to exhibit higher thermosensitivity compared to normal healthy cells, making them more susceptible to hyperthermia treatments. Various nanostructures, such as gold nanorods, silica-gold composites, solid gold nanoshells, core-shell gold nanoshells, and carbon nanotubes, can be employed in hyperthermia-based cancer therapy. These nanostructures exploit their unique properties to effectively target and destroy cancer cells through localized heating, enhancing the efficacy of treatment while minimizing damage to surrounding healthy tissue.

Nanosensor

Generally speaking, a nanosensor is composed of a biosensitive layer that contains biological recognition elements, either covalently linked to a transducer or integrated within it. The primary goal of the interaction between the target analyte and the bioreceptor is to induce physicochemical changes that can be translated into a quantifiable outcome, such as an electrical signal. Various nanomaterials, including polymer-based nanocomposite materials, carbon nanotubes (CNTs), gold nanoparticles (Au NPs), and quantum dots (QDs), have been employed in the development of nanosensors for detecting pesticides. One notable application involves biological receptors such as acetylcholinesterase (AChE) and choline oxidase (ChOx) enzymes, which serve as the basis for highly sensitive nanosensors capable of detecting carbamate and organophosphorus pesticides at low concentrations. These nanosensors leverage the specificity of the enzyme-substrate interactions to provide accurate and rapid detection, enhancing the ability to monitor pesticide levels in various environments (Kumari et al., 2023).

Nanorobots

Nanorobots are miniaturized devices designed to perform tasks comparable to those of conventional machines, with applications spanning various fields such as industry, medicine, and more. One promising aspect of nanorobots is their potential role in enhancing energy efficiency through the development of nanomotors. In medicine, nanorobots have shown promise in addressing infertility issues by functioning as engines that enhance sperm movement when attached to them. These robots operate at macro- or micro-scale, with the capability to manipulate objects at the nanoscale with precision. Initially, their practical use in medicine focused on identifying and eliminating cancer cells, marking a significant advancement in targeted cancer therapy. However, one of the most fascinating potential applications of nanorobots may be in dentistry, where they could assist in diagnostics, treatment, and oral health monitoring. Overall, the integration of nanorobots in phytochemistry, dentistry, and medicine signifies a transformative shift toward more precise and effective therapeutic interventions (Sujatha et al., 2010).

Current Fabrication Methods

The physicochemical properties of the polymer and the medication to be loaded determine the most suitable approach for creating nanoparticles. The following are the main processes used to produce nanoparticles from pre-made polymers.

Emulsion-Solvent Evaporation Method

Emulsification-solvent evaporation is a two-phase process essential for the preparation of nanospheres. The first phase involves emulsifying the polymer solution into an aqueous phase, followed by the second phase, in which the polymer solvent is evaporated, resulting in the precipitation of the polymer as nanospheres. These nanoparticles are then collected through ultracentrifugation, lyophilized for storage, and washed with distilled water to remove any remaining stabilizer or free drug. Despite their therapeutic potential, phytochemicals often encounter significant challenges, such as poor water solubility, limited penetration of physiological barriers, and difficulty reaching their target site, especially when administered orally. Their effectiveness *in vivo* is further compromised by rapid metabolism, excretion, and enzymatic and microbial digestion. To address these challenges, various nanotechnological approaches have been developed, leading to the creation of nanosized phytochemical-loaded delivery systems. For instance, di-benzoyl-methane, a structural analogue of curcumin, and turmeric have been nanoformulated using nanoemulsion techniques. This method has also been applied to encapsulate tannins, stilbenes, and flavonoids, which have demonstrated antioxidant properties *in vitro*. Additionally, carotenoids and bioactive lipids have been incorporated into nanoemulsions, enhancing their bioaccessibility and stability against autoxidation (Zuccari & Alfei, 2023).

Double Emulsion and Evaporation Method

Double emulsions can encapsulate water-soluble and water-insoluble pharmaceuticals, cosmetics, foods, and other high-value products. Since single emulsions allow drugs to rapidly partition into the external aqueous phase, double emulsion-based techniques are often employed for encapsulating hydrophilic compounds, which typically have low encapsulation efficiency. The primary challenge when utilizing double emulsions is optimizing various process factors to produce a homogeneous droplet size and maintain control over emulsion production. These emulsions can encapsulate a range of hydrophilic and hydrophobic phytochemical medications, including anticancer, anti-inflammatory, antibiotic, protein, and amino acid formulations (Iqbal, 2015).

Emulsion Diffusion Method

To maintain the initial thermodynamic equilibrium of both liquids, the encapsulating polymer is dissolved in a solvent that is only slightly water-miscible (such as benzyl alcohol or propylene carbonate) and then saturated with water. Next, depending on the oil-to-polymer ratio, the solvent phase that is saturated with polymer and water is emulsified in an aqueous solution containing a stabilizer. This process causes the solvent to diffuse to the exterior phase, forming nanospheres or nanocapsules. Finally, the solvent is removed by filtering or evaporating it according to its boiling point. This method offers several advantages, including excellent encapsulation efficiency (typically around 70%), simplicity, ease of scale-up, consistent batch-to-batch quality, no requirement for homogenization, and a narrow size distribution. By providing enhanced mechanical, physicochemical, biological, bioavailability, morphological, or release characteristics, the application of nanotechnology in conjunction with antibacterial phytochemicals can help achieve increased antibacterial efficacy against antibiotic-resistant bacteria (ARB). This approach involves the use of phytochemical-based nanomaterials, particularly polymeric nanofibers and NPs, in the treatment of ARB. It highlights the various types of phytochemicals incorporated into different nanomaterials, the processes involved in their creation, and the outcomes of studies evaluating their antibacterial effectiveness (Sandhiya et al. 2020; Iqbal et al., 2015).

Solvent Displacement Method

In solvent displacement, a premade polymer precipitates from an organic solution, and the organic solvent diffuses into the aqueous medium, either with or without a surfactant. A semipolar water-miscible solvent, such as acetone or ethanol, is used to dissolve the polymers, drugs, and/or lipophilic surfactants. This solution is then injected or poured into an aqueous solution containing a stabilizer while being stirred magnetically. The rapid diffusion of the solvent leads to the instantaneous formation of NPs. Subsequently, the solvent is extracted from the suspensions under reduced pressure. The rate at which the organic phase is added to the aqueous phase plays a crucial role in determining the particle size (Pathak et al., 2019).

Conclusion

The intersection of phytochemicals, nanotechnology, and anticancer applications offers significant potential for advancing cancer treatment. Phytochemicals, known for their health benefits, including anticancer properties, can be delivered more effectively through nanotechnology. Nanoformulations enhance the solubility, bioavailability, and targeted action of phytochemicals, improving their therapeutic efficacy while minimizing off-target effects. The fabrication process of nanoformulations is crucial, as it influences factors such as biocompatibility, drug release, and stability. Techniques such as emulsification and nanoprecipitation enable researchers to tailor nanoformulations to meet the specific needs of anticancer therapies. This targeted delivery approach may increase the therapeutic index of anticancer drugs, reducing systemic toxicity and improving patient outcomes. However, successfully translating nanoformulated phytochemicals into clinical practice requires addressing challenges such as scalability, long-term safety, and regulatory compliance. Collaboration across disciplines, including scientists, clinicians, and nanotechnologists, will be essential for advancing this field. Continued research and development could lead to innovative, safer, and more effective cancer treatments, contributing to the evolution of precision medicine. The convergence of phytochemicals, nanotechnology, and anticancer applications represents a promising frontier in cancer therapy, with the potential to significantly impact patient care.

References

Afzal, O., Altamimi, A. S. A., Nadeem, M. S., Alzarea, S. I., Almalki, W. H., Tariq, A., Mubeen, B., Murtaza, B. N., Iftikhar, S., Riaz, N., & Kazmi, I. (2022). Nanoparticles in drug delivery: From history to therapeutic applications. *Nanomaterials*, 12(24), 4494.

Ambreen, S., Lubna, A., Sampita, P., Saad, S. A., Mohamed, R., Umme, H., Sultan, A., Mohammed, M. G., & Faiyaz, S. (2022). Integrating nanotechnology with naturally occurring phytochemicals in neuropathy induced by diabetes. *Journal of Molecular Liquids*, 350, 118189.

An, H., Deng, X., Wang, F., Xu, P., & Wang, N. (2023). Dendrimers as nanocarriers for the delivery of drugs obtained from natural products. *Polymers*, 15(10), 2292.

Ashraf, M. A. (2020). Phytochemicals as potential anticancer drugs: Time to ponder nature's bounty. *Biomedical Research International*, 2020, 8602879.

Chavda, V. P., Vihol, D., & Mehta, B. (2022). Phytochemical-loaded liposomes for anticancer therapy: An updated review. *Nanomedicine: Nanotechnology, Biology, and Medicine*, 17(8), 547–568.

David, J., Mc, Clements, D. J., & Ozturk, B. (2022). Utilization of nanotechnology to improve the application and bioavailability of phytochemicals derived from waste streams. *Journal of Agricultural and Food Chemistry*, 70(23), 6884–6900.

Fang, M., Chen, M., Liu, L., & Li, Y. (2017). Applications of quantum dots in cancer detection and diagnosis: A review. *Journal of Biomedical Nanotechnology*, 13, 1–16.

Gunasekaran, T., Haile, T., Nigusse, T., & Dhanaraju, M. D. (2014). Nanotechnology: An effective tool for enhancing bioavailability and bioactivity of phytomedicine. *Asian Pacific Journal of Tropical Biomedicine*, 4(Suppl 1), S1–S7.

Iqbal, M., Zafar, N., Fessi, H., & Elaissari, A. (2015). Double emulsion solvent evaporation techniques used for drug encapsulation. *International Journal of Pharmaceutics*, 496, 284–302.

Khan, T., Ali, M., Khan, A., Nisar, P., Jan, S. A., Afridi, S., & Shinwari, Z. K. (2020). Anticancer plants: A review of the active phytochemicals, applications in animal models, and regulatory aspects. *Biomolecules*, 10(1), 47.

Kim, B., Park, J. E., Im, E., Cho, Y., Lee, J., Lee, H. J., Sim, D. Y., Park, W. Y., Shim, B. S., & Kim, S. H. (2021). Recent advances in nanotechnology with nano-phytochemicals: Molecular mechanisms and clinical implications in cancer progression. *International Journal of Molecular Sciences*, 22(7), 3571.

Kumari, R., Suman, K., Karmakar, S., Mishra, V., Lakra, S. G., Saurav, G. K., & Mahto, B. K. (2023). Regulation and safety measures for nanotechnology-based agri-products. *Frontiers in Genome Editing*, 5, 1200987.

Sujatha, V., Suresh, M., & Mahalaxmi, S. (2010). Nanorobotics: A futuristic approach. *SRM University Journal of Dental Sciences*, 1(1), 86–90.

Manickam, V., Sundar, V., Panchangam, R. L., Amiti, S. K., & Tamizhselvi, R. (2021). Nanotechnology in delivery and targeting of phytochemicals. In V. Yata, S. Ranjan, N. Dasgupta, & E. Lichtfouse (Eds.), *Nanopharmaceuticals: Principles and Applications* (Vol. 2, pp. 155–185). Springer.

Pathak, C., Vaidya, F. U., & Pandey, S. M. (2019). Mechanism for development of nanobased drug delivery system. In *Applications of Targeted Nano Drugs and Delivery Systems* (pp. 35–67). Elsevier.

Sandhiya, V., & Udhumansha, U. (2020). A review on herbal drug loaded into pharmaceutical carrier techniques and its evaluation process. *Future Journal of Pharmaceutical Sciences*, 20, 6.

Shoeb, E., Badar, U., Venkataraman, S., & Hefferon, K. (2021). Frontiers in bioengineering and biotechnology: Plant nanoparticles for anti-cancer therapy. *Vaccines*, 9(8), 830.

Singh, S., Sharma, B., Kanwar, S. S., & Kumar, A. (2016). Lead phytochemicals for anticancer drug development. *Frontiers in Plant Science*, 7, 1667.

Wang, S., Su, R., Nie, S., Sun, M., Zhang, J., Wu, D., & Moustaid-Moussa, N. (2014). Application of nanotechnology in improving bioavailability and bioactivity of diet-derived phytochemicals. *Journal of Nanoscience and Nanotechnology*, 25(4), 363–376.

Yang, T., Ji, R., Deng, X. X., Du, F. S., & Li, Z. C. (2014). Glucose-responsive hydrogels based on dynamic covalent chemistry and inclusion complexation. *Soft Matter*, 15, 2671–2678.

Yousefi, M., Narmani, A., & Jafari, S. M. (2020). Dendrimers as efficient nanocarriers for the protection and delivery of bioactive phytochemicals. *Advanced Colloid and Interface Science*, 278, 102125.

Yunus, Y., Khan, M., & Vasanti, S. (2017). Liposomes containing phytochemicals for cancer treatment: An update. *International Journal of Current Pharmaceutical Research*, 9(1), 20–24.

Zuccari, G., & Alfei, S. (2023). Development of phytochemical delivery systems by nano-suspension and nano-emulsion techniques. *International Journal of Molecular Sciences*, 24(12), 9824.

Chapter 18

The Impact of Nanophytoherbals in Cosmetics and Skin Regeneration

Garima Kapoor[1]
Lakshmi Maurya[1]
Rubina Bhutani[2]
and Navidha Aggarwal[3,*]
[1]KIET School of Pharmacy, KIET Group of Institutions, Ghaziabad, Uttar Pradesh, India
[2]School of Medical and Allied Sciences, GD Goenka University, Gurgaon, Haryana, India
[3]M.M. College of Pharmacy, Maharishi Markandeshwar (Deemed to be University), Mullana, Ambala, India

Abstract

The formulation and production of cosmeceuticals have undergone a significant and paradigm-shifting transformation, somewhat reminiscent of the extensive nanotechnology revolution. Today, the development and expansion of the pharmaceutical industries are greatly supported by the nano-formulated cosmeceuticals sector. The main focus of this chapter is the use of nanocarriers to deliver cosmetic ingredients to target areas such as skin, hair, and nails. This chapter highlights different types of nanocarriers that can enhance the delivery of cosmetics. It also discusses nanotechnology approaches in skin regeneration and their toxicological effects, drawing on relevant literature. The introduction of nanoparticles into the cosmetics industry has significantly improved the quality and sophistication of the final products. However, this revolution also carries health risks, as these tiny particles can penetrate intact skin barriers and potentially cause adverse effects. Nanotechnology-based cosmetics include sunscreens, hair cleansers, nail polish, and wrinkle-reducing agents. Given the explosive growth of the cosmetics industry and the integration of nanotechnology, scientific investigation is essential to assess the effectiveness, safety, and application of cosmeceuticals.

Keywords: delivery system, formulation, nanocarriers, nano cosmeceuticals, nanotechnology

---

* Corresponding Author's Email: navidhabansal16@gmail.com.

In: Phyto-Nanomedicine
Editors: Hitesh Chopra, Vinod Kumar Gauttam, Ajmer Singh Grewal et al.
ISBN: 979-8-89530-317-7

Abbreviations

NP	Nanoparticles
LP	Liposomes
SLN	Solid lipid nanoparticles
ACIs	Active cosmetic ingredients
NCs	Nano cosmeceuticals
NE	Nano emulsion
ROS	Reactive oxygen species
FD&C	Federal Food, Drug and Cosmetic
SPF	Sun protection factor
ECM	Extracellular matrix

Introduction

Nanotechnology is widely applied in fields such as dermatology, medicine, biomedical engineering, and cosmetics to create, produce, and characterize particles and devices with molecular dimensions ranging from 1 to 100 nm (Lu & Fuchs, 2014). The internal structural rearrangement of these materials leads to unique physical properties, such as an increased surface area, which alters their interaction with biological systems. This change significantly impacts the formulation and delivery systems of pharmaceutical and cosmeceutical preparations. Cosmeceuticals are produced and formulated using various advanced delivery methods, including liposomes (LP), solid lipid nanoparticles (SLNs), niosomes, gold nanoparticles, nanoemulsions (NE), and nanosomes. These systems optimize the stability of vitamins, antioxidants, and other natural or synthetic ingredients, especially unsaturated fatty acids, and improve the delivery of active cosmetic ingredients (ACIs) to their targets. These delivery techniques can also enhance the biocompatibility of drugs with other excipients, prolong their action, and increase carrier loading capacity. Cosmeceuticals are a blend of pharmaceutical formulations and personal care products. They outperform traditional cosmetics in terms of stability and efficacy, offering measurable results in treating various skin and hair conditions, from common dermatological issues like pigmentation and dryness to more complex problems such as wrinkles and photoaging. When formulated with nanoparticle technology or delivered in nano-sized carriers, these cosmeceuticals are referred to as "nanocosmeceuticals." David Baird asserts that nano cosmetics will be the first commercially viable brand using this advanced delivery technology, which is already present in long-lasting fragrances, skincare, and hair care products. The growth of nanocosmeceuticals (NCs) has steadily increased over the past decade. The use of NCs for delivering active cosmetic agents offers several advantages, including controlled release, targeted delivery, and occlusive dressing of moisturizing ingredients, which significantly enhances skin hydration. NCs can regulate the release of active ingredients from their carrier by incorporating different components and excipients in varying ratios and preparation methods that interact chemically or physically. Despite their many benefits, NCs also have some drawbacks due to their high reactivity. This reactivity can increase the formation of reactive oxygen species (ROS), which are the primary cause of damage to proteins, nucleic acids, and cellular membranes, and can also lead to inflammation. Elevated ROS levels, also known as oxidative stress, are believed to contribute to various clinical conditions, including carcinogenesis, neurodegenerative diseases, and aging. The human skin is the body's first line of defense against external stimuli and injuries. Wound healing and aging are two major processes that occur due to skin exposure to damage. Tissue renewal and regeneration have therefore become areas of significant clinical interest. Scaffolds, nanomaterials, and bioactive compounds have been used to support tissue homeostasis. Single-molecule nanoparticles, such as metals or metal oxides, have been shown to act as effective antibacterial agents and promote the healing of skin lesions and wounds. For example, gold and silver nanoclusters, ranging from 1.1 to 1.6 nm, have been found to enhance skin regeneration *in vivo* in rat models. *In vitro* studies have shown that gold clusters are particularly efficient, promoting cell proliferation and absorption, likely due to enhanced cellular metabolism. These nanoclusters also promote cell migration, a key phase in skin regeneration, and exhibit anti-inflammatory properties as ROS scavengers. Gold NPs (AuNPs) are highly biocompatible and can reduce inflammation, penetrate skin tissues, and support granulation tissue growth. Similarly, silver NPs (AgNPs) stimulate the growth of fibroblasts and keratinocytes by inhibiting respiratory pathways, contributing to faster wound healing and reduced scarring. Additionally, AgNPs can suppress the innate immune response, further accelerating wound healing and reducing scar formation.

Nanocarriers for Delivery of Cosmeceuticals

According to the FD&C Act, cosmetics are substances intended for application to the human body for cleansing, beautifying, or altering appearance. This broad category includes products such as hair care items, makeup, moisturizers, and fragrances. The incorporation of nanocarriers into cosmetic formulations has the potential to revolutionize the skincare industry by offering safer and more effective solutions. This is achieved through enhanced delivery mechanisms, improved stability, and greater efficacy (Chauhan & Chauhan, 2023; Nanda et al., 2020). Nanotechnology, a breakthrough of the 21st century, is transforming the cosmetic industry by introducing nanomaterials with sizes ranging from 1 to 100 nm. These particles provide increased stability, targeted delivery, and enhanced skin penetration. Nanocosmeceuticals, such as nanoliposomes and nanoemulsions, exemplify the transformative potential of nanotechnology, reshaping cosmetic formulations to offer improved effectiveness and personalized skincare solutions, as illustrated in Table 1 (Nanda et al., 2020).

Benefits of Nanocarriers in Cosmetics

- *Enhanced penetration*: Nanocarriers enable deeper penetration of active ingredients into the skin, ensuring improved efficacy by reaching target areas more effectively.
- *Improved stability*: Encapsulating sensitive cosmetic actives within nanocarriers protects them from degradation, oxidation, and UV radiation, thereby extending product shelf life.

Table 1. Advantages, disadvantages, and marketed preparations of different nano-carriers

Name of the carrier	Advantage	Disadvantage	Applications	Marketed preparations
Liposomes (S. Jain, Sapee, & Jain, 1998)	• Easy to synthesize, • Enhanced absorptions • Low risk • Higher absorption • Continuous delivery of ingredients • Biocompatible, nontoxic, and biodegradable	• Low loading capacity, • Physically and chemically instability, • Minimum reproducibility.	• Vitamins • Sunscreen • Fragrance • Sunblock creams, Antiaging creams, • Carotenoids, Conditioners • and shampoos	• Rehydrating Liposome Day cream • Liposome Face & Neck Lotion • Liposome Concentrate • C-Vit Liposomal Serum • Moisture Liposome Eye Cream • Dermosome • Capture Totale
Nanoemulsions	• Rapid penetration, • Merging textures, • Hydrating power • Delivery of lipophilic compound	• High cost, • Stability problems	• Skin care products • Controlled delivery systems. • Deodorants, • Sunscreens, • Hair care products. • Sunblock cream • Exfoliant scrub • Body firming lotion,	• Vital Nanoemulsions A-VC • Precision-Solution • Hyaluronic Acid and Nanoemulsion • Intensive Hydration Toner • Phyto-Endorphin Hand Cream • Vitacos Vita-Herb Nona-Vital Skin Toner (Dhapte-Pawar et al., 2020)
Niosomes	• Improving • Improving Bioavailability • Enhancing skin penetration • Deliver both hydrophilic hydrophobic compounds	• High cost, • Stability problems, • Vulnerability to oxidation	• Beauty creams • Hair related cosmetics	• Eusu Niosome Makam Pom Whitening Facial cream • Shampooing Floral Repair • Masque Floral Repair • Anti-Age Response Cream • Mayu Niosome Base Cream
Solid lipid nanoparticles (Ahmad, 2021)	• Low toxicity • More stable • Nanoscale geometry, • Skin penetration • Minimum toxicity, • Site dependent activity, • Higher bioavailability	• Side effects • Restrict patient compliance.	• Acne • Skin Mycoses • Psoriasis • Dermatitis • Hair growth	• NanoLipid Repair CLR • SURMER Crème • Olivenol Augenpflegebalsam

Name of the carrier	Advantage	Disadvantage	Applications	Marketed preparations
Gold and silver nanoparticles	• Antimicrobial properties • Noncytotoxic, • Biocompatible, • Highly stable, • Inert • High drug-loading capacity	• Toxicity • High cost • Stability problems	• Deodorant, • Facial creams, • Antiaging products, • Moisturizer creams • Face pack, • Lotions and creams.	• ChantecailleNano Gold Energizing Eye Serum • AmeiziiNano Gold Foil Liquid • LR Nano Gold and Silk Day Cream • O3+ 24 K Gold Gel Cream Orogold • 24K Nano Ultra Silk Serum (Dhapte-Pawar et al., 2020)
Dendrimers	• Transport to liver and macrophages • Hydrophobic and hydrophilic medicines can	• Toxicity • Stability	• Sunblock cream, • Shampoos, • Antiacne creams, • Hair gels, • Utilized for hair, nails, and skin • Vitamins A and B6	• Revlon (Das et al., 2018) • Carbosiloxane • Dendrimer • Keratin-peptide/ • dendrimer • Hydroxyl-functionalized • dendritic macromolecule

- *Targeted delivery*: Nanocarriers can be designed to deliver active ingredients to specific skin layers or address particular concerns like wrinkles, pigmentation, or hydration.
- *Reduced irritation*: By controlling the release rate of active ingredients, nanocarriers lower the risk of skin irritation that may occur with high concentrations of actives.
- *Versatility*: Nanocarriers allow for the incorporation of both hydrophilic and hydrophobic active ingredients, broadening the scope of cosmetic products that can benefit from their application.

Applications of Nanocarriers in Cosmetics

- *Anti-aging formulations*: Nanocarriers deliver antioxidants, peptides, and retinoids, which help combat signs of aging by promoting collagen production and reducing oxidative stress.
- *Sunscreen products*: Nanoencapsulation improves the stability and efficacy of UV filters, providing better sun protection while reducing the whitening effect typical of traditional sunscreens.
- *Skin lightening agents:* Nanocarriers allow for controlled release of agents like vitamin C and niacinamide, promoting even skin tone and reducing hyperpigmentation.
- *Moisturizers*: Nanocarrier-based formulations with hyaluronic acid and ceramides enhance skin hydration and restore the skin's barrier function, making them highly effective in moisturizing products.
- *Hair care products*: Nanocarriers can deliver nutrients and conditioning agents deep into the hair shaft, improving hair strength, shine, and manageability.

Nanotechnology is driving innovation in cosmetics, offering advanced nanosystems such as liposomes and nanoemulsions that enhance stability, penetration, and controlled release of active compounds. As cosmeceuticals grow with nanotechnology, they offer solutions for various skin and hair concerns, such as hyperpigmentation and hair damage (Pooja & Kulhari, 2024). Nanocarriers provide a promising route for innovation, set to transform the cosmetics industry with safer, more effective, and customized skincare solutions (El-Deeb et al., 2020).

Applications of Nanotechnology in Cosmetics

Nanotechnology in cosmetics utilizes nanomaterials, ranging from 1 to 100 nm, to improve product performance, appearance, and efficacy (Fytianos et al., 2020). These materials, such as zinc oxide, titanium dioxide, AuNPs, and liposomes, offer unique advantages including enhanced delivery of active ingredients, novel textures, and superior sun protection (Krutmann et al., 2021; Mihranyan et al., 2012; Jain et al., 2010; Raj et al., 2012). For instance, NPs can amplify the effectiveness of sunscreens and contribute to more appealing textures in cosmetic products. While nanotechnology offers potential benefits, such as increased efficacy, consumer satisfaction, and product differentiation, several challenges remain. These include unclear regulatory guidelines, concerns about the long-term health and environmental impacts of nanomaterials, and ethical issues related to nanoscale manipulation. As cosmetic dermatology continues to advance, it will be crucial to understand the safety, efficacy, and long-term effects of NP-based products to ensure their role in promoting health and innovation in cosmetic science (Nafisi et al., 2017; Lo & Fauzi, 2021; Liu et al., 2019).

Titanium Dioxide and Zinc Oxide

Sunscreens, which protect the skin from harmful sun radiation, are formulated to block UVB, UVA-2, and UVA-1 rays. Inorganic UV radiation filters, such as TiO_2 and ZnO, are commonly used due to their effectiveness in shielding the skin. TiO_2 is particularly superior at blocking UVB rays, while ZnO is more effective against UVA rays. Together, these particles provide broad-spectrum UV protection. TiO2 is the most popular inorganic nanoparticle in sunscreens, mainly because it offers a higher sun protection factor (SPF) at the nanoscale. Its transparency at this scale allows for greater protection and a more restorative effect compared to its non-nano counterparts. The enhanced properties of TiO_2 are largely due to its large surface-area-to-volume ratio at the nano level, which increases its molecular carrying capacity when the particles are smaller than 10^{-20} nm. Additionally, both ZnO and TiO2 in nanoparticle form demonstrate significant advantages over larger-scale materials, making them highly effective in modern sunscreen formulations (Yadwade et al., 2021).

Gold Nanoparticles

Many skincare products, including salves and lotions, now incorporate gold due to its beneficial properties. When gold particles in these products range in size from 5 to 400 nm, they are referred to as colloidal gold or nanogold. The size and surface area of these particles influence their color, which can vary from purple to scarlet. Gold NPs can take on various shapes, such as cubes, triangles, stars, clusters, nanospheres, nanorods, and nanoshells. Their stability and biocompatibility have made them highly suitable for skincare and cosmetic applications (Cizauskaite & Bernatoniene, 2018). Additionally, their well-known antibacterial and anti-aging properties have significant benefits for the cosmetics industry and wound healing. Gold-based NPs play a vital role in repairing skin damage, enhancing smoothness, elasticity, and overall skin appearance. Gold also has calming properties, making it an effective treatment for conditions such as sunburn, skin hypersensitivity, and inflammation, which makes it useful in various makeup and skincare formulations (Hameed et al., 2019).

Silver Nanoparticles

Silver NPs are among the most effective antimicrobial agents available. They can also be used in combination with silver-based compounds to control bacterial growth in various formulations. However, using silver in cosmetics may present challenges, as silver can precipitate in silver-based mixtures. These issues can be addressed by utilizing silver NPs, which offer enhanced stability and effectiveness. Despite the use of colloidal silver in cosmetic products, concerns about the safety of its nanostructure remain. In the U.S., many cosmetics lack antibacterial properties due to the absence of clear FDA regulations. Silver NPs, when added to cosmetic formulations, have been shown to maintain the stability of the mixture for at least a year, without signs of sedimentation (Effiong et al., 2019).

Lip Cosmetics

Lipstick and lip gloss are two widely used cosmetics. Lipsticks formulated with NPs enhance lip softness by preventing water loss from the trans-epidermal region, helping to keep the lips hydrated. NPs based on silica also contribute to a more even distribution of pigments in the formulation, preventing the pigments from migrating into the fine lines of the lips. This results in a smoother, more uniform appearance and improves the overall look of the cosmetic product (Huber & Burfeindt, 2019).

Micellar Nanoparticles

Micellar nanoparticle-based cosmetics are one of the latest trends in the beauty industry. Various brands, both international and local, are adopting this nanoparticle technology as an innovative approach to enhance the efficacy and quality of cosmetics. L'Oréal S.A., a prominent company in this field, offers two products that utilize micellar NPs, resulting in a nanoemulsion system. These products successfully create a stable and transparent nanoemulsion with oil-micelle dispersion, featuring an average particle size of less than 100 nm. In this nanoemulsion system, the oily phase consists of at least one oil with a molecular weight exceeding 400, which is dispersed in an aqueous phase (Lauterbach et al., 2015). Additionally, the formulation must include at least one selected anionic surfactant, with the weight ratio of the oily phase to the surfactant ranging from 2 to 10%. A higher proportion of oil in the formulation enhances both transparency and the cosmetic effects of the product. Moreover, micellar-based cosmetics are beneficial for various applications, including hair, skin, eyes, scalp, and mucous membranes (Dubey et al., 2022).

Potentially Active Chemical Constituents

Phytoconstituents are gaining popularity as ingredients in cosmetic formulations due to their ability to protect the skin from harmful external and internal agents and to aid in the treatment of various skin conditions (Hivechi et al., 2021). When the skin is exposed to sunlight and other environmental factors, ROS are generated. These ROS can interact with DNA, fatty acids, and proteins, leading to oxidative damage and a weakened antioxidant defense system. Such damage disrupts the skin's natural regulatory mechanisms, accelerating the aging process and increasing the risk of skin cancer. Signs of aging include wrinkles, roughness, a loss of elasticity, and uneven pigmentation. Herbal extracts are known for their anti-aging, healing, softening, and revitalizing properties, making them effective for addressing these concerns. Certain photoprotective phytoconstituents, such as resveratrol, green tea extract, curcumin, quercetin, and silymarin, are utilized in the formulation of herbal cosmetics that have the potential to reduce the risk of skin cancer and delay the aging process (Lu et al., 1993). Botanical extracts exhibit multifunctional properties, including photoprotection, anti-aging, moisturizing, antioxidant, astringent, and antibacterial effects (Kaur et al., 2007). Key chemical classes in these extracts include polyphenols, monoterpenes, flavonoids, organosulfides, and indoles, all of which contain natural compounds (Katiyar et al., 2000). After conducting a thorough literature review on herbs that act as photoprotectives, specific herbs have been selected based on their characteristics, availability, estimation methodologies, stability, and the efficacy of the resulting formulations, as well as findings from previous studies (Ahuja & Bajpai, 2024).

Nature of Phytoconstituents

Solubility is a crucial factor in the development of innovative formulations. The selection of the optimal formulation is determined by the nature of the phytoconstituent, specifically whether it is lipophilic or hydrophilic. Table 2 presents the chemical composition and solvent solubility of significant photoprotective phytoconstituents (Kuttan et al., 1987).

Nano-herbals in Skin Regeneration

Although skin regeneration and healing have advanced significantly in recent years, numerous obstacles remain to further enhance this progress. One such challenge is the careful selection of skin care products that contain active compounds (Hajleh et al., 2020). Nanofiber scaffolds have garnered attention for creating innovative drug-like skin care products, as they show great promise for both clinical and laboratory applications (Munʃoz et al., 2022). Both natural and synthetic scaffolds and fibers are commonly employed for skin regeneration and repair. These fibrous scaffolds are mechanically stable and can perform biological functions in the embedded environment (Gosiewska et al., 2001). The scaffold's design, choice of biomaterial, and interactions between the material and cells are the main factors determining mechanical stability, including the effective delivery of drugs or other beneficial substances. Biological function is regulated by signals from the extracellular matrix (ECM), neighboring cells, and growth factors (Reddi, 2000). ECM molecules surround the cells, controlling cellular functions and providing mechanical support. The primary goal of nanofiber scaffold design is to create an ideal structure that can temporarily replace the natural extracellular matrix until host cells can regenerate a new natural matrix (Alberts et al., 2002). Drug loading and delivery are additional uses for nanofiber scaffolds, showing promise for skin regeneration and healing. The drug delivered by the scaffold has a longer half-life due to the mechanical support provided by the scaffolds, addressing a common challenge in drug delivery. Two key concepts in skin regeneration and repair are the ability of surrounding cells to regenerate and the effective transport of skin drugs to target locations (Morganti et al., 2020). The cells that envelop injured tissue or participate in the tissue's self-healing process can proliferate into molecules that resemble the original tissue.

Table 2. Chemical profile, solubility, and mechanism in the treatment of important photoprotective phytoconstituents

Phytoconstituent	Structure	Solubility	Mechanism
Curcumin (Nakamura et al., 1998)	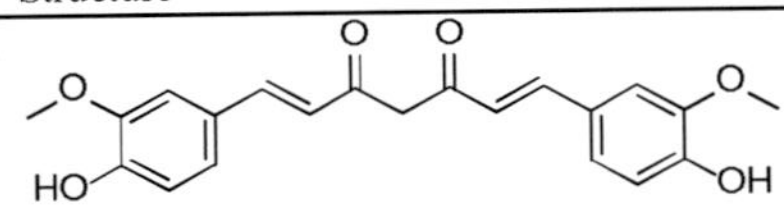	Soluble in Acetone, ethanol, DMSO, dimethyl formamide	Reduce ROS by preventing protein kinase C from activating Increase the amount of glutathione and GST activity Reduce arachidonic acid and lipid peroxidation Suppresses the activity of ornithine decarboxylase (ODC)
Resveratrol (Afaq et al., 2003)	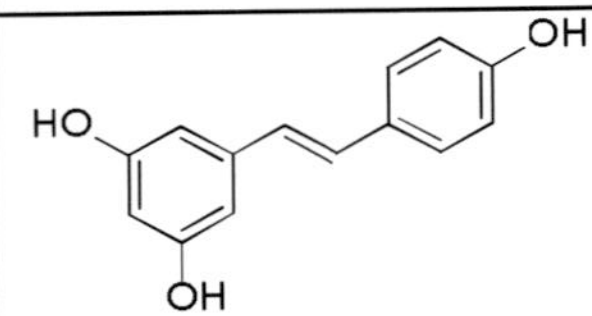	Soluble in ether, chloroform, ethanol, acetic acid, acetone.	Reduces the activities of COX-2 and ODC prevents elevated lipid peroxidation levels
Quercetin (Erden Inal et al., 2001)	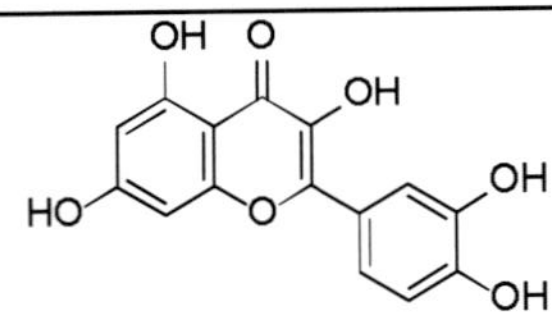	Soluble in isopropyl myristate, oleyl alcohol, propylene glycol monolaurate, propylene glycol monocaprylate (PGMC).	Antioxidant, glutathione peroxidase, reductase, catalase, and dismutase
Genistein	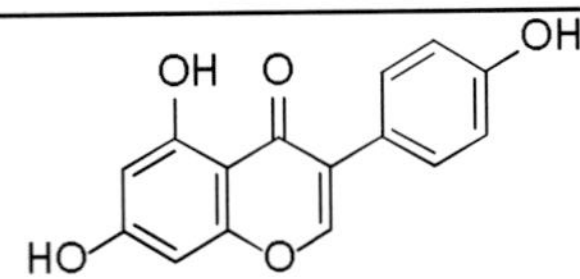	Ethanol, DMSO, dimethyl formamide.	Inhibits H2O2 production Inhibits hypersensitivity Reduction of edema
Silibinin/Silymarin	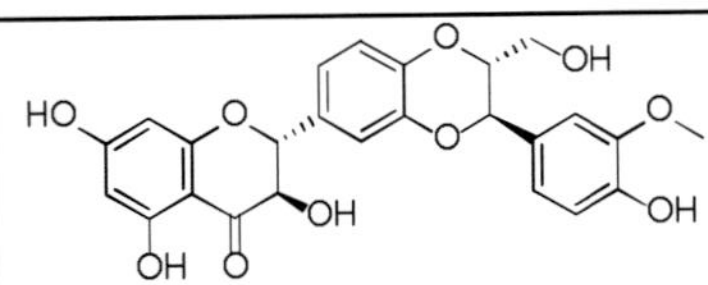	Soluble in gastric fluid, intestinal fluid, dioxane.	Inhibits skin edema, sunburn, and cell apoptosis, resists catalase activity, resists COX-2 activities

Phytoconstituent	Structure	Solubility	Mechanism
Ascorbic acid (Khan et al., 2016)	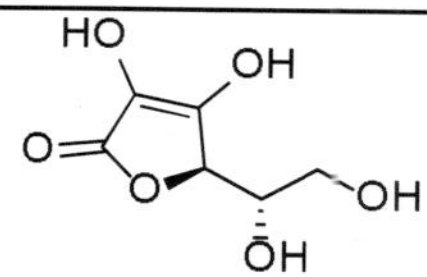	Soluble in water, ethanol, glycerol, propylene glycol.	Inhibits solar radiations induced p53, antioxidant enhancer
Green tea polyphenols/ catechins (Katiyar et al., 2001)	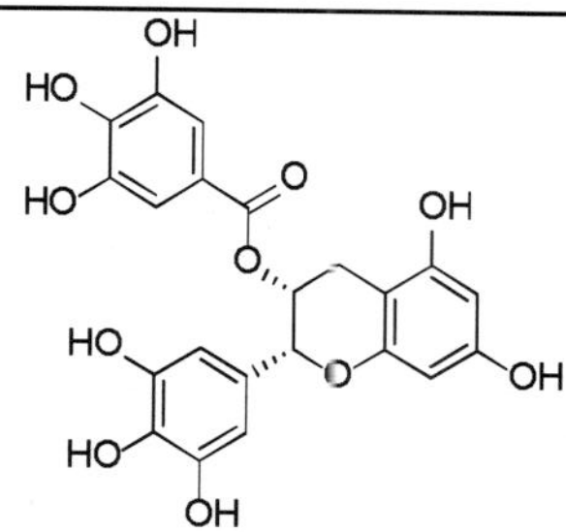		Reduction cyclobutane-pyrimidine dimers. Resists cutaneous edema and erythema.

The 3D molecular structure of living cells in a natural ECM consists primarily of two types of multifibrils at the nanoscale: proteins and proteoglycans. Therefore, the hierarchical organization of structures, along with nanoscale intermolecular binding interactions within the cellular environment, will enhance the morphology and functionality of the cells (Beznoska et al., 2019). Studies have indicated the effectiveness of nanofiber scaffolds in promoting skin repair and regeneration. To improve cell-matrix interactions, it is important to develop more biomimetic nanofiber scaffolds with nanoscale molecular architectures, larger surface areas for adsorbing proteins and skin medications, and multiple binding sites for cell membrane receptors (Lu & Fuchs, 2014). For all the above reasons, creating an appropriate nanofiber scaffold is critical in developing scaffolds that promote skin healing and regeneration (Bellu et al., 2021).

Toxicity Profile of Nano Cosmeceuticals

According to the concept of cosmeceuticals, prescriptions are not required since they do not possess any therapeutic properties (Zhu et al., 2006). These widely available products may have some short- and long-term adverse effects, which could restrict their use. Factors influencing these side effects include concentration, duration, and mode of administration. Cosmetics designed for application on the lips or surrounding areas may pose a risk of systemic toxicity if accidentally consumed, such as sticks, glosses, and coloring agents (Zhang et al., 2010). Cosmetics meant for application on the lips or areas that define them have the potential to cause systemic toxicity if accidentally consumed. Sticks, glosses, and coloring agents are examples of these (Oberdörster et al., 2005). The negative effects of cosmeceuticals are influenced by several variables: some are associated with the formulation qualities of the active components, others relate to the chemical makeup of the cosmeceutical agent, and others depend on factors such as surface area, coating composition, particle size, and tendency to aggregate (Aldawsari et al., 2015). If the surfaces of the organ and the nanostructure are similar, there may be a heightened risk of adverse effects (Yah et al., 2012). A typical correlation exists between increased surface area-to-volume ratio and heightened biological and chemical reactivity (Sayes et al., 2004). Consequently, poorly soluble NPs can exhibit strong toxicities and have been linked to breast cancer (Zhang, 2018). Further research is necessary to fully understand the toxicities associated with fullerenes, although preliminary indications suggest that their toxic effects may be related to their ability to oxidize cells. Following pulmonary exposure, ultrafine titanium dioxide particles can cause lung tissue damage and inflammatory responses. Although metallic nanoparticles possess antibacterial properties, their use has been linked to reductions in weight, spleen index, and red blood cell count in experimental animals. Additionally, because these NPs can cross the placenta, they are not considered safe for use during pregnancy. Formulations containing zinc and titanium oxides may lead to membrane damage by generating free radicals, particularly when exposed to UV radiation (Sen et al., 2009).

Future Prospectives

Cosmetics have evolved into nano cosmetics, and the development of technology along with the introduction of novel bioactive substances that can target cellular and tissue levels will be key to the industry's future success. Both consumers and the industry are increasingly vocal about their demands for cutting-edge treatments. Nano cosmetics represent advanced drug delivery technologies, offering administration methods that can mitigate the negative effects associated with traditional dosage forms. Scientific claims and research findings propose a distinct method for promoting targeted delivery in specific areas with multifaceted therapeutic effects. Utilizing herbal remedies, nano cosmetics effectively treat a variety of skin conditions, including psoriasis, bacterial and fungal infections, hyperpigmentation, pemphigus, and skin cancer (Buzea et al., 2007). The biomedical sector is expanding, addressing the medical needs of affected individuals. Clinical responses are required to evaluate newer nanocosmetics with innovative carriers, as suggested by scientific data investigations. Smart cosmetics, or nanoformulations, yield novel nanocosmetics with enhanced performance, reduced adverse effects, and improved bioavailability. They are considered a newer category, eco-friendly, and researched for skincare conditions like aging and hyperpigmentation, reflecting consumer preferences. Patents related to nanocosmetics that incorporate herbal components offer promising avenues for further investigation. The development of quick, cost-effective, safe, and biocompatible green processes has shown significant potential for producing biogenic colloidal gold and AgNPs (Poon & Burd, 2004). The creation of biogenic NPs involves several underlying molecular pathways, many of which remain to be elucidated. Investigating these pathways may be crucial for enhancing yield and modifying the synthesis of these NPs. Furthermore, innovative methods for creating and utilizing important metabolites for wound healing will be highlighted in synthesizing such NPs. Regulating the size and shape of the produced NPs will benefit from these techniques. These strategies will improve the wound healing capacity of biogenic NPs and enhance the management of wound infections. As noted, there is currently limited research on the ability of green-synthesized NPs to promote wound healing. Therefore, in-depth investigations into the molecular mechanisms involving multiple pathways are necessary, as understanding the involvement of these pathways will help determine how these nanomedicines can be uniquely effective for wound healing. Additional research is required to explore other medicinal plants for the green synthesis of NPs, aiming to create more affordable, biocompatible, and effective metal NPs. The primary toxicity associated with chemically manufactured NPs can be mitigated by using green-synthesized metal NPs, which often require further coating with biocompatible polymers and surfactants. However, more research is needed to understand the protein corona effect concerning biogenic NPs. This innovative technology holds the potential to develop new therapeutic agents that combine the benefits of medicinal plants, NPs, and wound healing. The use of biogenic Au and AgNPs in wound healing is relatively novel, but preliminary *in vivo* findings have been highly encouraging and promising.

Conclusion

Regenerative medicine still faces significant challenges in wound healing and skin rejuvenation, but nanotechnology has substantially advanced the field. Recent discoveries of NPs have opened new avenues for treating wounds, promoting tissue regeneration, and reversing aging-related morphogenetic changes. The use of these novel products, either alone or in combination, has greatly expanded due to regulated drug delivery mediated by nanodevices, biocompatibility, antimicrobial properties, and protection of affected areas. These factors contribute to excellent performance, safety, and ease of administration. The skincare sector has gained popularity worldwide, driven by the affordability of these products and their superior cosmetic results. By strategically managing natural materials, the industry is exploring uncharted territories in the cosmetics market while promoting contemporary health and beauty features. To overcome the limitations of traditional treatment methods, novel carriers such as liposomes, NPs, nanosponges, and nanocapsules found in nanocosmetics are emerging as innovative and effective strategies to treat dermal infections. The growing popularity of nanomedicines in the medical industry is propelled by their ability to provide targeted delivery, reduce dosage frequency, and enhance patient compliance, resulting in improved therapeutic outcomes. Furthermore, both lipophilic and hydrophilic medications can be encapsulated in nanoformulations, preventing drug degradation at specific locations. Preclinical research based on robust evidence is becoming increasingly vital before commercialization to enhance the efficacy of cosmetic products. The advancements in nanotechnology have paved the way for new delivery methods, known as nanomedicines, which can effectively address dermatological disorders while overcoming the limitations of traditional therapeutic approaches. Additionally, scientists and researchers are facing challenges related to the regulatory aspects of stability and safety standards, which need to be addressed before entering the pharmaceutical market. Thanks to nanocarriers, herbal remedies can now be applied topically with enhanced efficacy, reduced toxicity, and controlled release. Therefore, the application of nanotechnologies holds considerable promise for improving wound healing and rejuvenation, sustaining skin cell populations in challenging environments, and implementing therapeutic options currently utilized in clinical settings.

References

Afaq, F., Adhami, V. M., & Ahmad, N. (2003). Prevention of short-term ultraviolet B radiation-mediated damages by resveratrol in SKH-1 hairless mice. *Toxicology and applied pharmacology*, *186*(1), 28–37.

Ahmad, J. (2021). Lipid nanoparticles based cosmetics with potential application in alleviating skin disorders. *Cosmetics*, *8*(3), 84.

Bellu, E., Medici, S., Coradduzza, D., Cruciani, S., Amler, E., & Maioli, M. (2021). Nanomaterials in Skin Regeneration and Rejuvenation. *International journal of molecular sciences*, *22*(13), 7095.

Buzea, C., Pacheco, I. I., & Robbie, K. (2007). Nanomaterials and nanoparticles: sources and toxicity. *Biointerphases*, *2*(4), MR17–MR71.

Chauhan, A., & Chauhan, C. (2023). Emerging trends of nanotechnology in beauty solutions: A review. *Materials Today: Proceedings*, *81*, 1052-1059.

Cizauskaite, U., & Bernatoniene, J. (2018). Innovative natural ingredients-based multiple emulsions: The effect on human skin moisture, sebum content, pore size and pigmentation. *Molecules*, *23*(6), 1428.

Das, N., Sharma, P. A., Seth, A., Maheshwari, R., Tekade, M., Shrivastava, S. K., & Tekade, R. K. (2018). An overview of dendrimers and their biomedical applications. *Dendrimers for Drug Delivery*, 135-206.

Dhapte-Pawar, V., Kadam, S., Saptarsi, S., & Kenjale, P. P. (2020). Nanocosmeceuticals: Facets and aspects. *Future Science OA*, *6*(10), FSO613.

Dubey, S. K., Dey, A., Singhvi, G., Pandey, M. M., Singh, V., & Kesharwani, P. (2022). Emerging trends of nanotechnology in advanced cosmetics. *Colloids and surfaces B: Biointerfaces*, *214*, 112440.

Effiong, D. E., Uwah, T. O., Jumbo, E. U., & Akpabio, A. E. (2019). Nanotechnology in cosmetics: basics, current trends and safety concerns—A review. *Advances in Nanoparticles*, *9*(1), 1-22.

El-Deeb, N. M., Abo-Eleneen, M. A., Al-Madboly, L. A., Sharaf, M. M., Othman, S. S., Ibrahim, O. M., & Mubarak, M. S. (2020). Biogenically synthesized polysaccharides-capped silver nanoparticles: immunomodulatory and antibacterial potentialities against resistant Pseudomonas aeruginosa. *Frontiers in Bioengineering and Biotechnology*, *8*, 643.

Erden Inal, M., Kahraman, A., & Köken, T. (2001). Beneficial effects of quercetin on oxidative stress induced by ultraviolet A. *Clinical and experimental dermatology*, *26*(6), 536-539.

Fytianos, G., Rahdar, A., & Kyzas, G. Z. (2020). Nanomaterials in cosmetics: Recent updates. *Nanomaterials*, *10*(5), 979.

Hameed, A., Fatima, G. R., Malik, K., Muqadas, A., & Fazal-ur-Rehman, M. (2019). Scope of nanotechnology in cosmetics: dermatology and skin care products. *J. Med. Chem. Sci*, *2*(9).

Hivechi, A., Milan, P. B., Modabberi, K., Amoupour, M., Ebrahimzadeh, K., Gholipour, A. R., Sedighi, F., Amini, N., Bahrami, S. H., Rezapour, A., Hamidi, M., & Delattre, C. (2021). Synthesis and characterization of exopolysaccharide encapsulated PCL/gelatin skin substitute for full-thickness wound regeneration. *Polymers*, *13*(6), 854.

Huber, B., & Burfeindt, J. (2019). Nanotechnology in cosmetics. *Nanocosmetics: From Ideas to Products*, 17-25.

Jain, K., Kesharwani, P., Gupta, U., & Jain, N. K. (2010). Dendrimer toxicity: Let's meet the challenge. *International journal of pharmaceutics*, *394*(1-2), 122-142.

Jain, S., Sapre, R., & Jain, N. K. (1998). Proultraflexible lipid vesicles for effective transdermal delivery of norgesterol, proceedings of 25th conference of CRS.

Katiyar, S. K., Afaq, F., Perez, A., & Mukhtar, H. (2001). Green tea polyphenol (–)-epigallocatechin-3-gallate treatment of human skin inhibits ultraviolet radiation-induced oxidative stress. *Carcinogenesis*, 22(2), 287-294.

Kaur, I. P., & Agrawal, R. (2007). Nanotechnology: a new paradigm in cosmeceuticals. *Recent patents on drug delivery & formulation*, *1*(2), 171-182.

Khan, H., Akhtar, N., Khan, H. M. S., Arshad, A. I., Naeem, M., Sohail, M., ... & Nawaz, Z. (2016). Synergistic effects of ascorbyl palmitate and sodium ascorbyl phosphate loaded in multiple emulsions on facial skin melanin and erythema content. *Biomed Res*, *27*(2), 570-576.

Krutmann, J., Schalka, S., Watson, R. E. B., Wei, L., & Morita, A. (2021). Daily photoprotection to prevent photoaging. *Photodermatology, photoimmunology & photomedicine*, *37*(6), 482-489.

Kuttan, R., Sudheeran, P. C., & Josph, C. D. (1987). Turmeric and curcumin as topical agents in cancer therapy. *Tumori Journal*, *73*(1), 29-31.

Lauterbach, A., & Müller-Goymann, C. C. (2015). Applications and limitations of lipid nanoparticles in dermal and transdermal drug delivery via the follicular route. *European Journal of Pharmaceutics and Biopharmaceutics*, *97*, 152-163.

Liu, Y., Zhou, S., Gao, Y., & Zhai, Y. (2019). Electrospun nanofibers as a wound dressing for treating diabetic foot ulcer. *Asian Journal of Pharmaceutical Sciences*, *14*(2), 130-143.

Lo, S., & Fauzi, M. B. (2021). A review of the current update of collagen nanomaterials—fabrication, characterisation and its applications. *Pharmaceutics*, *13*(3), 316.

Lu, C., & Fuchs, E. (2014). Sweat gland progenitors in development, homeostasis, and wound repair. *Cold Spring Harbor perspectives in medicine*, *4*(2), a015222.

Lu, Y. P., L. Chang, R., Huang, M. T., & H. Conney, A. (1993). Inhibitory effect of curcumin on 12-O-tetradecanoylphorbol-13-acetate-induced increase in ornithine decarboxylase mRNA in mouse epidermis. *Carcinogenesis*, *14*(2), 293-297.

Mihranyan, A., Ferraz, N., & Strømme, M. (2012). Current status and future prospects of nanotechnology in cosmetics. *Progress in materials science*, *57*(5), 875-910.

Kaur, I. P., & Agrawal, R. (2007). Nanotechnology: a new paradigm in cosmeceuticals. *Recent patents on drug delivery & formulation*, *1*(2), 171–182. https://doi.org/10.2174/187221107780831888.

Nakamura, Y., Ohto, Y., Murakami, A., Osawa, T., & Ohigashi, H. (1998). Inhibitory effects of curcumin and tetrahydrocurcuminoids on the tumor promoter-induced reactive oxygen species generation in leukocytes *in vitro* and *in vivo*. *Japanese Journal of Cancer Research*, *89*(4), 361-370.

Nanda, A., Nanda, S., Nguyen, T. A., Rajendran, S., & Slimani, Y. (Eds.). (2020). *Nanocosmetics: fundamentals, applications and toxicity*. Elsevier.

Pooja, D., & Kulhari, H. (2024). *Nanotechnology Based Delivery of Phytoconstituents and Cosmeceuticals*. Springer.

Poon, V. K., & Burd, A. (2004). *In vitro* cytotoxicity of silver: implication for clinical wound care. *Burns*, *30*(2), 140-147.

Raj, S., Jose, S., Sumod, U. S., & Sabitha, M. (2012). Nanotechnology in cosmetics: Opportunities and challenges. *Journal of Pharmacy and Bioallied Sciences*, *4*(3), 186-193.

Sen, C. K., Gordillo, G. M., Roy, S., Kirsner, R., Lambert, L., Hunt, T. K., Gottrup, F., Gurtner, G. C., & Longaker, M. T. (2009). Human skin wounds: a major and snowballing threat to public health and the economy. *Wound repair and regeneration*, *17*(6), 763-771.

Yadwade, R., Gharpure, S., & Ankamwar, B. (2021). Nanotechnology in cosmetics pros and cons. *Nano Express*, *2*(2), 022003.

Yah, C. S., Iyuke, S. E., & Simate, G. S. (2012). A review of nanoparticles toxicity and their routes of exposures: transdermal delivery of insulin. *Iranian Journal of Pharmaceutical Sciences*, *8*(1), 299-314.

Zhang, X. D., Wu, H. Y., Wu, D., Wang, Y. Y., Chang, J. H., Zhai, Z. B., Meng, A. M., Liu, P. X., Zhang, L. A., & Fan, F. Y. (2010). Toxicologic effects of gold nanoparticles *in vivo* by different administration routes. *International journal of nanomedicine*, 5, 771-781.

Chapter 19

Applications of Nanophytoherbals in Respiratory Diseases

Raman Kumari[1,*]
Anuj Malik[1]
and Dinesh Kumar[2]
[1]M.M. College of Pharmacy, Maharishi Markandeshwar (Deemed to be University), Mullana, Ambala, Haryana, India
[2]School of Pharmacy, Deshbhagat University, Mandi Gobindgarh, Fathehgarh Sahib, Punjab, India

Abstract

Respiratory diseases, also referred to as pulmonary or lung conditions, include cystic fibrosis, chronic obstructive pulmonary disease (COPD), bronchial asthma, pulmonary fibrosis, and lung cancer. These disorders are recognized as progressive and incurable, ranking among the world's top five causes of death. Risk factors associated with these diseases include smoking, irreversible bronchoconstriction, alveolar degradation, and pulmonary vascular remodeling. Numerous synthetic compounds have been employed to treat various lung conditions, but they often come with life-threatening side effects. To mitigate the growing risk of respiratory illnesses, it is imperative to explore antibiotic alternatives as well as sustainable, economical, effective, and long-lasting approaches to address these widespread issues. In this context, the science of nanotechnology offers a promising avenue for combating respiratory diseases. Nanophyto-medicines are herbal formulations developed using nanotechnology, which utilizes phyto-chemically standardized herbal extracts or bioactive components. These plant-based antibiotics have fewer side effects and provide more effective therapeutic benefits compared to synthetic compounds. For instance, liposomes and polymeric NPs are examples of nano-based systems designed to enhance the stability and bioavailability of phytoconstituents, particularly in the treatment of long-term illnesses like lung cancer. Therefore, the combination of innovative drug delivery methods with herbal medicines proves effective in addressing severe chronic lung conditions.

Keywords: pulmonary diseases, herbal medicines, phytoconstitutents, liposomes, novel drug delivery systems

---

* Corresponding Author's Email: sinhmarraman07@gmail.com.

In: Phyto-Nanomedicine
Editors: Hitesh Chopra, Vinod Kumar Gauttam, Ajmer Singh Grewal et al.
ISBN: 979-8-89530-317-7

Abbreviations

RDs	Respiratory Diseases
NPs	Nanoparticles
NPs	Natural Products
SLNs	Solid Lipid Nanoparticles
CR	Curcumin
curcumin-SLNs	Curcumin Solid Lipid Nanoparticles
QT	Quercetin
SLM	Solid Lipid Microparticle
LM	Lipid Microparticle
Naringenin HPPCD	naringenin-hydroxypropyl-p-cyclodextrin
SD	Sprague-Dawley
GSH	Glutathione
MDA	malondialdehyde
LPS	Lipopolysaccharide
EMT	Epithelial-Mesenchymal Transition

Introduction

The upper respiratory tract comprises the larynx, trachea, oropharyngeal, and nasal cavities, while the lower respiratory tract contains the lungs, diaphragm, and bronchi, constituting the ventilatory system, also referred to as the human respiratory system (Hsia et al., 2016). The lungs play a crucial role in facilitating gas exchange, which is essential for sustaining life. Infections and ailments affecting the lungs and associated organs can hinder respiratory function (El-Kased, 2016). These respiratory diseases (RDs), which include conditions like lung cancer, lower respiratory tract infections, and obstructive pulmonary disease, significantly contribute to global disability and mortality. Risk factors for these disorders include smoking, irreversible bronchoconstriction, alveolar degradation, and pulmonary vascular remodeling (Wang et al., 2016). Modern developments in managing respiratory diseases involve a range of interventions, including vaccination, antibiotics, agonists, corticosteroids, ventilatory assistance, inhalation therapy, and lung surgery. The pressing need for potent and less harmful anti-infective agents arises from the emergence of new RDs and the rise of strains resistant to multiple drugs, as well as variations in pathogens, which undermine the efficacy of current treatments (Panahi et al., 2016; Behzadi & Leyva-Grado, 2019). To mitigate the escalating threat of RDs, it is essential to explore non-antibiotic alternatives and sustainable, cost-effective, and durable approaches. Nanotechnology emerges as a promising tool against RDs, enhancing drug delivery and targeting infections induced by multidrug-resistant pathogens (Hayat, 2018). Nanoparticles (NPs) possess antibacterial and antiviral properties, targeting multiple biomolecules and potentially halting the evolution of multidrug-resistant organisms (MDROs). NPs improve drug bioavailability, ensuring systematic release and reducing toxicity, with a focus on biodegradability for pulmonary-related nanodrugs. Particle size dictates deposition mechanisms, where NPs under 160 nm rely on diffusion, while larger particles use sedimentation and impaction (Sadikot et al., 2017). Natural products (NPs) are compounds generated by living organisms in their natural environment and serve as pivotal elements in drug discovery. These products stem from diverse sources, including minerals, terrestrial and marine life, plants, and animals. Plant-derived NPs are notable for their intricate, structurally diverse compounds tailored for specific biological functions. Phytochemicals, abundant in plants, contribute to their medicinal and organoleptic properties, gaining attention for their preventive and curative effects against ailments, including cancer, cardiovascular diseases, and respiratory conditions (Sorokina & Steinbeck, 2020). Despite being water-soluble, phytoconstituents face challenges in absorption due to their substantial molecular sizes and limited ability to pass through lipid membranes, which restricts their bioavailability and efficacy. Safety concerns arise from potential incompatibility with other ingredients and high systemic clearance, leading to low therapeutic blood levels and inconsistencies between *in vitro* and *in vivo* effects, which impede advancement through clinical trials (Lim et al., 2022). Nanomedicine aims to overcome these barriers, revolutionizing plant-based medication delivery by improving stability, solubility, and bioavailability through various nanoparticle delivery systems, including liposomes, dendrimers, metallic NPs, solid lipid nanoparticles (SLNs), nanocapsules, nanospheres, and nanogels (Mitchell et al., 2021).

Phytochemical Nanoformulations for Respiratory Complications

Curcumin (CR)

CR, a compound classified as a polyphenol primarily obtained from the rhizomes of *Curcuma longa* L. (turmeric), contributes to the yellow color of the rhizomes. It possesses antimicrobial, anticancer, and anti-inflammatory properties that impact both acute and chronic lung conditions. CR affects transcription factors and inflammatory cytokines, including TNF-α and IL-6, as well as enzymes associated with inflammatory disorders (Aggarwal & Harikumar, 2009). Adel et al., (2021) utilized hydroxypropyl β-cyclodextrin as a carrier and nanospray drying to produce proliposomes, revealing that proliposomal CR surpasses standard CR powder in terms of residence time in lung tissues, absorption rate, and overall quantity. Hu et al., (2018) developed large porous microparticles coated with CR to address bleomycin-induced lung fibrosis in rat models, demonstrating superior antifibrotic activity compared to regular CR powders, leading to reduced hydroxyproline levels, collagen-1 formation, and lung damage mitigation. In a study, administration of CR SLNs to animal models of asthma resulted in reduced airway hyper-responsiveness, lowered inflammatory cell infiltration, and suppression of T-helper-2-type cytokines, such as interleukin-4 and interleukin-13, in bronchoalveolar lavage fluid, compared to the asthma group that did not receive treatment (Wang et al., 2012). Zhang et al., (2019) administered CR synthesized with hydroxypropyl-γ-cyclodextrin directly to C57BL/6 mice exposed to a lethal dose of Klebsiella pneumoniae, resulting in decreased oxidative stress, inflammation, and mortality. Additionally, oral nebulized cyclodextrin-nano CR (200 μg/Kg) showed potential effectiveness in treating idiopathic pulmonary fibrosis (Kurniawan & Pawitan, 2022).

Quercetin (QT)

QT, a phenolic compound belonging to the flavonoid group, is abundantly found in various foodstuffs such as onions, apples, and broccoli, making it the most common flavonol constituent. QT exhibits considerable antioxidant activity through multiple mechanisms, including its ability to interact with reactive species and generate less reactive phenoxy radicals. In addition to activating the Nrf2 pathway, QT inhibits several protein kinases, enhancing the activity of antioxidant enzymes while suppressing the NF-κB pathway. This compound also prevents lung inflammation, redox imbalance, and the synthesis of matrix metalloproteinases MMP9 and MMP12, playing a significant role in their metabolism (Araújo et al., 2022). However, QT's therapeutic applicability is limited due to its lipophilicity, low aqueous miscibility, and poor absorption. Furthermore, the QT molecule undergoes extensive methylation in the body and contains a hydroxyl substituent with a catechol moiety. As a result of the body's rapid degradation of QT, high dosages must be administered frequently to achieve the desired therapeutic effect, which can lead to severe side effects (Scalia et al., 2013). To overcome these drawbacks, solid lipid microparticles (SLM) have been developed as a liposomal drug delivery technology. Two novel delivery systems have been created: one using lecithin and glyceryl behenate via the hot emulsion technique, and another utilizing soy lecithin and glyceryl trimyristate through the hot solvent diffusion method in QT-loaded SLM. The addition of a fatty acid molecule positively affects the structure of the microparticles, accelerating their disintegration rate. Additionally, the stability of QT was significantly enhanced when lipid microparticles of QT were prepared using tristearin and hydrogenated soybean phosphatidylcholine. Compared to QT alone, these lipid microparticles increased the protective action of the medication against oxidative damage. The formulation also demonstrated a sustained release in phosphate buffer. In summary, QT microparticles offer a promising delivery method with enhanced properties for QT inhalation (Scalia et al., 2013).

Naringenin

Citrus fruits are the primary source of naringenin, a versatile flavanone known for its potent bioactivity. Naringenin exhibits significant antioxidant, anti-inflammatory, anti-adipogenic, and cardioprotective properties. Its anti-inflammatory effects are particularly highlighted as a therapeutic advantage in treating lung diseases such as lung cancer, chronic obstructive pulmonary disease (COPD), asthma, and cystic fibrosis. Research has indicated that naringenin's pharmacological actions may be linked to its ability to ameliorate oxidative stress, serving as a potential underlying mechanism for its therapeutic effects (Chin et al., 2020). However, naringenin's low solubility in water and limited bioavailability have hindered its therapeutic potential. To enhance its pharmacodynamics and overall pharmacological properties, various nanoformulations are being developed. For instance, Guan et al. (2020) created a naringenin-hydroxypropyl-β-cyclodextrin (naringenin HPPCD) formulation specifically for pulmonary delivery (inhalation solution) to address these limitations. The pharmacokinetic profile of a 400 μg/kg formulation was studied in Sprague-Dawley (SD) rats using both intratracheal and intravenous injection methods, aiming to assess the formulation's effectiveness for pulmonary delivery. The *in vitro* permeability test utilized a human lung adenocarcinoma cell line known as Calu-3. The findings indicated that HPPCD acts as a sustained-release mechanism for naringenin, increasing the concentration of the compound in the fluid that lines the epithelium of Calu-3 cells. The pharmacokinetic profile of the naringenin-HPPCD inclusion demonstrated a rapid response and elevated lung levels when measured at different intervals. These results suggest that naringenin-HPPCD inclusion is a promising formulation approach for pulmonary administration (Guan et al., 2020).

Piperine

Piperine, a primary component and key constituent of the alkaloid class found in Piper nigrum fruits, has demonstrated dose-dependent effects on allergic reactions, including reduced sneezing, nose rubbing, and nasal redness (Haq et al., 2021). The substance exhibits immunomodulatory and antiallergic properties, as evidenced in rat models with ovalbumin-induced rhinitis. In these studies, piperine treatment led to significant improvements in sensitization-related symptoms, including sneezing, coughing, and nasal redness. Histological examination of the nasal mucosa revealed disruptions in bronchioles and alveoli, along with a noticeable reduction in redness. Additionally, piperine-containing plant extracts have shown enhanced antitussive effects (Khawas et al., 2017). In another study, administering piperine to mice resulted in a marked reduction in lung tumor growth associated with B16F-10 melanoma cells. Histological analysis revealed that piperine was 100% cytotoxic to melanoma cells, leading to a significant reduction in tumor mass. Mice treated with piperine exhibited tumor-free pleura and clear alveolar passages. Furthermore, a study investigating the efficacy of combining curcuminoids with piperine for treating sulfur mustard-induced chronic pulmonary issues measured serum levels of glutathione (GSH) and malondialdehyde (MDA). The results indicated a notable increase in GSH levels and a decrease in MDA levels, suggesting improvements in COPD and overall health-related quality of life (Panahi et al., 2016).

Resveratrol (RS)

Several plant species, including peanuts and grapes, contain the polyphenolic compound RS. In animal studies, RS has shown protective effects against lipopolysaccharide (LPS)-induced inflammation. It inhibits the TLR4/NF-κBp65/MAPKs signaling cascade and the NLRP3 inflammasome, effectively reducing LPS-induced acute lung inflammation (Wang et al., 2017). Additionally, RS mitigates the adverse effects of LPS on SIRT1 expression and inhibits the *in vivo* and *in vitro* activation of MAPKs and NF-κB. Moreover, RS attenuates inflammatory damage in the lungs resulting from spinal cord injury by suppressing NF-κB, enhancing SIRT1 expression, and significantly reducing neutrophil infiltration and the production of inflammatory mediators. In a mouse model of ovalbumin-induced asthma, RS effectively alleviated asthma symptoms by upregulating PTEN, reinstating INPP4A, decreasing MUC5AC expression and mucus overproduction, and downregulating TGF-β1. In addition, it suppresses epithelial-mesenchymal transition and TGF-β1/Smad signaling (Zhu et al., 2017).

Mechanism of Action of Plant-Based Natural Products

Inflammation of the human respiratory system is often a response to both physical injuries and microbiological diseases, particularly those caused by bacteria and viruses (Delclaux & Azoulay, 2003). During inflammation, various substances, including leukotrienes, tumor necrosis factor (TNF-α), nitric oxide, interleukins (IL-6, IL-5, IL-4, IL-1β), histamine, and prostaglandins, are released from inflammatory cells such as eosinophils, lymphocytes, and macrophages, leading to changes in lung function (Timalsina et al., 2021). Natural products have the potential to serve as agents with anti-inflammatory properties, targeting various aspects of respiratory inflammation, such as oxidative stress, fibroblast activation, extracellular matrix accumulation, epithelial-mesenchymal transition (EMT), and inflammatory injury. This makes them promising candidates for innovative respiratory treatments (Gong et al., 2014). Chemical agents that act as lung anti-inflammatory agents typically regulate redox status, inhibit adhesion and growth factors, enhance TIMP-1 expression, block NF-κB and MAPK pathways, suppress bacterial and viral activities, control the protease/anti-protease balance, and curb cytokine production (Wang et al., 2020). For instance, flavonoids like eriodictyol inhibit the production of inflammatory cytokines such as IL-1β, IL-6, and TNF-α while regulating the Nrf2 pathway in the lungs (Zhu et al., 2015). Other flavonoids, including luteolin and kaempferol, decrease the activation of MAPK and NF-κB pathways induced by LPS, along with neutrophil inflammation, KC, TNF-α, superoxide dismutase (SOD), and ICAM-1, thereby reducing lipid peroxidation and oxidative damage in lung tissues (Kuo et al., 2011; Chen et al., 2012). An experiment utilizing a mouse model demonstrated the anti-inflammatory effects of curcumin in combating lung inflammation caused by Klebsiella pneumonia. The study revealed that curcumin significantly reduces lung inflammation by regulating nitric oxide (NO), malondialdehyde (MDA), and myeloperoxidase (MPO) activities, decreasing TNF-α levels, and reducing bacterial load in lung tissue. Furthermore, it effectively suppresses neutrophil infiltration into the lungs. While the gold-standard antibiotic augmentin inhibits lung pathogens, the results indicated that curcumin may serve as a valuable adjuvant treatment for acute lung infections, either alone or in conjunction with specific antibiotics, as an immunomodulatory or anti-inflammatory agent (Bansal & Chhibber, 2010). Research has also indicated that quercetin possesses potent anti-inflammatory effects, achieved by blocking enzymes such as lipoxygenase, phospholipase A2 (via arachidonic acid), thromboxane, and cyclooxygenase, while modulating iNOS to inhibit NO formation (Santangelo et al., 2007). Sakuranetin, another natural product, has been shown to suppress MMP-12-positive and MMP-9-positive cells, NF-κB, and reduce M-CSF, IL-5, RANTES, TNF-α, eosinophils, and IL-1β in the lungs of elastase-treated mice (Taguchi et al., 2015). Compounds like optosine, dicentrine, gallocatechin gallate, berberine, berbamine, and epigallocatechin have demonstrated efficacy in suppressing viral replication and reducing virally induced respiratory inflammation (Chakravarti et al., 2021). Additionally, research has investigated whether 1,8-cineol, derived from essential oil extracted from Eucalyptus globulus leaves, could decrease the expression of the NF-κB target gene MUC2 (Greiner et al., 2013). The compound 3-methoxy-catalposide suppresses iNOS and COX-2 production in RAW264.7 cells stimulated by LPS. It reduces levels of NO and prostaglandin E2 (PGE2) and significantly inhibits the activation of inflammatory genes such as IL-1β, IL-6, and TNF-α, along with NF-κB activation and AP-1 nuclear translocation (Ryu et al., 2017). Rutin, matte flavonoside G, apigenin, and other compounds have demonstrated the ability to suppress the influenza virus in infections caused by bacteria and viruses by damaging viral membranes, preventing virus entry into cells, and blocking neuraminidase (Omrani et al., 2021). Tetragalloylquinic acid, derived from Galphimia glauca, is an effective anti-asthmatic medication when administered orally (5 mg/kg). It functions by inhibiting thromboxane formation *in vitro*, as well as bronchial constriction induced by platelet-activating factor (PAF), and bronchial hyperreactivity caused by PAF and allergen activation. Similarly, Picrorhiza kurroa demonstrated efficacy at a similar dose in preventing bronchial obstruction triggered by allergens and PAF (Dorsch & Wagner, 1991). Two alkaloids, stachydrine and synephrine, derived from the dried peel of ripe Citrus reticulata fruits, activate β-2 adrenergic receptor signaling, resulting in significant relaxation of contractions induced by acetylcholine chloride (ACh) in isolated guinea pig trachea. They also exhibit collaborative defense against histamine-induced experimental asthma by extending the latency period. Their combined bronchodilatory and antitussive properties explain their use as anti-asthmatic therapies in traditional Chinese medicine, with stachydrine being particularly effective in reducing coughing induced by citric acid (Shi et al., 2009). Therefore, natural substances possess the ability to alleviate inflammation and respiratory ailments by inhibiting bacteria and viruses, as well as by modulating the balance between proteases and antiproteases, oxidative stress, and the NF-κB and MAPK pathways. Natural products rich in terpenes, flavonoids, and alkaloids represent a valuable resource for chemotherapy drugs with positive effects on chronic respiratory conditions (Table 1).

Table 1. Natural products targeting different cell signaling pathways

Natural Product	Nature	Mechanism of action
Apigenin	Flavonoid	Anti-inflammatory by lowering TNF-α, IL-17A, and interleukin (IL)-6 levels
Curcumin	Alkaloid	Reduces hyperresponsiveness and inflammation of the allergic airways by preventing the NF-κB signaling pathway from being activated.
Ellagic acid	Polyphenol	Treatment for inflammatory lung disease suppressed NF-kB and AP-1 signaling and decreased the COX-2-induced worsening of inflammation.
Kaempferol	Flavonoid	Inhibit lipopolysaccharide-induced acute lung damage and strengthen the NF-kB and MAPK pathways. Also, a main protease inhibitor for SARS-CoV-2.
Luteolin	Flavone	Inhibits NF-κB and MAPK pathways, prevents macrophages from producing nitric oxide, inhibits TNF-α and interleukin-6 generated by LPS and reduces inflammation caused by neutrophils.
Lycopene	Carotenoid hydrocarbon	Trigger apoptosis and inhibit growth and metastasis of lung cancer cells
Naringenin	Flavonoid	Anti-inflammatory via inhibition of pulmonary Ikappa Balpha degradation and NF-kappa-B DNA-binding activity
Naringin	Flavanone glycoside	Reduction of IL-4, IL-5, IL-13, and INF-δ levels
Quercetin	Flavonoid	Suppresses IL-6, nitric oxide, IL-10, IL 1β and serum necrosis factor α. Antioxidant and anti-inflammatory
Resveratrol	Polyphenolic compound	Modulate many cell signaling molecules to make tumor cells more susceptible to chemotherapeutic drugs (Prasher et al., 2020).

Applications of Nanophytoherbals in Respiratory Diseases

The application of nanotechnology in pulmonary medicine exemplifies its potential for effective drug delivery, especially for nucleic acid-based therapies. Inhaled medications are rapidly absorbed by the lung epithelium, coating the respiratory tract. This method allows precise control over particle size, facilitating deep lung administration, modulating phagocytic absorption, and preventing removal by resident macrophages. Nanotechnology plays a crucial role in oral and intravenous pulmonary treatments, particularly for overcoming multidrug resistance in leukemia. By modifying surface characteristics, nanotechnology enhances biocompatibility, minimizes thrombosis, and alters cell adhesion, thereby improving the performance of stents and valves. Additionally, nanoparticle-based thrombolytic agents have been shown to enhance clot removal effectiveness. In the context of lung and blood disorders, nano-scaffold techniques have demonstrated the ability to regulate the proliferation and differentiation of progenitor and stem cells (Adetunji et al., 2021). Phytomedicines are gaining popularity due to their natural origins and low risk of adverse effects. However, despite showing remarkable *in vitro* activity, herbal powders and extracts often exhibit limited efficacy *in vivo* due to challenges like poor solubility, inconsistent particle size, inadequate absorption, and rapid clearance. To overcome these obstacles, numerous nanotechnology approaches have been explored to enhance the administration of herbal treatments, including nanospheres, liposomes, and phytosomes (Abhinav et al., 2016). These methods have shown promise in improving the bioavailability and bioactivity of phytomedicines by reducing particle size, incorporating polymers, employing nano-structured carrier systems, and modifying surface properties (Sharma et al., 2017). Surface modification techniques can involve the use of hydrophilic, stabilizing, and mucoadhesive polymers or surfactants, which can enhance nanoparticle stability and absorption by altering zeta potential (Tiwari et al., 2012). Research has demonstrated that incorporating nanotechnology can significantly improve the biological efficacy of phytomedicines, leading to the development of nano phytomedicines. Lung cancer is the most prevalent cancer worldwide, and various plant extracts and essential oils have shown efficacy against it through multiple mechanisms, including reducing tumor size, decreasing cell viability, and modulating cytokines. Certain plant components have been found to affect Cyt c levels, alter cell cycle phases, and upregulate proteins associated with cell death. Moreover, natural products can inhibit the phosphorylation of AXL and activate apoptotic pathways within lung cancer cells, such as p-JNK, Akt/mTOR, Bax, and Bcl2. These compounds also influence cell morphology, decrease migration and proliferation, produce oxidative markers, and alter levels of p-eIF2α, GRP78, IgG, and carcinoembryonic antigen (CEA), positioning plant extracts as promising candidates for lung cancer treatment, particularly in combination with conventional anticancer therapies (Memarzia et al., 2023). Nanotechnology has the potential to significantly enhance drug delivery and nucleic acid-based therapies to pulmonary disease sites. The therapeutic approach of inhalation allows direct access to the respiratory tract lining and lung epithelium, facilitating deep lung delivery while controlling phagocytic absorption and local macrophage particle removal. Furthermore, the incorporation of nanotechnology into oral and intravenous pulmonary drug delivery can enhance treatment efficacy through precise cell targeting and controlled bioavailability. In hematology, nanotechnology is promising in combating drug resistance in leukemia by preventing drug evacuation from cancer cells and enabling effective siRNA distribution to lymphocytes, thus preventing apoptosis during sepsis. Devices like stents and valves can be made more biocompatible through strategic surface modifications that control cell adhesion and activation while reducing thrombosis. Additionally, nanoparticle-based thrombolytic agents hold great promise for improving clot removal effectiveness. The utilization of nano-scaffold strategies can also regulate the differentiation and proliferation of progenitor and stem cells in both pulmonary and blood-related diseases (Buxton, 2009). The gradual delivery of drugs to lung tissues using nanocarrier systems can improve patient adherence and reduce dosing frequency. In contrast to oral or intravenous methods, inhalable nanocarriers provide a viable alternative that minimizes the side effects associated with elevated drug concentrations in the bloodstream. However, the development of such systems necessitates thorough evaluation of potential long-term concerns related to excipient toxicity and nanoscale carriers. The small size and customizable surface properties of nanomaterials offer opportunities for innovation in targeted treatment platforms for lung cells and controlled drug release. Combining nanotechnology with pulmonary drug delivery can enhance treatment outcomes, optimize drug targeting and release, and address biological and physical barriers to improve needle-free inhalation vaccinations (Upadhyay & Ganguly, 2015). Natural products like zingerone, mangiferin, glycyrrhizin, curcumin, turmerones, and gingerols represent important sources of unique and biologically active compounds for treating common respiratory disorders. Although these compounds show encouraging biological properties, there is a lack of comprehensive clinical and toxicological studies to support their efficacy and safety. Techniques such as bioassay-guided isolation, virtual screening, metabolomics, molecular modeling, high-throughput screening, natural product library research, and database analysis can be employed to investigate these aspects. Understanding the mechanisms of bioactive compounds, refining lead compounds, conducting toxicology evaluations, formulating products, assessing pharmacokinetics, determining dosage regimens, and employing targeted drug delivery methods remain vital in the ongoing exploration and enhancement of respiratory medications. The emergence of modern techniques, including biogenic metal-based nanoparticles in nanomedicine, marks a significant advancement. This approach has already shown efficacy in drug delivery through nebulizers, producing particle sizes capable of reaching the alveoli for rapid and efficient treatment with minimal therapeutic doses (Oriola & Oyedeji, 2022).

Conclusion

Recently, there has been increasing interest in exploring the health advantages of natural plant-based products for the purpose of discovering new drugs. This section provides thorough insights into the use of natural products and their plant-derived components, which are formulated into nanodrugs to treat pulmonary ailments. Utilizing nano-sized formulations of these plant compounds offers a significant advantage in improving their pharmaceutical qualities, addressing issues such as solubility and bioavailability. Numerous nanoformulations containing plant-derived compounds have demonstrated promising effectiveness compared to their original states, particularly in treating lung inflammatory conditions. However, further studies should prioritize evaluating their efficacy through clinical trials and consider additional factors, such as potential side effects and toxicity associated with these plant compound-loaded nanostructures.

References

Abhinav, M., Neha, J., Anne, G., & Bharti, V. (2016). Role of novel drug delivery systems in bioavailability enhancement: At a glance. *International Journal of Drug Delivery Technology*, *6*(1), 7-26.

Adel, I. M., ElMeligy, M. F., Abdelrahim, M. E., Maged, A., Abdelkhalek, A. A., Abdelmoteleb, A. M., &Elkasabgy, N. A. (2021). Design and characterization of spray-dried proliposomes for the pulmonary delivery of curcumin. *International journal of nanomedicine*, 2667-2687.

Adetunji, C. O., Inobeme, A., Olaniyan, O. T., Ajayi, O. O., Olaniyan, S., & Adetunji, J. B. (2021). Application of nanodrugs derived from active metabolites of medicinal plants for the treatment of inflammatory and lung diseases: recent advances. *Medicinal Plants for Lung Diseases: A Pharmacological and Immunological Perspective*, 609-622.

Aggarwal, B. B., & Harikumar, K. B. (2009). Potential therapeutic effects of curcumin, the anti-inflammatory agent, against neurodegenerative, cardiovascular, pulmonary, metabolic, autoimmune and neoplastic diseases. *The international journal of biochemistry & cell biology*, *41*(1), 40-59.

Araújo, N. P. D. S., de Matos, N. A., Oliveira, M., de Souza, A. B. F., Castro, T. D. F., Machado-Júnior, P. A., & Bezerra, F. S. (2022). Quercetin improves pulmonary function and prevents emphysema caused by exposure to cigarette smoke in male mice. *Antioxidants*, *11*(2), 181.

Bansal, S., & Chhibber, S. (2010). Curcumin alone and in combination with augmentin protects against pulmonary inflammation and acute lung injury generated during Klebsiella pneumoniae B5055-induced lung infection in BALB/c mice. *Journal of medical microbiology*, *59*(4), 429-437.

Behzadi, M. A., & Leyva-Grado, V. H. (2019). Overview of current therapeutics and novel candidates against influenza, respiratory syncytial virus, and Middle East respiratory syndrome coronavirus infections. *Frontiers in microbiology*, *10*, 1327.

Buxton, D. B. (2009). Nanomedicine for the management of lung and blood diseases. *Nanomedicine*, *4*(3), 331-339.

Chakravarti, R., Singh, R., Ghosh, A., Dey, D., Sharma, P., Velayutham, R., & Ghosh, D. (2021). A review on potential of natural products in the management of COVID-19. *RSC advances*, *11*(27), 16711-16735.

Chen, X., Yang, X., Liu, T., Guan, M., Feng, X., Dong, W., & Sun, Z. (2012). Kaempferol regulates MAPKs and NF-κB signaling pathways to attenuate LPS-induced acute lung injury in mice. *International immunopharmacology*, *14*(2), 209-216.

Chin, L. H., Hon, C. M., Chellappan, D. K., Chellian, J., Madheswaran, T., Zeeshan, F., & Dua, K. (2020). Molecular mechanisms of action of naringenin in chronic airway diseases. *European journal of pharmacology*, *879*, 173139.

Delclaux, C., & Azoulay, E. (2003). Inflammatory response to infectious pulmonary injury. *European Respiratory Journal*, *22*(42 suppl), 10s-14s.

Dorsch, W., & Wagner, H. (1991). New antiasthmatic drugs from traditional medicine? *International Archives of Allergy and Immunology*, *94*(1-4), 262-265.

El-Kased, R. F. (2016). Natural antibacterial remedy for respiratory tract infections. *Asian Pacific Journal of Tropical Biomedicine*, *6*(3), 270-274.

Gong, J. H., Cho, I. H., Shin, D., Han, S. Y., Park, S. H., & Kang, Y. H. (2014). Inhibition of airway epithelial-to-mesenchymal transition and fibrosis by kaempferol in endotoxin-induced epithelial cells and ovalbumin-sensitized mice. *Laboratory investigation*, *94*(3), 297-308.

Greiner, J. F. W., Müller, J., Zeuner, M. T., Hauser, S., Seidel, T., Klenke, C., & Kaltschmidt, C. (2013). 1, 8-Cineol inhibits nuclear translocation of NF-κB p65 and NF-κB-dependent transcriptional activity. *Biochimica et Biophysica Acta (BBA)-Molecular Cell Research*, *1833*(12), 2866-2878.

Guan, M., Shi, R., Zheng, Y., Zeng, X., Fan, W., Wang, Y., & Su, W. (2020). Characterization, *in vitro* and *in vivo* evaluation of naringenin-hydroxypropyl-β-cyclodextrin inclusion for pulmonary delivery. *Molecules*, *25*(3), 554.

Haq, I. U., Imran, M., Nadeem, M., Tufail, T., Gondal, T. A., & Mubarak, M. S. (2021). Piperine: A review of its biological effects. *Phytotherapy research*, *35*(2), 680-700.

Hsia, C. C., Hyde, D. M., & Weibel, E. R. (2016). Lung structure and the intrinsic challenges of gas exchange. *Comprehensive physiology*, *6*(2), 827.

Hu, Y., Li, M., Zhang, M., & Jin, Y. (2018). Inhalation treatment of idiopathic pulmonary fibrosis with curcumin large porous microparticles. *International Journal of Pharmaceutics*, *551*(1-2), 212-222.

Khawas, S., Nosáľová, G., Majee, S. K., Ghosh, K., Raja, W., Sivová, V., & Ray, B. (2017). *In vivo* cough suppressive activity of pectic polysaccharide with arabinogalactan type II side chains of Piper nigrum fruits and its synergistic effect with piperine. *International Journal of Biological Macromolecules*, *99*, 335-342.

Kuo, M. Y., Liao, M. F., Chen, F. L., Li, Y. C., Yang, M. L., Lin, R. H., & Kuan, Y. H. (2011). Luteolin attenuates the pulmonary inflammatory response involves abilities of antioxidation and inhibition of MAPK and NFκB pathways in mice with endotoxin-induced acute lung injury. *Food and Chemical Toxicology*, *49*(10), 2660-2666.

Lim, C. L., Raju, C. S., Mahboob, T., Kayesth, S., Gupta, K. K., Jain, G. K., &Nissapatorn, V. (2022). Precision and advanced nano-phytopharmaceuticals for therapeutic applications. *Nanomaterials*, *12*(2), 238.

Memarzia, A., Saadat, S., Asgharzadeh, F., Behrouz, S., Folkerts, G., &Boskabady, M. H. (2023). Therapeutic effects of medicinal plants and their constituents on lung cancer, *in vitro*, *in vivo* and clinical evidence. *Journal of Cellular and Molecular Medicine*, *27*(19), 2841-2863.

Mitchell, M. J., Billingsley, M. M., Haley, R. M., Wechsler, M. E., Peppas, N. A., & Langer, R. (2021). Engineering precision nanoparticles for drug delivery. *Nature reviews drug discovery*, *20*(2), 101-124.

Muzammil, S., Hayat, S., Fakhar-E-Alam, M., Aslam, B., Siddique, M. H., Nisar, M. A., & Wang, Z. (2018). Nanoantibiotics: Future nanotechnologies to combat antibiotic resistance. *Front. Biosci*, *10*(2), 352-374.

Omrani, M., Keshavarz, M., Nejad Ebrahimi, S., Mehrabi, M., McGaw, L. J., Ali Abdalla, M., &Mehrbod, P. (2021). Potential natural products against respiratory viruses: a perspective to develop anti-COVID-19 medicines. *Frontiers in pharmacology*, *11*, 586993.

Oriola, A. O., & Oyedeji, A. O. (2022). Plant-derived natural products as lead agents against Common Respiratory Diseases. *Molecules*, *27*(10), 3054.

Panahi, Y., Ghanei, M., Hajhashemi, A., &Sahebkar, A. (2016). Effects of curcuminoids-piperine combination on systemic oxidative stress, clinical symptoms and quality of life in subjects with chronic pulmonary complications due to sulfur mustard: a randomized controlled trial. *Journal of dietary supplements*, *13*(1), 93-105.

Prasher, P., Sharma, M., Mehta, M., Paudel, K. R., Satija, S., Chellappan, D. K., & Dua, K. (2020). Plants derived therapeutic strategies targeting chronic respiratory diseases: Chemical and immunological perspective. *Chemico-biological interactions*, *325*, 109125.

Ryu, H. W., Lee, S. U., Lee, S., Song, H. H., Son, T. H., Kim, Y. U., & Oh, S. R. (2017). 3-Methoxy-catalposide inhibits inflammatory effects in lipopolysaccharide-stimulated RAW264. 7 macrophages. *Cytokine*, *91*, 57-64.

Sadikot, R. T., Kolanjiyil, A. V., Kleinstreuer, C., & Rubinstein, I. (2017). Nanomedicine for treatment of acute lung injury and acute respiratory distress syndrome. *Biomedicine hub*, *2*(2), 1-12.

Santangelo, C., Vari, R., Scazzocchio, B., Di Benedetto, R., Filesi, C., & Masella, R. (2007). Polyphenols, intracellular signalling and inflammation. *Annali-istitutosuperiore di sanita*, *43*(4), 394.

Scalia, S., Haghi, M., Losi, V., Trotta, V., Young, P. M., & Traini, D. (2013). Quercetin solid lipid microparticles: a flavonoid for inhalation lung delivery. *European Journal of Pharmaceutical Sciences*, *49*(2), 278-285.

Scalia, S., Trotta, V., Traini, D., Young, P. M., Sticozzi, C., Cervellati, F., &Valacchi, G. (2013). Incorporation of quercetin in respirable lipid microparticles: Effect on stability and cellular uptake on A549 pulmonary alveolar epithelial cells. *Colloids and Surfaces B: Biointerfaces*, *112*, 322-329.

Sharma, R., Hazra, J., & Prajapati, P. K. (2017). Nanophytomedicines: A novel approach to improve drug delivery and pharmacokinetics of herbal medicine. *Bio Bull*, *3*(1), 132-5.

Shi, Q., Liu, Z., Yang, Y., Geng, P., Zhu, Y. Y., Zhang, Q., & Bai, G. (2009). Identification of anti-asthmatic compounds in Pericarpium citrireticulatae and evaluation of their synergistic effects. *Acta Pharmacologica Sinica*, *30*(5), 567-575.

Sorokina, M., & Steinbeck, C. (2020). Review on natural products databases: where to find data in 2020. *Journal of cheminformatics*, *12*(1), 20.

Taguchi, L., Pinheiro, N. M., Olivo, C. R., Choqueta-Toledo, A., Grecco, S. S., Lopes, F. D., & Prado, C. M. (2015). A flavanone from Baccharis retusa (Asteraceae) prevents elastase-induced emphysema in mice by regulating NF-κB, oxidative stress and metalloproteinases. *Respiratory research*, *16*, 1-15.

Timalsina, D., Pokhrel, K. P., & Bhusal, D. (2021). Pharmacologic Activities of Plant-Derived Natural Products on Respiratory Diseases and Inflammations. *BioMed Research International*, *2021*(1), 1636816.

Tiwari, G., Tiwari, R., Sriwastawa, B., Bhati, L., Pandey, S., Pandey, P., & Bannerjee, S. K. (2012). Drug delivery systems: An updated review. *International journal of pharmaceutical investigation*, *2*(1), 2.

Upadhyay, S., Ganguly, K., & Palmberg, L. (2015). Wonders of nanotechnology in the treatment for chronic lung diseases. *Journal of Nanomedicine & Nanotechnology*, *6*(6), 1.

Vitria Kurniawan, S. (2022). Curcumin nanoformulation for pulmonary drug delivery. *Research Journal of Pharmacognosy*, *9*(4), 73-81.

Wang, C., Zhou, J., Wang, J., Li, S., Fukunaga, A., Yodoi, J., & Tian, H. (2020). Progress in the mechanism and targeted drug therapy for COPD. *Signal Transduction and Targeted Therapy*, *5*(1), 248.

Wang, G., Hu, Z., Fu, Q., Song, X., Cui, Q., Jia, R., & Yin, Z. (2017). Resveratrol mitigates lipopolysaccharide-mediated acute inflammation in rats by inhibiting the TLR4/NF-κBp65/MAPKs signaling cascade. *Scientific reports*, *7*(1), 45006.

Wang, H., Naghavi, M., Allen, C., Barber, R. M., Bhutta, Z. A., Carter, A., & Bell, M. L. (2016). Global, regional, and national life expectancy, all-cause mortality, and cause-specific mortality for 249 causes of death, 1980–2015: a systematic analysis for the Global Burden of Disease Study 2015. *The lancet*, *388*(10053), 1459-1544.

Wang, W., Zhu, R., Xie, Q., Li, A., Xiao, Y., Li, K., & Wang, S. (2012). Enhanced bioavailability and efficiency of curcumin for the treatment of asthma by its formulation in solid lipid nanoparticles. *International journal of nanomedicine*, 3667-3677.

Zhang, B., Swamy, S., Balijepalli, S., Panicker, S., Mooliyil, J., Sherman, M. A., & Suresh, M. V. (2019). Direct pulmonary delivery of solubilized curcumin reduces severity of lethal pneumonia. *The FASEB Journal*, *33*(12), 13294.

Zhu, G. F., Guo, H. J., Huang, Y. A. N., Wu, C. T., & Zhang, X. F. (2015). Eriodictyol, a plant flavonoid, attenuates LPS-induced acute lung injury through its antioxidative and anti-inflammatory activity. *Experimental and therapeutic medicine*, *10*(6), 2259-2266.

Zhu, X. D., Lei, X. P., & Dong, W. B. (2017). Resveratrol as a potential therapeutic drug for respiratory system diseases. *Drug design, development and therapy*, 3591-3598.

Chapter 20

The Clinical Status of Phytonanoherbal Therapies

Navidha Aggarwal[1]
Sunayna Choudhary[1]
Preeti[2]
Davinder Kumar[3]
and Shiva Tushir[4,*]

[1]M.M. College of Pharmacy, Maharishi Markandeshwar (Deemed to be University), Mullana, Ambala, Haryana, India
[2]Gurugram Global College of Pharmacy, Farruknagar, Gurugram, Haryana, India
[3]College of Pharmacy, PGIMS, Pt. B. D. Sharma University of Health Sciences, Rohtak, Haryana, India
[4]Department of Pharmacy, Panipat Institute of Engineering and Technology, Panipat, Haryana, India

Abstract

This chapter introduces the rapidly evolving field of phytonanoherbal therapies, where traditional herbal medicine converges with advanced nanotechnology and computational analysis. It aims to provide a comprehensive overview of the current clinical applications, while also highlighting emerging trends and addressing key challenges in the field. The chapter paves the way for an in-depth exploration of the transformative potential of these therapies in shaping the future of alternative medicine. It progresses by examining the clinical landscape of phytonanoherbal treatments, with a focus on recent innovations at the crossroads of herbal medicine and nanotechnology. Key attention is given to novel therapeutic approaches and the strategic application of analytical tools for in-depth evaluation. Additionally, the chapter reviews findings from ongoing clinical trials and research efforts, assessing the efficacy and safety of phytonanoherbal therapies, thereby contributing to the broader discussion on their role in modern healthcare.

Keywords: nanotechnology, clinical studies, nanoformulation, drug development, clinical trial

* Corresponding Author's Email: klershiva@gmail.com.

In: Phyto-Nanomedicine
Editors: Hitesh Chopra, Vinod Kumar Gauttam, Ajmer Singh Grewal et al.
ISBN: 979-8-89530-317-7

Abbreviations

CD-PEG	Cyclodextrin-polyethylene glycol
EMA	European Medicines Agency
ERL	Eudragit® LPO
FDA	Food and Drug Administration
PCL	Poly-ε-caprolactone
PEG	Polyethylene glycol
PEI	Polyethylenimine
PLA	Poly-lactic acid
PLGA	Polylactic-co-glycolic acid
SLNs	Solid lipid nanoparticles
TMC	Trimethylated chitosan
TPGS	Tocopheryl polyethylene glycol 1000 succinate
UV	Ultraviolet

Introduction

Nanotechnology is a multidisciplinary field that integrates science and engineering to create materials and systems at the nanoscale, with a focus on manipulating atoms, molecules, and macromolecular structures. (Sahoo and Labhasetwar, 2003). The term "nano" originates from the Greek word for "dwarf." A nanometer (nm) is one billionth of a meter, approximately the width of six carbon atoms or ten water molecules. When materials are reduced to the nanoscale, their chemical and physical properties—such as strength, conductivity, and reactivity—undergo significant changes. Nanotechnology plays a crucial role across various disciplines, utilizing nanoparticles to tackle key challenges in healthcare, environmental sustainability, and technological advancement. In drug delivery, nanoparticles improve medication solubility, bioavailability, and controlled release, while reducing systemic toxicity. In cancer therapy, they enable precise targeting of cancer cells, minimizing harm to healthy tissue. Nanoparticles also enhance imaging sensitivity in techniques such as MRI and CT scans and serve as probes in biomedical sensors for detecting biological and environmental analytes. In regenerative medicine, they aid in tissue repair and organ regeneration. Cosmetics utilize nanoparticles for improved product effectiveness and enhanced UV protection. In electronics, nanoparticles increase conductivity and enable device miniaturization in applications like sensors and batteries. Additionally, they act as catalysts in industrial processes, improve water purification systems, and enhance energy storage and conversion in renewable technologies (Beniwal et al., 2022; Kumar, 2023).

Nanoformulations

A nanoformulation refers to any active pharmaceutical ingredient that has been reduced to the nanometer scale. Several types of nanoformulations are used in pharmaceutical applications, including liposomes, nanoparticles, nanocapsules, micelles, dendrimers, and nanoemulsions.

Each offers distinct advantages, such as improved drug delivery, controlled release, and enhanced bioavailability. These nanoformulations are essential for optimizing the therapeutic effectiveness of drugs while minimizing side effects.

- *Liposomes:* Liposomes are spherical vesicles made up of phospholipid bilayers. They have the ability to encapsulate hydrophilic drugs within their aqueous core and hydrophobic drugs within their lipid bilayers.
- *Polymeric nanoparticles*: Polymeric nanoparticles are composed of synthetic or natural polymers such as poly(lactic-co-glycolic acid) (PLGA), polyethylene glycol (PEG), and chitosan. These nanoparticles provide controlled drug release and protect the encapsulated drugs.
- *Micelles*: Micelles are formed through the self-assembly of amphiphilic molecules in aqueous solutions, creating a core-shell structure. This structure allows the solubilization of hydrophobic drugs within the core, enhancing their bioavailability.
- *Dendrimers:* Dendrimers are highly branched, tree-like macromolecules characterized by their unique structure. They can encapsulate drugs within their inner core or conjugate medications on their surface, enabling controlled release and targeted distribution.
- *Nanoemulsions:* Nanoemulsions are colloidal dispersions consisting of nanoscale oil droplets stabilized by surfactants. They are utilized to encapsulate hydrophobic drugs, enhancing their solubility.
- *Solid lipid nanoparticles (SLNs):* SLNs are biocompatible lipid nanoparticles that remain solid at room temperature. They offer controlled release and protection for pharmaceuticals, especially for lipophilic drugs.
- *Nanocrystals:* Nanocrystals are pure drug nanoparticles stabilized by surfactants or polymers. They enhance the solubility and bioavailability of medications, particularly for those that are weakly water-soluble.
- *Nanogels:* Nanogels are three-dimensional networks made up of hydrogel nanoparticles. They can encapsulate drugs within their mesh structure, allowing for sustained release over time.
- *Carbon nanotubes*: Carbon nanotubes are cylindrical structures made of carbon that possess remarkable mechanical, electrical, and thermal properties. They can be functionalized to encapsulate drugs for targeted delivery and imaging applications.
- *Metal nanoparticles*: Metal nanoparticles, such as gold, silver, and iron oxide, possess unique physicochemical properties. They can be utilized for drug delivery, imaging, and therapeutic applications (Chopra et al., 2023).

Nanomedicine Development

The development of nanomedicine is a multi-stage process that includes research and discovery, preclinical development, formulation optimization, toxicology and safety assessments, clinical translation, regulatory approval, commercialization, and continuous innovation (Figure 1). It begins with foundational research on nanomaterials and drug delivery technologies, followed by preclinical testing to evaluate safety and efficacy. Formulations are optimized for stability and targeted specificity, with comprehensive toxicity studies conducted. Successful candidates then advance to clinical trials, where their safety and efficacy are further assessed through various phases. Regulatory approval is sought to enable commercialization and market access, while post-marketing surveillance ensures ongoing safety in real-world applications. This process is continuously fueled by research and innovation, aiming to address unmet medical needs and improve patient outcomes.

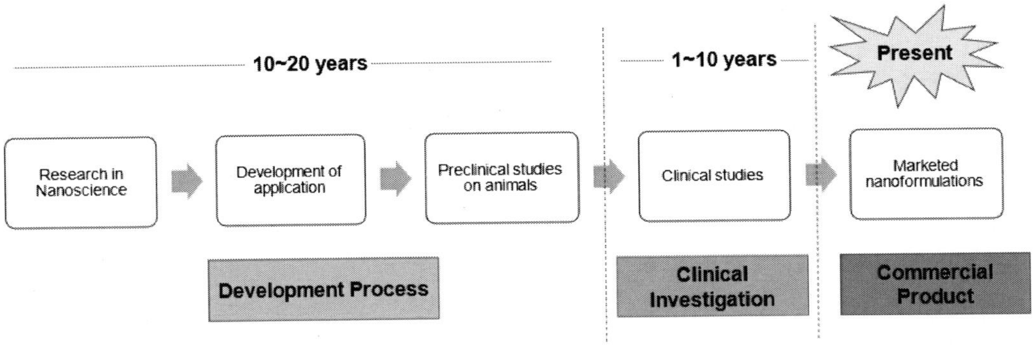

Figure 1. Different stages of nanomedicine development.

Phytonanoherbal

Traditional herbal therapies have several disadvantages (Yuan, 2016), but nanotechnology offers solutions (Nasrollahzadeh et al., 2019), leading to the emergence of a new field known as phytonanoherbals. The use of natural resources, particularly plants and herbs, for medicinal purposes is an ancient practice (Garg et al., 2024; Pan et al., 2014), and these remedies are trusted by a large segment of the population. In developing countries, many people rely on plants and herbs for their healthcare needs, giving rise to the field of phytopharmaceuticals (Alexander et al., 2016). In recent years, the convergence of nanotechnology and herbal medicine has resulted in the emergence of phytonanoherbal therapies, representing a promising new frontier in healthcare. This field merges the therapeutic properties of botanical extracts with the precision and versatility of nanoscale materials. Phytonanoherbal therapies have the potential to effectively manage a variety of disorders and tackle challenges associated with biopharmaceuticals through the application of nanotechnology (Wang et al., 2003). Research on specific phytoconstituents or plant extracts (Boora et al., 2014), focusing on parameters such as solubility and permeation, helps in formulating targeted phytonanoherbals. For instance, the problem of low bioavailability in compounds like curcumin (Gorgani et al., 2017; Satyavert et al., 2021), piperine, and rutin can be addressed through the fabrication of polymeric phytonanoherbals (Munjal et al., 2023). Various types of phytonanoherbal patents related to diverse pharmacological activities have been reported in the literature (Matos et al., 2015). Over the last decade, there has been a significant increase in the approval of phytonanoherbal patents (Grabowski, 2002). The advancement of sustainable phytonanoherbals designed to target specific sites and improve bioavailability has fueled the increase in patent approvals, with curcumin-based products representing the highest number (Mollaoglu-Korkmaz et al., 2013; Chatzinasiou et al., 2019).

Regulatory Aspect Related to Phytonanoherbals

Before phytonanoherbals can enter the market, it is crucial to consider their regulatory aspects (Interstate Technology & Regulatory Council, 2009). Various parameters must be assessed, including the safety of specific formulations (Aucouturier et al., 2001), as reflected in safety profile data (Holtmeier, 2011), as well as the therapeutic equivalency and pharmacokinetic properties of these products (El Desoky et al., 1993). Regulatory guidelines differ by country (Burgers et al., 2003) but must also conform to international standards (World Health Organization, 2007). Nanotechnology-based delivery systems have the potential to enhance the biological activity of herbal medicines and address existing challenges (Bonifacio et al., 2014). Despite the progress made, significant obstacles remain in translating these technologies into clinical practice. A major challenge is testing innovative methods to regulate the interactions between nanomaterials and biological systems. The development of multifunctional systems to address diverse biological and therapeutic needs, as well as the feasibility of scaling up processes to rapidly introduce new therapeutic strategies to the market, pose additional challenges in the advancement of nanotechnology-based drug delivery systems (Sharma et al., 2011). Furthermore, evaluating the effectiveness of nanoparticle targeting and ensuring compliance with global standards for toxicological and biocompatibility profiles are critical challenges that must be overcome.

Clinical Implications Related to Phytonanoherbals

The current status of phytonanoherbal therapies represents a groundbreaking approach at the intersection of nanotechnology and herbal medicine, offering significant potential for healthcare advancement. Notable research, such as that by Lauro et al. (2019) and Dewi et al. (2011), has provided important insights into the clinical efficacy and diverse applications of these innovative interventions. These studies indicate that the enhanced bioavailability and targeted delivery of phytochemicals at the nanoscale could play a crucial role in precision medicine and improving therapeutic outcomes. However, translating these promising preclinical findings into practical clinical applications poses several challenges. An overview of various *in vivo* and *in vitro* scientific studies on phytonanoherbals is summarized in Table 1. The integration of nanotechnology and herbal medicine has sparked a transformative paradigm in healthcare, leading to the emerging field of phytonanoherbal therapies. Recent research highlights the efficacy, safety profiles, and potential applications of these therapies, which harness the therapeutic potential of botanical compounds at the nanoscale. This innovative approach promises to enhance precision and effectiveness, revolutionizing modern medicine.

Clinical Trials Related to Phytonanoherbals

Clinical studies conducted in a scientific manner provide a robust framework for the assay and validation of phytopharmaceuticals (van Beek et al., 2009). Monographs for herbs intended for use as phytopharmaceuticals should include a comprehensive safety profile to identify any associated toxic effects, thereby enabling a more thorough understanding of their clinical status.

Drug delivery continues to be a significant challenge in pharmaceutical sciences, as drug molecules encounter numerous obstacles after administration, whether parenterally or orally. Once in the body, drugs are subjected to a variety of harsh internal conditions, and various physiological and biological barriers can lead to suboptimal concentrations of the administered drug at the target disease site. Despite the widespread use of herbs, the optimization and acceptance of phytopharmaceuticals lag behind that of allopathic medicines. While nanotechnology presents numerous advantages in the medical field, it also introduces certain drawbacks that must be addressed (Shubhika, 2013). Clinical researchers have raised concerns regarding the high cost of nanotechnology, the challenges associated with scaling up production, and the potential inhalation of nanoparticles (Firth et al., 2019). Inhalation can lead to severe lung diseases (Lee et al., 2015) and other conditions that disrupt homeostasis or may even result in death (Strandberg et al., 2010). The use of nanostructured systems in herbal medicine has been widely proposed as a way to enhance the benefits of plant extracts (Bonifacio et al., 2014). These systems can facilitate the prolonged release of active ingredients, reduce dosage requirements, minimize adverse effects, and enhance therapeutic efficacy. A summary of clinical trials on phytonanoherbals is provided in Table 2.

Challenges in Phytonanoherbal Therapies

One of the main challenges in developing phytonanoherbal formulations is their complex pharmacokinetics. While nanotechnology presents opportunities for controlled release and targeted delivery, understanding how these formulations interact with the human body remains a significant hurdle. Liao et al., (2023) emphasize the necessity of a comprehensive understanding of pharmacological dynamics to optimize therapeutic strategies. Furthermore, standardization and quality control present considerable obstacles. The inherent variability in herbal extracts and potential batch-to-batch differences complicate efforts to ensure the reproducibility and reliability of therapeutic outcomes. Addressing these issues necessitates robust quality control measures and standardized manufacturing processes. Regulatory frameworks also play a vital role in the integration of phytonanoherbal therapies into mainstream healthcare. The lack of clear guidelines and standardized protocols for evaluating the safety and efficacy of phytonanoherbal formulations hinders their widespread acceptance. It is essential to establish regulatory frameworks that balance innovation with patient safety to navigate the regulatory landscape and build confidence among healthcare practitioners and consumers. The current status of phytonanoherbal therapies reflects a growing interest in the synergy between nanotechnology and herbal medicine. Research by Lauro et al., (2019) and Dewi et al., (2011) showcases promising outcomes, highlighting the potential of these therapies to address complex health challenges. These interventions offer improved therapeutic efficacy, reduced side effects, and targeted delivery, making them appealing for various medical applications. However, several obstacles remain that impede their integration into conventional healthcare. One major challenge in developing phytonanoherbal formulations is the intrinsic complexity of herbal extracts, which typically contain a variety of bioactive compounds. Understanding the synergistic interactions and potential synergies at the nanoscale is vital for optimizing therapeutic formulations. The study by Liao et al., (2023) emphasizes the necessity for a deeper understanding of the pharmacokinetics of nanoscale phytochemicals to effectively navigate these complexities.

Table 1. *In vivo/in vitro* studies of various phytonanoherbals

Phytoconstituents/Plant name	Type of nanoformulation	Disease/Treatment	*In vivo/in vitro* studies	Reference
Aerval anata	Silver-copper nanoparticles	Cytotoxic activity	HeLa cell lines	(Thirumoorthy et al., 2024)
Aphanamixis polystachya (leaf extract)	Liposomal nanoparticles	Neuroprotective	Mice	(Shariare et al., 2020)
Artemether	Polymeric nanorods	Evaluation studies	Targeted delivery of antimalarial drugs	(Bhide & Jindal, 2021)
Berbamine	Lipid based nanoparticles	Metastatic cancer	*In vitro* and *in vivo* studies (on C57BL/6 mice)	(Parhi et al., 2017)
Berberine	Gold nanoparticles	Breast cancer	MTT assay	(Chiu et al., 2021)
Berberine	Polymeric nanoparticles	Dissolution and bioavailability studies	*In vitro* studies	(Jia et al., 2018)
Carvacrol	Polyethylenimine (PEI)-coated nanoparticles	Antimicrobial activity	Against Escherichia coli, Listeria monocytogenes, Salmonella enterica and Staphylococcus aureus	(Niza et al., 2020)
Cassia fistula	Gold nanoparticles	Antidiabetic	Induction of diabetes by intraperitoneal injection of STZ in Wistar rats	(Daisy & Saipriya, 2012)
Chrysin	Chitosan nanoparticles	Pancreatic and lung adenocarcinoma	Inhibition of mitochondrial complex II and ubiquinone oxidoreductase	(Ragab et al., 2022)
Coenzyme Q10	Trimethylated chitosan (TMC) poly(d,l-lactide-co-glycolide) (PLGA) nanoparticles (TMC/PLGA–NP)	Neuroprotective and brain drug delivery carrier in AD	APP/PS1 transgenic mice	(Wang et al., 2010)
Curcumin	BTN-PEG-PCL nanoparticles	Anticancer	On human breast adenocarcinoma (MCF-7), human embryonic kidney (HEK293), and human umbilical vein endothelial (HUVEC) cell lines	(Dezfouli et al., 2022)
Curcumin	Eudragit® RLPO (ERL)	*In vitro* release studies	Viability of Caco-2 cells	(Umerska et al., 2018)
Curcumin	Magnetic nanoparticles	Triple-negative breast cancers	MTT assay	(Ashkbar et al., 2020)
Curcumin	Monomethyl poly (ethylene glycol)-poly (ε-caprolactone)-poly (trimethylene carbonate) (also called MPEG-P(CL-co-TMC)) micelles	Colon cancer	CT26 cells	(Yang et al., 2015)
Curcumin	Nanocapsules stabilized by bovine serum albumin-capped gold nanoclusters (BSA-AuNCs)	Tumor cell theranosis	*In vitro* studies	(Fu et al., 2018)

Table 1. (Continued)

Phytoconstituents/Plant name	Type of nanoformulation	Disease/Treatment	*In vivo/in vitro* studies	Reference
Curcumin	Nanospheres	Cutaneous wound repair	Human umbilical cord-derived mesenchymal stem cells (MSCs)	(Kim et al., 2020)
Curcumin	PEGylated PLGA nanoparticles	Anticancer	Triple-negative breast cancer cells	(Prabhuraj et al., 2020)
Curcumin	PLA NPS within alginate/gelatin hydrogels	Immunomodulation	Cultures of NIH3T3 fibroblast cells	(Zamboni et al., 2022)
Curcumin	PLA-PEG copolymer	Treatment of liver inflammation	Streptozotocin induced diabetic rats	(El-Naggar et al., 2019)
Curcumin	Polycaprolactone (PCL) + Curcumin (Cur) + amine functionalized Santa Barbara Amorphous (NH2-SBA-15) nanofiber	Wound healing	Swiss 3T6 cell lines	(Rathinavel et al., 2021)
Curcumin	Silver nanoparticles	Hepatoprotective	CCl4- induced hepatotoxicity in mice	(Ebaid et al., 2021)
Curcumin and docetaxel	Poly lactide-co-glycolide (PLGA) nanoparticles	Treatment of glioma	Overcome blood brain barrier	(Seko et al., 2021)
Curcumin and nisin	Poly lactic acid nanoparticle	Cardioprotective	Isoproterenol induced myocardial infarction in guinea pigs	(Nabofa et al., 2018)
Cymbopogon martini essential oil	Poly-ε-caprolactone (PCL) nanoparticles	Antioxidant and antimicrobial activity	Against DPPH free radical assay, S. aureus and E. coli	(Jummes et al., 2020)
Epigallocatechin gallate	p(HEMA-co-GMA) membranes	Prevented bacterial colonization and adhesion	Against S. aureus CCUG 10778	(Acet et al., 2023)
Essential oils from Mentha spicata	Gold and silver nanoparticles	Cytotoxic activity	MTT assay on HEPG-2cell line	(Moosavy et al., 2023)
Fagonia cretica	Zinc oxide nanoparticles	Antibacterial, antifungal, cytotoxic, protein kinase inhibitory, and antidiabetic activity	Against K. pneumonae, E. coli, B. subtilis; A. flavus, F. solani;brine shrimps	(Kiani et al., 2022)
Hesperetin	Nanocrystals	Regenerative dentistry	Oninflamed human dental pulp stem cells and monocytes (U937)	(Alipour et al., 2023)
Huperzine A	Nanoemulsion modified with lactoferrin	Neuroprotective in AD	hCMEC/D3 cells (*In vitro* model)	(Jiang et al., 2019)
Lagenaria siceraria	Zinc oxide nanoparticles	Antimalarial	Against malarial vectors and parasites	(Kalpana et al., 2020)
Lingzhi extracts	PLGA nanoparticles	In corneal wound healing	In corneal epithelial cells	(Tsai et al., 2021)
Liquorice	Silver nanoparticles	Wound healing and antibacterial activity	Against E. coli and methicillin-resistant S. aureus (MRSA)	(Mohammed et al., 2023)

Phytoconstituents/Plant name	Type of nanoformulation	Disease/Treatment	*In vivo/in vitro* studies	Reference
Mentha pulegium and Ficus carica extracts	Silver oxide nanoparticles	Antibacterial activity	Against E. coli	(Shahzad Shirazi et al., 2022)
Paclitaxel	Biotinylated and non-biotinylated PEG-PLA nanoparticles	Anticancer activity	*In vitro* brain tumor (glioma) cells (BT4C)	(Pulkkinen et al., 2008)
Paclitaxel	Folate decorated paclitaxel loaded poly(lactide) (PLA)–tocopheryl polyethylene glycol 1000 succinate (TPGS) nanoparticles	Anti-cancer	*In vitro* effect on HeLa cell lines and *in vivo* effect on colorectal tumor growth in nude mouse	(Thu et al., 2015)
Paclitaxel	Peptide (TLYP-1-NP) -functionalized PEG–PLA nanoparticles	Glioma therapy	In both human umbilical vein endothelial cells and rat C6 glioma cells	(Hu et al., 2013)
Peppermint oil	Nanoemulsion loaded polycaprolactone nanofibrous dermal patches	Antimicrobial and antibiofilm activity	Skin disorders	(El-Naggar et al., 2023)
Plantago lanceolata extract	Silver nanoparticles	Antibacterial activity	Against Agrobacterium tumefaciens, Proteus vulgaris, S. aureus, and E. coli	(Shah et al., 2021)
Proanthocyanidins from grape extracts	Poly-lactic acid (PLA) nanoparticle	Higher encapsulation efficiency	*In vitro* release studies	(Fernández et al., 2016)
Quercetin	Chitosan nanoparticles	Antioxidant activity	*In vitro* studies	(Zhang et al., 2008)
Quercetin	PLA nanoparticles	Anti-cancer	In human breast cancer cells	(Pandey et al., 2015)
Quercetin	PLGA nanoparticles and thermosensitive gel formulations	In burn wound healing	In Wistar rats	(Cetin et al., 2022)
Quercetin	Polylactides (PLAS) with a β-CD core	Antibacterial	Against Staphylococcus aureus, Escherichia coli and Klebsiella pneumoniae	(Kost et al., 2020)
Quercetin	Polymeric (Eudragit® S100) nanoparticles	Anticancer	CT26 murine colon carcinoma cells	(Sunoqrot & Abujamous, 2019)
Resveratrol	Methoxy poly(ethylene glycol)-poly(lactide) copolymer (also called MPEG-PLA) nanoparticles	Reduction of plasma degradation, hepatic metabolism and as anticancer	C57BL/6J mouse model with subcutaneous B16-F10 melanoma	(Yee et al., 2022)
Resveratrol	PLA-coated co-micellar nanosystem	Intra-articular treatment of arthritis	Freund's adjuvant into both knee joints of adult Wistar rats	(Kamel et al., 2019)
Selenium	Niosomes	Anticancer activity	MTT assay on human foreskin fibroblasts normal cell line	(Haddadian et al., 2022)
Silymarin	Eudragit® RS100 nanoparticles	Cholestasis-induced fibrosis	Livers of rats	(Younis et al., 2016)
Vincristine sulfate and verapamil hydrochloride	PLGA nanoparticles	Optimization of the incorporation of two hydrophilic drugs	Drug entrapment efficiency studies	(Song et al., 2008)
Zingiber officinale	Silver nanoparticles	Antidiabetic	Streptozotocin induced diabetes in rats	(Garg et al., 2016)

Table 2. Clinical status of various plants/phytoconstituents as nanoformulations

Phytoconstituents/ Plant Name	Nanoformulation	Disease	Clinical trial phase	Clinical trials ID
Abraxane (albumin-bound paclitaxel)	Albumin-bound paclitaxel	Metastatic breast cancer	Observational study	NCT02555696
Abraxane with Carboplatin	Albumin-bound paclitaxel	Advance non-small cell lung cancer	Phase 4	NCT02151149
Camptothecin (CRLX-101) and Capecitabine	Cyclodextrin-polyethylene glycol (CD-PEG) nanoparticles	Rectal cancer	Phase 1 Phase 2	NCT02010567
Capsaicin	Topical preparation of nanoparticle	Diabetic neuropathy	Phase 2 Phase 3	NCT01125215
CRLX101	Cyclodextrin-polyethylene glycol (CD-PEG) nanoparticles	Advanced or metastatic stomach, gastro-esophageal, or esophageal cancer	Phase 2	NCT01612546
CRLX101 (NLG207)	Cyclodextrin-polyethylene glycol (CD-PEG) nanoparticles	Advanced non-small cell lung cancer	Phase 2	NCT01380769
CRLX101 (NLG207)	Cyclodextrin-polyethylene glycol (CD-PEG) nanoparticles	Advanced solid tumours	Phase 1 Phase 2	NCT00333502
Curcumin (Lipocurc)	Liposomes	Advanced or metastatic cancer	Phase 1 Phase 2	NCT02138955
Curcumin/ Doxorubicin-encapsulating Nanoparticle (IMX-110)	Curcumin/Doxorubicin-loaded EGFR-targeting Nanocells	Advanced solid tumours	Phase 1 Phase 2	NCT03382340
Curcumin® (CUC-01) and Paclitaxel	-	Advanced and metastatic breast cancer	Phase 2	NCT03072992
Docetaxel	[89Zr]-Df-CriPec®	Solid tumors	Phase 1	NCT03712423
Docetaxel	CriPec® docetaxel	Advanced epithelial ovarian cancer who are resistant to prior platinum-based chemotherapy	Phase 2	NCT03742713
Docetaxel	CriPec® technology- An amphiphilic methoxy-poly(ethylene glycol)-b-poly[N-(2-hydroxypropyl) methacrylamide lactate] also called as (mPEG-b-pHPMAmLacn) block copolymers	Solid tumors	Phase 1	NCT02442531
Docetaxel	Intravesical Nanoxel®M- Polymeric nanoparticles	Bacilliuscalmette-guerin refractory non-muscle invasive bladder cancer	Phase 3	NCT02982395
Docetaxel	Liposome encapsulated	Solid tumors	Phase 1	NCT01151384
Docetaxel	Nanosomal lipid suspension	Advanced solid tumours Triple negative breast cancer patients	Phase 1 Phase 3	NCT01957995 NCT03671044

Docetaxel	Polymeric micelle	Esophageal carcinoma	Phase 2	NCT03585673
Docetaxel	Polymeric micelle	Recurrent or metastatic head and neck squamous cell carcinoma	Phase 2	NCT02639858
Docetaxel	Polymeric nanoparticles	Advanced solid malignancies	Phase 1	NCT01103791
Docetaxel and Taxotere	Polymeric nanoparticles	Advanced solid tumour	Phase 1	NCT02274610
Fenugreek	Transdermal patch	Antinociceptive	Randomized Controlled Trial	(Ansari et al., 2019)
Nab-paclitaxel (with Sitravatinib and Tislelizumab)	-	Metastatic triple-negative breast cancer (TNBC)	Phase 2	NCT04734262
Nab-paclitaxel with Gemcitabine and Cisplatin	Albumin-bound nanoparticles of paclitaxel	Metastatic transitional cell carcinoma of urothelial tract	Phase 2	NCT03051373
NK105 (Paclitaxel)	Polymeric micellar nanoparticle	Metastatic or recurrent breast cancer	Phase 3	NCT01644890
Paclitaxel	ABI-007 (A cremophor-free, protein stabilized nanoparticles of paclitaxel)	Metastatic breast cancer	Phase 2 Phase 3	NCT00046514 NCT00046527
Paclitaxel	Liposomes	Metastatic breast cancer	Phase 4	NCT02142790
Paclitaxel	Micellar nanoparticles and Cremophor® EL	Ovarian cancer	Phase 3	NCT00989131
Paclitaxel (ABI-007), Carboplatin with Herceptin®	Albumin-bound Paclitaxel	Advanced breast cancer	Phase 2	NCT00093145
Paclitaxel with Cisplatin	Liposomes	Squamous non-small-cell lung cancer	Phase 4	NCT02996214
Quercetin	PLGA-PEG NPs	Squamous cell carcinoma	Phase 2	NCT05456022
Vinorelbine (Navelbine; vinca alkaloid) and Erlotinib	-	Non-small cell lung cancer	Phase 1	NCT00702182
Vinorelbine tartrate	Liposomal injection	Advanced malignancy	Phase 1 Phase 2	NCT02925000
Zein (a natural, biocompatible, and biodegradable polymer)	Nanoparticles	Glycaemic control	Not applicable	NCT05560412

Another significant obstacle is the scalability and reproducibility of manufacturing processes. Ensuring consistent quality across batches is essential for the reliability and safety of phytonanoherbal formulations. To address these challenges, standardization efforts must be guided by stringent quality control measures, which are crucial for fostering broader clinical acceptance. Although the potential of phytonanoherbal therapies is evident, their integration into conventional medical practices hinges on establishing clear regulatory pathways. Regulatory frameworks must adapt to accommodate the unique characteristics of these therapies, balancing innovation with safety and efficacy considerations. Collaborative efforts among researchers, regulatory bodies, and industry stakeholders are essential for defining standardized protocols to assess the safety and efficacy of phytonanoherbal formulations. The current status of phytonanoherbal therapies is promising, with considerable potential benefits for healthcare. However, overcoming challenges related to pharmacokinetics, manufacturing standardization, and regulatory frameworks is critical to realizing their full clinical potential. The referenced studies contribute to ongoing discussions about these challenges and opportunities, guiding future research and development efforts in the field.

Worldwide Market Analysis and Industry Forecast for Phytonanoherbals

The global market for phytonanoherbal therapies is currently experiencing a transformative phase, characterized by a growing interest in and recognition of their potential within the healthcare sector. Industry reports and research studies indicate that the market is on a positive trajectory, driven by several factors (Jadhav et al., 2020; Gunjan et al., 2015). The rising demand for natural and plant-based therapies, coupled with advancements in nanotechnology, is fostering innovation in phytonanoherbal interventions.

Research and development activities are increasing, with companies actively investing in the exploration of nanoscale formulations derived from medicinal plants. The Asia-Pacific region, known for its rich tradition of herbal medicine, is emerging as a key player in this market, with heightened investment in research and commercialization efforts. North America and Europe also maintain a strong market presence, focusing on the integration of phytonanoherbal therapies into comprehensive healthcare practices.

The phytonanoherbal market offers a diverse range of products, including nanoparticles encapsulating herbal extracts, nanocrystals, and nanoemulsions. (Jadhav et al., 2020; Gunjan et al., 2015). These formulations aim to enhance the bioavailability, stability, and targeted delivery of phytochemicals, catering to the evolving needs of consumers and healthcare professionals. However, the market faces significant challenges, particularly the absence of standardized regulations and guidelines for development and commercialization. While regulatory bodies are starting to acknowledge the necessity for specific frameworks for these products, a comprehensive global approach is still required.

Market analysis indicates that the phytonanoherbal sector encompasses a variety of applications, including pharmaceuticals, nutraceuticals, and cosmetics (Khan et al., 2019; Tilburt et al., 2008). The therapeutic potential of these interventions extends beyond traditional herbal medicine, with pharmaceutical companies investigating their use for targeted drug delivery and improved efficacy. Increasing consumer awareness of natural and plant-based products is driving market growth, in alignment with a global trend toward wellness and preventive healthcare.

Collaborations and partnerships between pharmaceutical companies, herbal product manufacturers, and nanotechnology firms are becoming increasingly common. These strategic alliances aim to leverage combined expertise, expedite product development, and tackle challenges related to scalability and standardization (Kumar et al., 2023; Sarmah et al., 2022). Despite this progress, hurdles persist, including the lack of universally accepted standards for quality control and manufacturing processes, as well as regulatory uncertainties regarding product claims and labeling.

The future outlook for the phytonanoherbal therapies industry is promising, with significant growth anticipated. Ongoing research, technological advancements, and a rising consumer preference for natural healthcare solutions are expected to drive market expansion. The integration of advanced technologies, such as artificial intelligence and machine learning, is likely to enhance the development and optimization of phytonanoherbal formulations (Singh et al., 2021; Nanbban et al., 2022). Additionally, startups and niche players are contributing to market growth, although they face challenges related to scalability and market penetration.

Conclusion

This chapter offers a thorough exploration of ongoing clinical trials and research studies to provide insights into the real-world performance of these therapies. The global fusion of traditional herbal medicine with modern nanotechnology has resulted in the creation of innovative pharmacological treatments that hold the potential to enhance health outcomes. By integrating natural remedies and herbal extracts with advanced nanocarrier systems, these therapies are anticipated to greatly improve the efficacy and applicability of existing drug delivery methods, making them more relevant and effective in today's medical practice.

References

Acet, Ö., Dikici, E., Acet, B. Ö., Odabaşı, M., Mijakovic, I., & Pandit, S. (2023). Inhibition of bacterial adhesion by epigallocatechin gallate attached polymeric membranes. *Colloids and Surfaces B: Biointerfaces*, *221*, 113024.

Alexander, A., Patel, R. J., Saraf, S., & Saraf, S. (2016). Recent expansion of pharmaceutical nanotechnologies and targeting strategies in the field of phytopharmaceuticals for the delivery of herbal extracts and bioactives. *Journal of Controlled Release*, 241, 110-124.

Alipour, M., Sharifi, S., Samiei, M., Shahi, S., Aghazadeh, M., & Dizaj, S. M. (2023). Synthesis, characterization, and evaluation of Hesperetin nanocrystals for regenerative dentistry. *Scientific Reports*, *13*(1), 2076.

Ansari, M., Sadeghi, P., Mahdavi, H., Fattahi-Dolatabadi, M., Mohamadi, N., Asadi, A., & Sharififar, F. (2019). Fenugreek dermal patch, a new natural topical antinociceptive medication for relieving the postherniotomy pain, a double-blind placebo controlled trial. *Journal of Complementary and Integrative Medicine*, *16*(3), 20180082.

Ashkbar, A., Rezaei, F., Attari, F., & Ashkevarian, S. (2020). Treatment of breast cancer *in vivo* by dual photodynamic and photothermal approaches with the aid of curcumin photosensitizer and magnetic nanoparticles. *Scientific Reports*, *10*(1), 21206.

Aucouturier, J., Dupuis, L., & Ganne, V. (2001). Adjuvants designed for veterinary and human vaccines. *Vaccine, 19*(17-19), 2666-2672.

Barkat, M. A., Goyal, A., Barkat, H. A., Salauddin, M., Pottoo, F. H., & Anwer, E. T. (2021). Herbal medicine: Clinical perspective and regulatory status. *Combinatorial chemistry & high throughput screening*, 24(10), 1573-1582.

Beniwal, M., Jain, N., Jain, S., & Aggarwal, N. (2022). Design, synthesis, anticancer evaluation and docking studies of novel 2-(1-isonicotinoyl-3-phenyl-1 H-pyrazol-4-yl)-3-phenylthiazolidin-4-one derivatives as Aurora-A kinase inhibitors. *BMC chemistry*, 16(1), 61.

Bhide, A. R., & Jindal, A. B. (2021). Fabrication and evaluation of artemether loaded polymeric nanorods obtained by mechanical stretching of nanospheres. *International Journal of Pharmaceutics*, *605*, 120820.

Bonifacio, B. V., da Silva, P. B., Ramos, M. A. D. S., Negri, K. M. S., Bauab, T. M., & Chorilli, M. (2014). Nanotechnology-based drug delivery systems and herbal medicines: a review. *International journal of nanomedicine*, 9, 1-15.

Boora, F., Chirisa, E., & Mukanganyama, S. (2014). Evaluation of nitrite radical scavenging properties of selected Zimbabwean plant extracts and their phytoconstituents. *Journal of Food Processing* (1), 918018.

Boukhatem, M. N., & Setzer, W. N. (2020). Aromatic herbs, medicinal plant-derived essential oils, and phytochemical extracts as potential therapies for coronaviruses: future perspectives. *Plants*, *9*(6), 800.

Burgers, J. S., Cluzeau, F. A., Hanna, S. E., Hunt, C., & Grol, R. (2003). Characteristics of high-quality guidelines: evaluation of 86 clinical guidelines developed in ten European countries and Canada. *International journal of technology assessment in health care*, *19*(1), 148-157.

Cetin, N., Menevse, E., Celik, Z. E., Ceylan, C., Rama, S. T., Gultekin, Y., Tekin, T., & Sahin, A. (2022). Evaluation of burn wound healing activity of thermosensitive gel and PLGA nanoparticle formulation of quercetin in Wistar albino rats. *Journal of Drug Delivery Science and Technology*, 75, 103620.

Chatzinasiou, L., Booker, A., MacLennan, E., Mackonochie, M., & Heinrich, M. (2019). Turmeric (Curcuma longa L.) products: What quality differences exist? *Journal of Herbal Medicine*, 17, 100281.

Chiu, C. F., Fu, R. H., Hsu, S. H., Yu, Y. H., Yang, S. F., Tsao, T. C. Y., Chang, K. B., Yeh, C. A., Tang, C. M., & Huang, S.-C. (2021). Delivery capacity and anticancer ability of the berberine-loaded gold nanoparticles to promote the apoptosis effect in breast cancer. *Cancers*, *13*(21), 5317.

Chopra, H., Goyal, R., Agarwal, N., Mishra, D., & Gautam, R. K. (2023). Edible Mushroom assisted synthesis and applications of metal nanoparticles: A comprehensive review. *Journal of Integrated Science and Technology*, *11*(1) ,427-427.

Council, T. I. T. R. (2009). Phytotechnology Technical and Regulartory Guidance and Decision Trees. *Phytotechnologies.*

Daisy, P., & Saipriya, K. (2012). Biochemical analysis of Cassia fistula aqueous extract and phytochemically synthesized gold nanoparticles as hypoglycemic treatment for diabetes mellitus. *International Journal of Nanomedicine*, 1189-1202.

Dewi, M. K., Chaerunisaa, A. Y., Muhaimin, M., & Joni, I. M. (2022). Improved activity of herbal medicines through nanotechnology. *Nanomaterials*, 12(22) ,4073.

Dezfouli, E. A., Kiaie, S. H., Danafar, H., Nomani, A., & Sadeghizadeh, M. (2022). BTN-PEG PCL nanoparticles for targeted delivery of curcumin: *In vitro* and in Ovo assessment. *Journal of Drug Delivery Science and Technology*, *74*, 103382.

Ebaid, H., Habila, M., Hassan, I., Al-Tamimi, J., Omar, M. S., Rady, A., & Alhazza, I. M. (2021). Curcumin-containing Silver Nanoparticles Prevent Carbon Tetrachloride- induced Hepatotoxicity in Mice. *Combinatorial Chemistry & High Throughput Screening*, *24*(10),1609-1617.

El Desoky, E., Meinshausen, J., Bühl, K., Engel, G., Harings-Kaim, A., Drewelow, B., & Klotz, U. (1993). Generation of pharmacokinetic data during routine therapeutic drug monitoring: Bayesian approach vs. pharmacokinetic studies. *Therapeutic drug monitoring*, *15*(4),281-288.

El-Naggar, M. E., Abdelgawad, A. M., Abdel-Sattar, R., Gibriel, A. A., & Hemdan, B. A. (2023). Potential antimicrobial and antibiofilm efficacy of essential oil nanoemulsion loaded polycaprolactone nanofibrous dermal patches. *European Polymer Journal*, *184*, 111782.

El-Naggar, M. E., Al-Joufi, F., Anwar, M., Attia, M. F., & El-Bana, M. A. (2019). Curcumin-loaded PLA-PEG copolymer nanoparticles for treatment of liver inflammation in streptozotocin-induced diabetic rats. *Colloids and Surfaces B: Biointerfaces*, *177*, 389-398.

Fernández, K., Aburto, J., von Plessing, C., Rockel, M., & Aspé, E. (2016). Factorial design optimization and characterization of poly-lactic acid (PLA) nanoparticle formation for the delivery of grape extracts. *Food Chemistry*, *207*, 75-85.

Firth, J., Torous, J., Stubbs, B., Firth, J. A., Steiner, G. Z., Smith, L., & Sarris, J. (2019). The "online brain": how the Internet may be changing our cognition. *World Psychiatry*, 18(2), 119-129.

Fu, C., Ding, C., Sun, X., & Fu, A. (2018). Curcumin nanocapsules stabilized by bovine serum albumin-capped gold nanoclusters (BSA-AuNCs) for drug delivery and theranosis. *Materials Science and Engineering: C*, *87*, 149-154.

Garg, P., Aggarwal, N., Garg, V., Dutt, R., Singh, R. P., Kumar, V., Chopra, H., Al-Mazroua, H. A., Attia, S. M., Ahmad, S. F., & Bin Emran, T. (2024). Assessment of Antidepressant Activity of Stem of Jasminum multiflorum Andrews and Jasminum mesnyi Hance by Modulating Neurochemicals and Reducing Oxidative Stress. *Journal Of Biological Regulators and Homeostatic Agents*, 38(2), 1649-1661.

Garg, A., Pandey, P., Sharma, P., & Shukla, A. (2016). Synthesis and characterization of silver nanoparticle of ginger rhizome (Zingiber officinale) extract: synthesis, characterization and anti diabetic activity in streptozotocin induced diabetic rats. *European Journal of Biomedical and Pharmaceutical Sciences*, *3*(7), 605-611.

Gorgani, L., Mohammadi, M., Najafpour, G. D., & Nikzad, M. (2017). Piperine—the bioactive compound of black pepper: from isolation to medicinal formulations. *Comprehensive reviews in food science and food safety*, 16(1), 124-140.

Grabowski, H. (2002). Patents, innovation and access to new pharmaceuticals. *Journal of International Economic Law*, 5(4), 849-860.

Gunjan, M., Naing, T. W., Saini, R. S., Ahmad, A., Naidu, J. R., & Kumar, I. (2015). Marketing trends & future prospects of herbal medicine in the treatment of various disease. *World Journal of Pharmaceutical Research*, 4(9), 132-155.

Haddadian, A., Robattorki, F. F., Dibah, H., Soheili, A., Ghanbarzadeh, E., Sartipnia, N., Hajrasouliha, S., Pasban, K., Andalibi, R., Ch, M. H., Azari, A., Chitgarzadeh, A., Kashtali, A. B., Mastali, F., Noorbazargan, H., & Mirzaie, A. (2022). Niosomes-loaded selenium nanoparticles as a new approach for enhanced antibacterial, anti-biofilm, and anticancer activities. *Scientific Reports*, *12*(1), 21938.

Holtmeier, W., Zeuzem, S., Preiss, J., Kruis, W., Böhm, S., Maaser, C., Raedler, A., Schmidt, C., Schnitker, J., Schwarz, J., Zeitz, M., & Caspary, W. (2011). Randomized, placebo-controlled, double-blind trial of Boswellia serrata in maintaining remission of Crohn's disease: good safety profile but lack of efficacy. *Inflammatory bowel diseases*, 17(2), 573-582.

Hu, Q., Gao, X., Gu, G., Kang, T., Tu, Y., Liu, Z., Song, Q., Yao, L., Pang, Z., Jiang, X., Chen, H., & Chen, J. (2013). Glioma therapy using tumor homing and penetrating peptide-functionalized PEG–PLA nanoparticles loaded with paclitaxel. *Biomaterials*, *34*(22), 5640-5650.

Jadhav, C. A., Vikhe, D. N., & Jadhav, R. S. (2020). Global and domestic market of herbal medicines: A review. *Research Journal of Science and Technology*, 12(4), 327-330.

Jia, J., Zhang, K., Zhou, X., Zhou, D., & Ge, F. (2018). Precise dissolution control and bioavailability evaluation for insoluble drug berberine via a polymeric particle prepared using supercritical CO2. *Polymers*, *10*(11), 1198.

Jiang, Y., Liu, C., Zhai, W., Zhuang, N., Han, T., & Ding, Z. (2019). The optimization design of lactoferrin loaded HupA nanoemulsion for targeted drug transport via intranasal route. *International Journal of Nanomedicine*, 14, 9217-9234.

Jummes, B., Sganzerla, W. G., da Rosa, C. G., Noronha, C. M., Nunes, M. R., Bertoldi, F. C., & Barreto, P. L. M. (2020). Antioxidant and antimicrobial poly-ε-caprolactone nanoparticles loaded with Cymbopogon martinii essential oil. *Biocatalysis and Agricultural Biotechnology*, *23*, 101499.

Kalpana, V. N., Alarjani, K. M., & Rajeswari, V. D. (2020). Enhancing malaria control using Lagenaria siceraria and its mediated zinc oxide nanoparticles against the vector Anopheles stephensi and its parasite Plasmodium falciparum. *Scientific Reports*, *10*(1), 21568.

Kamel, R., Abbas, H., & Shaffie, N. M. (2019). Development and evaluation of PLA-coated co-micellar nanosystem of Resveratrol for the intra-articular treatment of arthritis. *International Journal of Pharmaceutics*, *569*, 118560.

Kiani, B. H., Ikram, F., Fatima, H., Alhodaib, A., Haq, I.-u., Ur-Rehman, T., & Naz, I. (2022). Comparative evaluation of biomedical and phytochemical applications of zinc nanoparticles by using Fagonia cretica extracts. *Scientific Reports*, *12*(1), 10024

Kim, D. W., Choi, C. H., Park, J. P., & Lee, S. J. (2020). Nanospheres Loaded with Curcumin Improve the Bioactivity of Umbilical Cord Blood-Mesenchymal Stem Cells via c-Src Activation During the Skin Wound Healing Process. *Cells*, *9*(6), 1467.

Khan, M. S. A., & Ahmad, I. (2019). Herbal medicine: current trends and future prospects. In *New look to phytomedicine* (pp. 3-13). Academic Press.

Kolenyak dos Santos, F., Helena Oyafuso, M., Priscila Kiill, C., Palmira Daflon-Gremiao, M., & Chorilli, M. (2013). Nanotechnology-based drug delivery systems for treatment of hyperproliferative skin diseases-a review. *Current Nanoscience*, *9*(1), 159-167.

Kumar, Rajiv. "Nanotechnology in herbal medicine: Challenges and future perspectives." In *Nanotechnology in Herbal Medicine*, pp. 515-548. Woodhead Publishing, 2023.

Kost, B., Svyntkivska, M., Brzeziński, M., Makowski, T., Piorkowska, E., Rajkowska, K., Kunicka-Styczyńska, A., & Biela, T. (2020). PLA/β-CD-based fibres loaded with quercetin as potential antibacterial dressing materials. *Colloids and Surfaces B: Biointerfaces*, *190*, 110949.

Lauro, M. R., Musumeci, T., Sansone, F., Puglisi, G., & Pignatello, R. (2019). Polymeric Colloidal Carriers for Natural Polyphenolic Compounds. In *Novel Drug Delivery Systems for Phytoconstituents*, pp. 261-282. CRC Press.

Lee, W. H., Loo, C. Y., Traini, D., & Young, P. M. (2015). Inhalation of nanoparticle-based drug for lung cancer treatment: Advantages and challenges. *Asian journal of pharmaceutical sciences*, 10(6), 481-489.

Liao, W., Li, Y., Wang, J., Zhao, M., Chen, N., Zheng, Q., Wan, L., Mou, Y., Tang, J., & Wang, Z. (2022). Natural products-based nanoformulations: A new approach targeting CSCs to cancer therapy. *International Journal of Nanomedicine*, 17, 4163.

Matos, M. J., Vazquez-Rodriguez, S., Uriarte, E., Santana, L., & Borges, F. (2015). Synthesis and pharmacological activities of non-flavonoid chromones: A patent review (from 2005 to 2015). *Expert Opinion on Therapeutic Patents*, 25(11), 1285-1304.

Munjal K., Ahmad, S., Gupta, A., Haye, A., Amin, S., Mir, S. R. (2020). Polyphenol-enriched fraction and the compounds isolated from *Garcinia indica* fruits ameliorate obesity through suppression of digestive enzymes and oxidative stress. *Pharmacognosy Magazine*, 16(70), S236-S245.

Munjal, K., Gautam, V. K., Goel, Y., Ahamad, J., & Mir, S. R. (2023). Qualitative diagnostic features of alkaloidal spices. In *Analysis of food spices* (1st ed., pp. 16). CRC Press.

Mitragotri, S., Burke, P. A., & Langer, R. (2014). Overcoming the challenges in administering biopharmaceuticals: Formulation and delivery strategies. *Nature Reviews Drug Discovery*, 13(9), 655-672.

Mohammed, H. A., Amin, M. A., Zayed, G., Hassan, Y., El-Mokhtar, M., & Saddik, M. S. (2023). *In vitro* and *in vivo* synergistic wound healing and anti-methicillin-resistant Staphylococcus aureus (MRSA) evaluation of liquorice-decorated silver nanoparticles. *The Journal of Antibiotics*, *76*(5), 291-300.

Mollaoglu-Korkmaz, S., Swarup, L., & Riley, D. (2013). Delivering sustainable, high-performance buildings: Influence of project delivery methods on integration and project outcomes. *Journal of Management in Engineering*, 29(1), 71-78.

Moosavy, M.-H., de la Guardia, M., Mokhtarzadeh, A., Khatibi, S. A., Hosseinzadeh, N., & Hajipour, N. (2023). Green synthesis, characterization, and biological evaluation of gold and silver nanoparticles using Mentha spicata essential oil. *Scientific Reports*, *13*(1), 7230

Nabofa, W. E. E., Alashe, O. O., Oyeyemi, O. T., Attah, A. F., Oyagbemi, A. A., Omobowale, T. O., Adedapo, A. A., & Alada, A. R. A. (2018). Cardioprotective Effects of Curcumin-Nisin Based Poly Lactic Acid Nanoparticle on Myocardial Infarction in Guinea Pigs. *Scientific Reports*, *8*(1), 16649.

Nanbban, R., & Kamaraj, R. (2022). Herbal product regulation and development in India. NeuroQuantology, 20(17), 381.

Niza, E., Božik, M., Bravo, I., Clemente-Casares, P., Lara-Sanchez, A., Juan, A., Klouček, P., & Alonso-Moreno, C. (2020). PEI-coated PLA nanoparticles to enhance the antimicrobial activity of carvacrol. *Food Chemistry*, *328*, 127131.

Nasrollahzadeh, M., Sajadi, S. M., Sajjadi, M., & Issaabadi, Z. (2019). An introduction to nanotechnology. *In Interface science and technology* (Vol. 28, pp. 1-27). Elsevier.

Pan, S. Y., Litscher, G., Gao, S. H., Zhou, S. F., Yu, Z. L., Chen, H. Q., Zhang, S. F., Tang, M. K., Sun, J. N., & Ko, K. M. (2014). Historical perspective of traditional indigenous medical practices: the current renaissance and conservation of herbal resources. *Evidence-Based Complementary and Alternative Medicine*, 2014(1), 525340.

Pandey, S. K., Patel, D. K., Thakur, R., Mishra, D. P., Maiti, P., & Haldar, C. (2015). Anti-cancer evaluation of quercetin embedded PLA nanoparticles synthesized by emulsified nanoprecipitation. *International Journal of Biological Macromolecules*, *75*, 521-529.

Parhi, P., Suklabaidya, S., & Kumar Sahoo, S. (2017). Enhanced anti-metastatic and anti-tumorigenic efficacy of Berbamine loaded lipid nanoparticles *in vivo*. *Scientific Reports*, *7*(1), 5806.

Prabhuraj, R. S., Bomb, K., Srivastava, R., & Bandyopadhyaya, R. (2020). Selection of superior targeting ligands using PEGylated PLGA nanoparticles for delivery of curcumin in the treatment of triple-negative breast cancer cells. *Journal of Drug Delivery Science and Technology*, *57*, 101722.

Pulkkinen, M., Pikkarainen, J., Wirth, T., Tarvainen, T., Haapa-aho, V., Korhonen, H., Seppälä, J., & Järvinen, K. (2008). Three-step tumor targeting of paclitaxel using biotinylated PLA-PEG nanoparticles and avidin–biotin technology: Formulation development and *in vitro* anticancer activity. *European Journal of Pharmaceutics and Biopharmaceutics*, *70*(1), 66-74.

Ragab, E. M., El Gamal, D. M., Mohamed, T. M., & Khamis, A. A. (2022). Therapeutic potential of chrysin nanoparticle-mediation inhibition of succinate dehydrogenase and ubiquinone oxidoreductase in pancreatic and lung adenocarcinoma. *European Journal of Medical Research*, *27*(1), 172.

Rathinavel, S., Korrapati, P. S., Kalaiselvi, P., & Dharmalingam, S. (2021). Mesoporous silica incorporated PCL/Curcumin nanofiber for wound healing application. *European Journal of Pharmaceutical Sciences*, *167*, 106021

Rathore, A. S., Saxena, N., Thakur, G., & Mishra, S. (2023). Artificial intelligence and machine learning applications in biopharmaceutical manufacturing. Trends in Biotechnology, 41(4), 497-510.

Sachan, A. K., & Gupta, A. (2015). A review on nanotized herbal drugs. *International journal of pharmaceutical sciences and research*, *6*(3), 961.

Ajazuddin, & Saraf, S. (2010). Applications of novel drug delivery system for herbal formulations. *Fitoterapia*, 81(7), 680-689.

Sarmah, D. (2022). Indian Herbal Drug Industry: Prospects and Current Scenario. *Current Trends in Pharmaceutical Research*, *9*(1).

Satyavert, Gupta, S., Choudhury, H., Jacob, S., Nair, A. B., Dhanawat, M., & Munjal, K. (2021). Pharmacokinetics and tissue distribution of hydrazinocurcumin in rats. *Pharmacological Reports, 73*(6), 1734-1743.

Seko, I., Tonbul, H., Tavukçuoğlu, E., Şahin, A., Akbas, S., Yanık, H., Öztürk, S. C., Esendagli, G., Khan, M., & Capan, Y. (2021). Development of curcumin and docetaxel co-loaded actively targeted PLGA nanoparticles to overcome blood brain barrier. *Journal of Drug Delivery Science and Technology*, *66*, 102867.

Shah, M. Z., Guan, Z.-H., Din, A. U., Ali, A., Rehman, A. U., Jan, K., Faisal, S., Saud, S., Adnan, M., Wahid, F., Alamri, S., Siddiqui, M. H., Ali, S., Nasim, W., Hammad, H. M., & Fahad, S. (2021). Synthesis of silver nanoparticles using Plantago lanceolata extract and assessing their antibacterial and antioxidant activities. *Scientific Reports*, *11*(1), 20754.

Shahzad Shirazi, M., Moridi Farimani, M., Foroumadi, A., Ghanemi, K., Benaglia, M., & Makvandi, P. (2022). Bioengineered synthesis of phytochemical-adorned green silver oxide (Ag2O) nanoparticles via Mentha pulegium and Ficus carica extracts with high antioxidant, antibacterial, and antifungal activities. *Scientific Reports*, *12*(1), 21509.

Shariare, M. H., Rahman, M., Lubna, S. R., Roy, R. S., Abedin, J., Marzan, A. L., Altamimi, M. A., Ahamad, S. R., Ahmad, A., Alanazi, F. K., & Kazi, M. (2020). Liposomal drug delivery of Aphanamixis polystachya leaf extracts and its neurobehavioral activity in mice model. *Scientific Reports*, *10*(1), 6938.

Sharma, A. T., Mitkare, S. S., & Moon, R. S. (2011). Multicomponent herbal therapy: A review. *International Journal of Pharmaceutical Sciences Review and Research*, 6, 185-187.

Singh, S., & Shukla, V. K. (2021). Current regulations for herbal medicines in India. *International Journal of Drug Regulatory Affairs*, 9(2), 30-34.

Kwatra, S. (2013). Nanotechnology and medicine—The upside and the downside. *International Journal of Drug Development and Research*, 5(1), 1-10.

Song, X., Zhao, Y., Wu, W., Bi, Y., Cai, Z., Chen, Q., Li, Y., & Hou, S. (2008). PLGA nanoparticles simultaneously loaded with vincristine sulfate and verapamil hydrochloride: Systematic study of particle size and drug entrapment efficiency. *International Journal of Pharmaceutics*, *350*(1), 320-329.

Sprong, N., Driessen, P. H., Hillebrand, B., & Molner, S. (2021). Market innovation: A literature review and new research directions. *Journal of Business Research*, 123, 450-462.

Strandberg, K. L., Rotschafer, J. H., Vetter, S. M., Buonpane, R. A., Kranz, D. M., & Schlievert, P. M. (2010). Staphylococcal superantigens cause lethal pulmonary disease in rabbits. *The Journal of Infectious Diseases*, 202(11), 1690-1697.

Sunoqrot, S., & Abujamous, L. (2019). pH-sensitive polymeric nanoparticles of quercetin as a potential colon cancer-targeted nanomedicine. *Journal of Drug Delivery Science and Technology*, *52*, 670-676.

Tilburt, J. C., & Kaptchuk, T. J. (2008). Herbal medicine research and global health: An ethical analysis. *Bulletin of the World Health Organization*, 86, 594-599.

Thirumoorthy, G., Balasubramanian, B., George, J. A., Nizam, A., Nagella, P., Srinatha, N., Pappuswamy, M., Alanazi, A. M., Meyyazhagan, A., Rengasamy, K. R. R., & Veerappa Lakshmaiah, V. (2024). Phytofabricated bimetallic synthesis of silver-copper nanoparticles using Aerva lanata extract to evaluate their potential cytotoxic and antimicrobial activities. *Scientific Reports*, *14*(1), 1270.

Thu, H. P., Nam, N. H., Quang, B. T., Son, H. A., Toan, N. L., & Quang, D. T. (2015). *In vitro* and *in vivo* targeting effect of folate decorated paclitaxel loaded PLA–TPGS nanoparticles. *Saudi Pharmaceutical Journal*, *23*(6), 683-688.

Tsai, I. L., Tsai, C.-Y., Kuo, L.-L., Woung, L.-C., Ku, R.-Y., & Cheng, Y.-H. (2021). PLGA nanoparticles containing Lingzhi extracts rescue corneal epithelial cells from oxidative damage. *Experimental Eye Research*, *206*, 108539.

Umerska, A., Gaucher, C., Oyarzun-Ampuero, F., Fries-Raeth, I., Colin, F., Villamizar-Sarmiento, M. G., Maincent, P., & Sapin-Minet, A. (2018). Polymeric nanoparticles for increasing oral bioavailability of curcumin. *Antioxidants*, *7*(4), 46.

van Beek, T. A., & Montoro, P. (2009). Chemical analysis and quality control of Ginkgo biloba leaves, extracts, and phytopharmaceuticals. *Journal of Chromatography A*, 1216(11), 2002-2032.

Wang, Z. L. (2003). New developments in transmission electron microscopy for nanotechnology. *Advanced Materials*, 15(18), 1497-1514.

World Health Organization. (2007). *Quality Assurance of Pharmaceuticals: A Compendium of Guidelines and Related Materials. Good Manufacturing Practices and Inspection*. Vol. 2. World Health Organization.

Wang, Z. H., Wang, Z. Y., Sun, C. S., Wang, C. Y., Jiang, T. Y., & Wang, S. L. (2010). Trimethylated chitosan-conjugated PLGA nanoparticles for the delivery of drugs to the brain. *Biomaterials*, *31*(5), 908-915.

Yang, X., Li, Z., Wang, N., Li, L., Song, L., He, T., Sun, L., Wang, Z., Wu, Q., Luo, N., Yi, C., & Gong, C. (2015). Curcumin-Encapsulated Polymeric Micelles Suppress the Development of Colon Cancer *In Vitro* and *In Vivo*. *Scientific Reports*, *5*(1), 10322.

Yee, Y. J., Benson, H. A. E., Dass, C. R., & Chen, Y. (2022). Evaluation of novel conjugated resveratrol polymeric nanoparticles in reduction of plasma degradation, hepatic metabolism and its augmentation of anticancer activity *in vitro* and *in vivo*. *International Journal of Pharmaceutics*, *615*, 121499.

Younis, N., Shaheen, M. A., & Abdallah, M. H. (2016). Silymarin-loaded Eudragit® RS100 nanoparticles improved the ability of silymarin to resolve hepatic fibrosis in bile duct ligated rats. *Biomedicine & Pharmacotherapy*, *81*, 93-103.

Yuan, Haidan, Qianqian Ma, Li Ye, and Guangchun Piao. "The traditional medicine and modern medicine from natural products." *Molecules* 21, no. 5 (2016), 559.

Zamboni, F., Ren, G., Culebras, M., O'Driscoll, J., O'Dwyer, J., Ryan, E. J., & Collins, M. N. (2022). Curcumin encapsulated polylactic acid nanoparticles embedded in alginate/gelatin bioinks for in situ immunoregulation: Characterization and biological assessment. *International Journal of Biological Macromolecules*, *221*, 1218-1227.

Zhang, Y., Yang, Y., Tang, K., Hu, X., & Zou, G. (2008). Physicochemical characterization and antioxidant activity of quercetin-loaded chitosan nanoparticles. *Journal of Applied Polymer Science*, *107*(2), 891-897.

Chapter 21

Integrating Nanotechnology with Herbal Medicine for Enhanced Therapeutics and an Overview of Regulatory Considerations

Anchal Sharma[1,*]
Arushi[1]
Bhumika Thakur[1]
Shiv Kumar[1]
Vinod Kumar Gauttam[1]
Kavita Munjal[2]
and Teena Vishwakarma[3]
[1]Shiva Institute of Pharmacy, Chandpur, Bilaspur, Himachal Pradesh, India
[2]Amity Institute of Pharmacy, Amity University, Noida, Uttar Pradesh, India
[3]I.E.S. Institute of Pharmacy, I.E.S. University, Bhopal, Madhya Pradesh, India

Abstract

Herbal remedies are increasingly being preferred over conventional medications for the relief of various disease symptoms. As a result, the pharmaceutical industry is actively focused on discovering novel therapeutic agents derived from medicinal plants. Approximately 25% of new molecular entities approved by the FDA are of plant origin. Nanomedicine has emerged as a major area of interest, bringing new challenges for the scientific community, industry, and regulatory bodies. To address unmet medical needs and improve human health and quality of life, innovative scientific and technological methods must be developed. Despite the numerous benefits of phytomedicines, they present several challenges, including toxicity, poor bioavailability, stability issues, and patient compliance. To overcome these limitations, herbal nanoformulations can be introduced. Several patented formulations highlight the interaction between nanotechnology and herbal products, as nanotechnology influences nearly every aspect of life, raising concerns about human safety. Consequently, there is an increasing need for the development of safety regulations for nanomaterials. This chapter explores various

* Corresponding Author's Email: anchalsharma69511@gmail.com.

In: Phyto-Nanomedicine
Editors: Hitesh Chopra, Vinod Kumar Gauttam, Ajmer Singh Grewal et al.
ISBN: 979-8-89530-317-7

nanoherbal formulations and provides an overview of safety and regulatory considerations in nanophytoherbal therapeutics.

Keywords: regulatory aspects, nanoherbal formulations, nanotechnology, stability, bioavailability, patient compliance

Abbreviations

WHO	World Health Organization
MRI	Magnetic Resonance Imaging
BBB	Blood Brain Barier
PPE	Personal Protective Equipment
FDA	Food and Drug Administration
EMA	European Medicines Agency
IRB	Institutional Review Board
NDDS	Novel Drug Delivery System

Introduction

The growing interest in herbal remedies reflects a broader trend toward natural and holistic approaches to healthcare. Many individuals view herbal medicines as gentler and safer alternatives to synthetic drugs, often because they are perceived as "natural" and have a long history of use in traditional medicine systems across the globe. This belief is further supported by an increasing number of clinical studies that validate the therapeutic efficacy of certain herbal remedies, adding scientific credibility to their use. However, while herbal remedies offer potential benefits, it's important to approach them with caution. The therapeutic properties of many herbs are well-documented, but they can also pose risks if not used correctly. For instance, the quality and consistency of herbal products can vary significantly due to less stringent regulation compared to pharmaceutical drugs. This variability can affect the safety and effectiveness of the remedies. Additionally, herbal medicines may not be suitable for everyone, particularly for individuals with specific health conditions or those taking other medications, as interactions can occur. Therefore, it's crucial to consult with a healthcare professional, such as a doctor or a qualified herbalist, before incorporating herbal remedies into one's healthcare regimen. This ensures that their use is safe, appropriate, and effective, aligning with the individual's overall health needs and treatment goals (Patel et al., 2012; Malik et al., 2015). Herbal treatments, in contrast to the commonly utilized allopathic method, contain thousands of elements that act in concert to combat ailments. In order to improve patient compliance and reduce the need for recurrent administration, phytotherapeutics require a scientific strategy to administer the components over time (Yadav et al., 2011). The preference for herbal or traditional medicine, particularly in the management of certain disorders or for holistic therapy, is indeed notable. While modern medicine excels in various aspects, including acute care and advanced treatments, traditional medicine systems offer alternative approaches that focus on holistic well-being and often present fewer adverse effects. Traditional medicine systems such as Ayurveda, Unani, Chinese medicine, and homeopathy have gained recognition globally for their approaches to health and healing. These systems typically utilize herbs, animals, and mineral resources to formulate remedies tailored to individual needs. The World Health Organization (WHO) defines herbal medicines as products containing parts of plants, other plant materials, or combinations thereof as active ingredients. The WHO has also recognized the importance of traditional medicine and encourages its integration into national healthcare systems where appropriate. India, in particular, boasts a rich tradition of herbal medicine, with approximately 2,500 species of plants found in the wild and around 150 species cultivated on a large scale. This underscores the significant role that herbal medicine plays in healthcare practices worldwide. This statistic reflects the enduring popularity and trust placed in traditional medicine systems, especially in regions where they have been integral to cultural and healthcare practices for centuries. While herbal and traditional medicines offer promising avenues for healthcare, it's crucial to ensure proper regulation, quality control, and integration with modern medical practices to maximize their efficacy and safety. Collaboration between traditional healers, modern healthcare practitioners, researchers, and policymakers is essential to harness the potential of traditional medicine while safeguarding public health and promoting evidence-based practices (Pandey et al. 2013). Creating innovative drug delivery systems for herbal components is one way to accomplish this. In order to improve patient compliance and reduce the need for recurrent administration, phytotherapeutics require a scientific strategy to administer the components over time. NDDS not only reduce the need for repeated administration to overcome non-compliance, but they also enhance therapeutic value by increasing bioavailability, reducing toxicity, and improving other variables. Herbal extracts have additional features that make them attractive to large pharmaceutical corporations for use in novel formulation methods. These benefits include the capacity to solve the primary problem of poor absorption and bulk dosage (Sungthongjeen et al., 1999). Nanotechnology has indeed brought transformative changes to various disciplines, with medicine being one of the most significantly impacted through the advent of nanomedicine. By harnessing the unique properties of materials at the nanoscale, researchers and medical professionals can develop innovative devices and dosage forms designed for a wide range of healthcare applications. Nanomedicine effectively bridges the gap between nanotechnology and medicine, providing groundbreaking solutions to numerous healthcare challenges. The applications of nanomedicine are vast, offering unprecedented opportunities for advancements in diagnostics, treatment, and overall patient care. Contribution of nanomedicine extends across different healthcare sectors, demonstrating its pivotal role in the future of medical technology (Figure 1).

Nanomedicine is a rapidly evolving field that leverages nanotechnology to develop nanocarriers—structures designed to encapsulate and deliver therapeutic agents such as drugs or genetic materials to specific targets within the body. These nanocarriers are typically constructed from safe materials, including synthetic biodegradable polymers, lipids, polysaccharides, and other biocompatible substances. These materials are selected for their ability to safely transport therapeutic payloads while minimizing potential adverse effects on the body. In the context of herbal medicines, which often consist of complex mixtures of bioactive compounds derived from plants, nanotechnology offers exciting possibilities for enhancing therapeutic efficacy. The integration of nanotechnology into herbal biomedical research presents a promising avenue for improving drug delivery systems, addressing challenges associated with herbal medicines, and potentially enhancing their therapeutic efficacy while minimizing side effects.

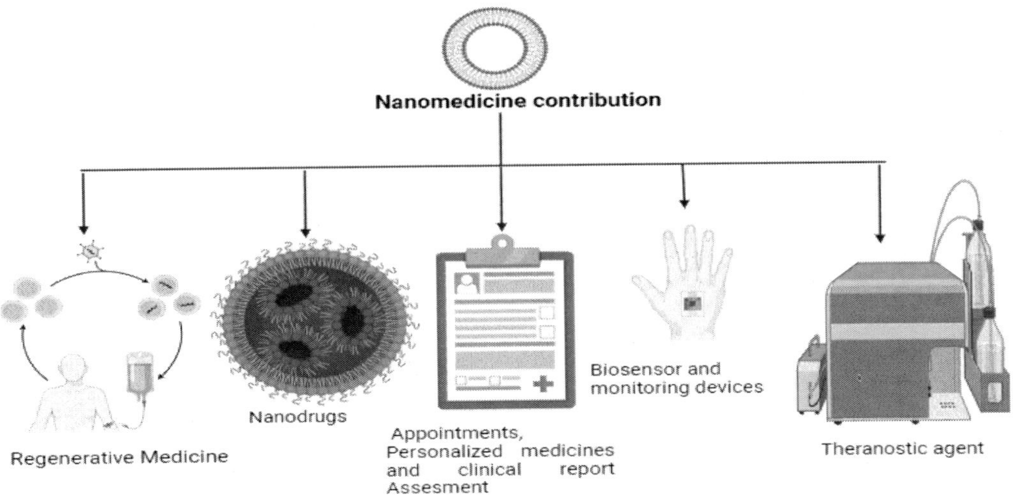

Figure 1. Contribution of nanomedicine in different healthcare sectors.

Herbal nanoparticles, which contain plant extracts or active isolates, are particularly promising because they may offer the same pharmacological potential as conventional drugs but with fewer side effects (Mamillapalli, 2016). Nanoparticles nanoparticles can be engineered to achieve specific characteristics, such as isolation, design, particle size, and morphology, to enhance the delivery of herbal medicines to specific body sites. This targeted approach aims to maximize therapeutic efficacy while reducing potential side effects. For instance, nanoparticulate systems can be used to direct herbal medications to specific organs like the kidneys, lungs, gastrointestinal system, and brain, thereby reducing dosage requirements and administration frequency. Nanoparticulate systems can also improve the delivery of hydrophobic or poorly water-soluble herbal molecules, overcoming limitations such as low bioavailability and increased systemic clearance (Lu et al., 2007; Vanduffel, 2001). However, despite these advantages, there are some limitations to the use of natural medicines, especially in situations like acute or life-threatening conditions, where conventional medicine may be more effective. Additionally, the self-medication of herbal medicines carries risks, such as the potential for overdose in the absence of well-defined dosage guidelines, the risk of toxicity due to incorrect plant identification, or improper preparation techniques. Moreover, the lack of stringent regulation of herbal medicines may lead to issues like adulteration, low-quality plant material, and inconsistent standards between batches and manufacturers (Munjal et al., 2023). The promising potential of herbal medicines observed *in vitro* does not always translate into successful therapeutic applications *in vivo*, primarily due to the low or unclear bioavailability of active phytochemical ingredients. Novel drug delivery techniques, including the use of nanoparticles, may provide solutions to these limitations by enhancing the effective and efficient delivery of these medications to targeted tissues and body systems. Nanoparticles offer unique physicochemical characteristics, such as high reactivity, a large surface area to mass ratio, a functionalizable structure, and an ultrasmall, programmable size. These features can enhance pharmacokinetic properties like solubility and bioavailability, as well as pharmacodynamic effects, and improve the physical and chemical stability of herbal medicines, potentially reducing the side effects associated with conventional medications (Nalini et al., 2017; Satyavert et al., 2021). The development of nanophytomedicines involves a variety of methods, such as solvent emulsification-diffusion, salting out, complex coacervation, co-precipitation, supercritical fluid technology, nanoprecipitation, and self-assembly processes, with solvent-based methods being among the most commonly used. A comprehensive safety assessment of novel topical herbal nanoformulations is crucial, considering potential toxicities related to both the herbal medication and components of the nanosystem. Additionally, the nanoparticles, alongside the herbal medications, may enter the bloodstream, potentially generating free radicals or causing unexpected interactions with immune system cells, posing further safety challenges (Tapadiya, 2017).

Safety Consideration in Nanophytoherbals Therapeutics

Nanophytoherbal therapeutics, which integrates nanotechnology with herbal medicine, presents a promising approach to enhance drug delivery and improve therapeutic outcomes. However, as with any emerging field, it comes with its own set of safety considerations that must be carefully addressed to ensure safe and effective use (Osman, 2019).

Toxicity of Nanoparticles

The toxicity of nanoparticles in nanophytoherbal formulations is a critical concern that necessitates thorough evaluation to ensure the safety of these innovative therapies. Nanoparticles, owing to their extremely small size and unique physicochemical properties, can pose significant risks that require careful consideration. One of the primary concerns is the increased surface area of nanoparticles, which, while beneficial for enhancing drug delivery, can also elevate their reactivity, potentially leading to heightened toxicity. The size-dependent cellular uptake of nanoparticles is another crucial factor, as it can influence cellular functions and contribute to adverse effects. Surface charge and coating stability are also pivotal, as they determine how nanoparticles interact with cells, impacting their potential toxicity (Oberdo, 2009). On a biological level, nanoparticles may provoke inflammatory responses and immunotoxic effects, potentially leading to oxidative stress and cellular damage (Holsapple et al., 2005). Furthermore, concerns about genotoxicity, mutagenicity, and the potential for long-term accumulation of nanoparticles in organs underscore the need for comprehensive *in vitro* and *in vivo* studies to fully assess these risks. Ethical considerations also play a significant role in the responsible development of nanophytoherbal formulations. Issues, such as informed consent, transparency about the components of nanoparticles, and the potential risks associated with their use, are integral to ensuring that research and development are conducted ethically (Kanwal et al., 2019). In conclusion, understanding and mitigating the toxicity of nanoparticles in nanophytoherbals requires a multifaceted approach. This approach should encompass dose-dependent effects, the biodegradability of nanoparticles, and strict adherence to regulatory standards to ensure that nanotechnology is safely integrated into herbal medicine formulations (Mukherjee et al., 2015). Toxicity assessments of nanoparticles are critical in ensuring their safe application, especially in nanophytoherbal formulations. Researchers typically employ both *in vitro* and *in vivo* models to evaluate the potential adverse effects of nanoparticles, carefully analyzing how these particles interact with biological systems before they can be considered for clinical studies or applications. These studies consider various factors such as size, surface charge, coating stability, and cellular uptake to understand their impact on cellular functions and overall toxicity. Regular updates and advancements in nanoparticle safety research are essential, as they contribute to ongoing efforts to understand and mitigate potential risks associated with nanoparticle use. These continuous evaluations help refine safety protocols, ensuring that new findings are integrated into safety assessments. Figure 2 illustrates the mechanisms by which the overuse of nanophytoherbals may induce cellular toxicity.

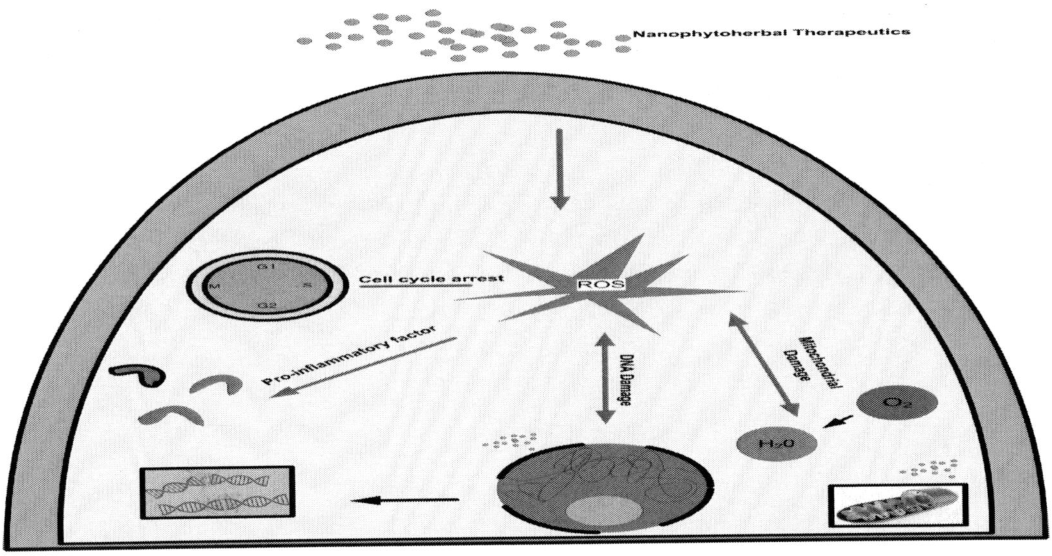

Figure 2. Mechanism of cell toxicity due to nanophytoherbal therapeutics.

Biodegradability and Biodistribution

Evaluating the biodegradability of nanoparticles is essential to prevent their accumulation in the body over time. The choice of materials for nanoparticles greatly influences their biodegradability, with natural materials often offering superior biocompatibility and biodegradability compared to synthetic alternatives. Modifying the nanoparticle surface, such as by functionalizing them with biodegradable polymers or coatings, can enhance their breakdown in biological environments. Some nanoparticles are designed to respond to specific enzymes within biological systems, allowing for targeted degradation and release of payloads, such as herbal compounds, at designated sites. Ideally, biodegradable nanoparticles should be metabolized into non-toxic byproducts that are efficiently cleared from the body via normal metabolic pathways, thereby reducing the risk of accumulation. It is also important to consider the environmental impact of nanoparticle degradation, ensuring that degradation products are environmentally benign (Rudrapal et al., 2022; Munjal et al., 2020). Additionally, studying the biodistribution of nanophytoherbal formulations is crucial to understand how and where nanoparticles are distributed within the body. Nanoparticle size, surface charge, and coating influence their interactions with biological entities and their distribution in the body. Biodistribution studies help determine the extent of nanoparticle accumulation in target organs or tissues, with targeted delivery systems aiming to enhance nanoparticle concentration at specific sites for improved therapeutic outcomes (Ray et al., 2023). Understanding whether nanoparticles can cross physiological barriers, like the blood-brain barrier (BBB), is crucial, as engineered nanoparticles with improved permeability can enable drug delivery to specific anatomical sites. Various imaging techniques, such as fluorescence microscopy, MRI, or radiolabeling, can be employed to track and visualize nanoparticle biodistribution in preclinical and clinical studies. The route of administration significantly affects biodistribution, and longitudinal studies are important for understanding how nanoparticle distribution evolves over time.

Interaction with Biological System

Understanding how nanoparticles interact with biological systems is crucial for developing various applications, including drug delivery systems like those used in nanophytoherbal therapeutics. These interactions can significantly influence the safety, efficacy, and overall performance of nanoparticles. Key aspects include the mechanism of cellular uptake, where nanoparticles often enter cells through endocytosis—either clathrin-mediated or caveolae-mediated—which affects the efficiency and rate of uptake. Factors such as nanoparticle size, shape, and surface properties also influence cellular penetration, with smaller nanoparticles often entering cells more effectively. Once inside, nanoparticles may localize in specific cellular compartments, such as endosomes or lysosomes; designing nanoparticles to escape these compartments or target particular organelles can enhance therapeutic effectiveness. Nanoparticles can trigger inflammatory responses and oxidative stress, potentially leading to cell damage, making it important to understand and mitigate these effects (Nagarajan et al., 2014). They should also be evaluated for blood compatibility to avoid adverse effects like haemolysis or coagulation, with surface modifications often employed to improve this compatibility (Lim et al., 2022). Additionally, when nanoparticles are exposed to biological fluids, proteins adsorb onto their surface, forming a protein corona that can influence their behavior and interactions with cells. Nanoparticles may be phagocytosed by macrophages, which affects their clearance from the body, and surface modifications can alter these interactions. Furthermore, nanoparticles can modulate immune responses, and understanding their impact on the immune system is crucial for predicting potential immunotoxicity. For drug delivery, overcoming physiological barriers such as BBB is essential, and some nanoparticles are specifically designed to penetrate these barriers for targeted delivery to specific tissues.

Immunogenicity and Allergic Reactions

Examining the immunogenicity of nanophytoherbal formulations is essential to ensure they do not provoke adverse immune responses. Immunogenicity refers to the potential of nanoparticles or herbal extracts, or their combination, to elicit an immune response, which could lead to allergic reactions or other immune-related issues. Several factors influence immunogenicity, including particle size, shape, surface properties, dosage, and administration route. Preclinical studies are crucial for assessing immunotoxicity by evaluating the impact of these formulations on immune cells and overall immune system function. Allergic reactions may arise from either the nanoparticles or the herbal components, necessitating testing for allergenicity using both *in vitro* and *in vivo* models. Standard allergy testing methods, such as skin patch tests, may be adapted for these formulations. Regulatory agencies mandate comprehensive safety assessments, including immunogenicity and allergy studies, before approving nanophytoherbal therapeutics for clinical use. These assessments are vital for understanding and ensuring the overall safety profile of these innovative therapeutics (Gomes et al., 2014).

Quality and Standardization of Herbal Extracts

The integration of nanotechnology with herbal medicine necessitates rigorous control over the herbal component to ensure consistency, efficacy, and safety. Proper identification of the plant species is crucial, as incorrect identification can lead to variations in therapeutic compounds and potential safety issues. Additionally, different plant parts may contain varying concentrations of active compounds, making it essential to standardize the extraction process to a specific plant part to ensure consistency in the formulation. Furthermore, the extraction techniques used must be standardized to guarantee reproducibility and consistency in the composition of the herbal extract, ensuring that the final nanophytoherbal product is both effective and safe.

Regulatory Compliance

Regulatory compliance is crucial for the development, production, and marketing of nanophytoherbals, ensuring that these products are safe, effective, and consistent. Key considerations include referencing established pharmacopoeial standards, such as those from USP and EP, to ensure compliance with recognized quality benchmarks for pharmaceuticals. Comprehensive preclinical and clinical studies are necessary to demonstrate the safety and efficacy of nanophytoherbals, which is essential for regulatory submissions (Mukherjee 2015). The preparation and submission of regulatory dossiers, which should include detailed information on the product's composition, manufacturing process, and safety and efficacy data, are required. Aligning with international standards and guidelines helps promote consistency and facilitates global market acceptance.

Ethical Considerations

In the development and application of nanophytoherbal therapeutics, ethical considerations are essential to ensure responsible research conduct, participant protection, and adherence to ethical medical practices. Key ethical aspects include: (i) providing participants with clear and comprehensive information about the nature, purpose, potential risks, and benefits of the research (Asmatulu et al., 2013); (ii) obtaining informed consent voluntarily, without coercion, and ensuring participants have the right to withdraw from the study at any time; (iii) ensuring scientific validity by designing studies that produce meaningful and valid data; (iv) disseminating results ethically with accurate and transparent reporting; (v) safeguarding participant privacy by handling personal information confidentially; and (vi) engaging in educational outreach to inform the public about nanophytoherbal therapeutics, their benefits, and the ethical considerations involved (Chakrapany and Chandan 2014).

Environmental Impact

The environmental impact of nanophytoherbal therapeutics involves evaluating the potential effects on ecosystems, natural resources, and overall sustainability associated with their development, production, and use (Liu 2015). Key considerations include: (i) understanding nanoparticle behavior in the environment, including their persistence, degradation, and potential transformation into other forms; (ii) investigating the impact of nanoparticles on soil microorganisms, which are crucial for ecological balance; (iii) considering implications for agricultural ecosystems if nanophytoherbal products are used in crop production; (iv) assessing the release of nanoparticles into the air during production and use; (v) implementing proper disposal methods for nanomaterial-containing waste to prevent environmental contamination; and (vi) exploring green synthesis methods that use eco-friendly materials and reduce hazardous substances (Howard 2015).

Scaling Up Production

Scaling up the production of nanophytoherbal therapeutics presents new safety challenges that must be carefully managed. To address potential occupational exposure to nanoparticles, it is essential to implement robust safety measures, including the use of personal protective equipment (PPE) and effective containment systems. Developing and adhering to safe handling procedures is crucial, alongside providing comprehensive training and education for personnel on proper handling, storage, and disposal of nanomaterials. Rigorous quality control measures should be maintained to ensure consistency and quality across different production scales. Advanced characterization techniques must be employed to monitor the physicochemical properties of nanoparticles, ensuring they meet safety and efficacy standards. Additionally, safe and environmentally friendly disposal methods should be developed for waste generated during production, including unused materials and by-products. Engaging with the local community to inform them about safety measures, emergency response plans, and the facility's safety commitment is also important (Bonifacio 2014).

Monitoring and Surveillance

Monitoring and surveillance of nanophytoherbal therapeutics involve systematic efforts to ensure safety, efficacy, and compliance with ethical and regulatory standards throughout their lifecycle. This includes regular health monitoring of personnel involved in production, handling, and administration to detect any potential health effects. Continuous monitoring of air and water quality around production facilities is crucial to identify and mitigate the release of nanoparticles into the environment (Sachan and Gupta, 2015). Patients in clinical trials or receiving these therapeutics require ongoing monitoring to evaluate safety, efficacy, and adverse reactions, with long-term follow-up studies essential for tracking health post-treatment. Ethics committees must oversee research to ensure ethical conduct, reviewing informed consent processes and documentation regularly. Additionally, conducting surveys and engaging with the local community to gather feedback on perceptions, concerns, and observed impacts is vital, alongside establishing open communication channels to address queries and provide information on safety measures (Javed, 2019).

Regulatory Considerations in Nanophytoherbal Therapeutics

Biological products derived from natural resources and non-biological medical products, which are synthesized, are both subjected to rigorous evaluation for safety, efficacy, bioequivalence, and therapeutic equivalence before market entry. Various countries have specific guidelines and regulatory controls for these products. WHO has established guidelines to aid in formulating national policies on traditional medicine, focusing on examining their potential usefulness, including safety and efficacy (WHO, Geneva, 1996). In India, the Drug and Cosmetics Act of 1940 governs traditional medicine, with implementation overseen by state governments. India, as a rich source of herbs, adheres to the standards outlined in the Indian National Health Policy, which emphasizes the need for proper standardization of drugs (Srikumar, 2006). The Department of AYUSH, Government of India, has introduced a central scheme for developing standard operating procedures and pharmacopoeial standards for Ayurvedic preparations (Kalaiselvan, 2010). However, regulations for herbal drug products in Europe and the United States are more stringent compared to those in India (Singh, 2011).

Pharmacovigilance of Herbal Medicine

The need for a robust safety monitoring system for herbal medicines is growing, as highlighted by Asiri (2008). Despite some reports of adverse drug reactions, ginseng is an example of a safe herbal product that is in high demand. However, this level of safety is not universally applicable to all herbal products. Therefore, pharmacovigilance is crucial to ensure the safety of herbal drugs for human health (Barnes, 2003). To achieve global harmonization, WHO has established specific guidelines addressing the safety, efficacy, and quality of herbal medicines. The Medicines and Healthcare Products Regulatory Agency in the UK has introduced the "yellow card" scheme to monitor the safety of herbal medicines. Globally, medicinal herbs are recognized as valuable therapeutic aids not only for treating diseases but also for maintaining overall health (Atmakuri, 2010).

Conclusion

The role of nanophytoherbals in pharmaceutical sciences and research has become increasingly significant. This book chapter underscores the importance of safety and regulatory considerations in the development and application of nanophytoherbals. Medicinal plants and their derived products are defined and regulated differently across countries, leading to varied approaches for licensing, dispensing, manufacturing, and marketing. To ensure the safety, quality, and efficacy of herbal products, adherence to WHO guidelines is crucial. Advances in analytical techniques, such as high-technology-oriented hyphenated methods, play a pivotal role in setting quality standards and specifications. These advancements enable manufacturers to obtain marketing approval from regulatory authorities, ensuring the therapeutic efficacy, safety, and shelf life of herbal drugs, thus benefiting the entire pharmaceutical industry.

References

Asiri, Y., Al-Dhawailie, A., Alqasoumi, S., Al-Yahya, M., & Rafatullah, S. (2008). Pharmacovigilance in herbal medicine: A paradigm to drug toxicity monitoring in conventional health care. *Hungarian medical journal 2*(3), 351-363.

Asmatulu, R., Zhang, B., & Asmatulu, E. (2013). Safety and ethics of nanotechnology. In *Nanotechnology safety* (pp. 31-41). Elsevier.

Atmakuri, L. R., & Dathi, S. (2010). Current trends in herbal medicines. *Journal of Pharmaceutical Research*, 3(1), 109-113.

Barnes, J. (2003). Pharmacovigilance of herbal medicines: A UK perspective. *Drug Safety*, 26(12), 829-851.

Bonifácio, B. V., Silva, P. B., Ramos, M. A., Negri, K. M., Bauab, T. M., & Chorilli, M. (2014). Nanotechnology-based drug delivery systems and herbal medicines: a review. *International Journal of Nanomedicine*, 9, 1–15.

Chakrapany, S., & Chandan, S. (2014). Nano carriers of novel drug delivery system for "Ayurveda Herbal Remedies" need of hour–A bird's eye view. *American Journal of PharmTech Research, 4*(2), 60-69.

Deepak Yadav, D. Y., SuruchiSuri, S. S., Choudhary, A. A., MohdSikender, M. S., Hemant, H., Beg, M. N., V. Garg V. G, Atlaf Ahmad A. A. & MohdAsif, M. A. (2011). Novel approach: herbal remedies and natural products in pharmaceutical science as nano drug delivery systems, *International Journal of Pharmacy and Technology,* 3(3), 3092-3116.

Gibson, J. M., Osman, K. K., Conroy-Ben, O., & Giang, A. (2023). Environmental Science for the Betterment of All. *Environmental Science & Technology, 57*(36), 13267-13269.

Gomes, A., Ghosh, S., Sengupta, J., Datta, P., & Gomes, A. (2014). Herbonanoceuticals: a new step towards herbal therapeutics. *Medicinal and Aromatic Plants, 3*(3), 162.

Holsapple, M. P., Farland, W. H., Landry, T. D., Monteiro-Riviere, N. A., Carter, J. M., Walker, N. J., & Thomas, K. V. (2005). Research strategies for safety evaluation of nanomaterials, Part II: Toxicological and safety evaluation of nanomaterials, current challenges and data needs. *Toxicological Sciences*, 88(1), 12–17.

Howard, J. (2015). Current occupational health and safety concerns. *Working Safety with Nanotechnology* OHS_HS240(no. m), 1–21.

Kalaiselvan, V., Shah, A. K., Patel, F. B., Shah, C. N., Kalaivani, M., & Rajasekaran, A. (2010). Quality assessment of different marketed brands of Dasamoolaristam, an Ayurvedic formulation. *International Journal of Ayurveda Research*, 1(1), 10.

Kanwal, Z., Raza, M. A., Manzoor, F., Riaz, S., Jabeen, G., Fatima, S., & Naseem, S. (2019). A comparative assessment of nanotoxicity induced by metal (silver, nickel) and metal oxide (cobalt, chromium) nanoparticles in Labeorohita. *Nanomaterials*, 9(2), 309.

Lim, C. L., Raju, C. S., Mahboob, T., Kayesth, S., Gupta, K. K., Jain, G. K., Dhobi, M., Nawaz, M., Wilairatana, P., & Nissapatorn, V. (2022). Precision and advanced nano-phytopharmaceuticals for therapeutic applications. *Nanomaterials*, 12(2), 238.

Liu, C.-X. (2015). Nanotechnology challenge: Safety of nanomaterials and nanomedicines. *Asian Journal of Pharmacodynamics and Pharmacokinetics*, 7(6), 17–31.

Lu, J., Liong, M., Sherman, S., Xia, T., Kovochich, M., Nel, A. E., Zink, J. I., & Tamanoi, F. (2007). Mesoporous silica nanoparticles for cancer therapy: Energy-dependent cellular uptake and delivery of paclitaxel to cancer cells. *Nanobiotechnology*, 3, 89-95.

Malik, J., Munjal, K., & Deshmukh, R. (2015). Attenuating effect of standardized lyophilized Cinnamomum zeylanicum bark extract against streptozotocin-induced experimental dementia of Alzheimer's type. *Journal of Basic and Clinical Physiology and Pharmacology*, 26(3), 275-285.

Mamillapalli, V. (2016). Nanoparticles for herbal extracts. *Asian Journal of Pharmaceutics*, 10(2), S54-S60.

Mukherjee, P. K., Bahadur, S., Chaudhary, S. K., Kar, A., & Mukherjee, K. (2015). Quality related safety issue-evidence-based validation of herbal medicine farm to pharma. In *Evidence-based validation of herbal medicine* (pp. 1-28). Elsevier.

Munjal, K., Ahmad, S., Gupta, A., Haye, A., Amin, S., & Mir, S. R. (2020). Polyphenol-enriched fraction and the compounds isolated from Garcinia indica fruits ameliorate obesity through suppression of digestive enzymes and oxidative stress. *Pharmacognosy Magazine*, 16(70), S236–S245.

Munjal, K., Gautam, V. K., Goel, Y., Ahamad, J., & Mir, S. R. (2023). Qualitative diagnostic features of alkaloidal spices. In *Analysis of Food Spices* (pp. 135–150). CRC Press.

Nalini, M., Lena, M., Sumathi, P., & Sundaravadivelan, C. (2017). Effect of phyto-synthesized silver nanoparticles on developmental stages of malaria vector, Anopheles stephensi and dengue vector, Aedes aegypti. *Egyptian Journal of Basic and Applied Sciences*, 4(3), 212–218.

Oberdörster, G. (2010). Safety assessment for nanotechnology and nanomedicine: Concepts of nanotoxicology. *Journal of Internal Medicine*, 267(1), 89–105.

Osman, E. M. (2019). Environmental and health safety considerations of nanotechnology. Biomedical *Journal of Scientific & Technical Research*, 19(4), 14501–14515.

Pandey, M. M., Rastogi, S., & Rawat, A. K. S. (2013). Indian traditional Ayurvedic system of medicine and nutritional supplementation. *Evidence-Based Complementary and Alternative Medicine*, 2013, 376327.

Patel, D. K., Kumar, R., Laloo, D., & Hemalatha, S. (2012). Natural medicines from plant sources used for therapy of diabetes mellitus: An overview of its pharmacological aspects. *Asian Pacific Journal of Tropical Disease*, 2(3), 239–250.

Ray, M. K., Mishra, A. K., Mohanta, Y. K., Mahanta, S., Chakrabartty, I., Kungwani, N. A., Panda, S. K., & Pudake, R. N. (2023). Nanotechnology as a promising tool against phytopathogens: A futuristic approach to agriculture. *Agriculture*, 13(9), 1856.

Sachan, A. K., & Gupta, A. (2015). A review on nanotized herbal drugs. *International Journal of Pharmaceutical Sciences and Research*, 6(3), 961.

Satyavert, Gupta, S., Choudhury, H., Jacob, S., Nair, A. B., Dhanawat, M., & Munjal, K. (2021). Pharmacokinetics and tissue distribution of hydrazinocurcumin in rats. *Pharmacological Reports*, 73(6), 1734–1743.

Shrikumar, S., Maheshwari, U., Sughanti, A., & Ravi, T. K. (2006). WHO guidelines for standardization of herbal drugs. *Pharminfo.net*, 2, 78–81.

Singh, A., Sharan, V. A., Kharab, V., & Bhandari, A. (2011). Current status on regulation of herbal medicine in Europe, United States, and India. *Journal of NaturaConscientia*, 2(3), 406–422.

Sungthongjeen, S., Pitaksuteepong, T., Somsiri, A., & Sriamornsak, P. (1999). Studies on pectins as potential hydrogel matrices for controlled-release drug delivery. *Drug Development and Industrial Pharmacy*, 25(12), 1271–1276.

Tapadiya, G. G. (2017). Impact of nanotechnology on global trade of herbal drugs: An overview. *International Journal of Green Pharmacy*, 11(03), S371-S376.

Vanduffel, W., Fize, D., Mandeville, J. B., Nelissen, K., Van Hecke, P., Rosen, B. R., Tootell, R. B., & Orban, G. A. (2001). Visual motion processing investigated using contrast agent-enhanced fMRI in awake behaving monkeys. *Neuron*, 32(4), 565–577.

World Health Organization. (1998). *Quality Control Methods for Medicinal Plant Materials*. World Health Organization.

Chapter 22

Safety and Regulatory Considerations in Nanophytoherbal Therapeutics: A Global Perspective on Preclinical and Clinical Evaluations

Abhinav Singhal*
and Vishnu Mittal
Guru Gobind Singh College of Pharmacy, Yamunanagar, Haryana, India

Abstract

This chapter focuses on conducting an in-depth analysis of the safety considerations associated with nanophytoherbal therapeutics, encompassing both preclinical and clinical aspects. The exploration extends to the regulatory landscape governing the development and commercialization of nanophytoherbal products, with particular emphasis on global perspectives and variations. The primary objectives of this study include evaluating the safety profiles of nanophytoherbal formulations through preclinical models, scrutinizing existing regulatory frameworks and guidelines relevant to nanophytoherbal therapeutics, proposing recommendations for standardizing safety assessments in nanophytoherbal research, and elucidating the implications of safety findings on the regulatory approval process. The methodology employs a systematic review of existing literature, incorporating data from preclinical studies, clinical trials, and regulatory documents. Comparative analyses are conducted to identify commonalities and variations in safety assessments across different nanophytoherbal formulations. The results highlight the diverse safety profiles among nanophytoherbals, emphasizing the need for standardized evaluation methods. Regulatory analyses reveal the dynamic nature of guidelines across regions, necessitating a nuanced approach to compliance. The key findings of the study propose directions for potential improvements in current safety assessment protocols, providing a basis for enhancing the overall quality and reliability of nanophytoherbal therapeutics. In conclusion, the research underscores the importance of standardized safety assessments to ensure the reliability of research outcomes and contributes to regulatory harmonization. The implications extend to both the scientific community and regulatory bodies, promoting a safer and more streamlined development process for nanophytoherbal therapeutics.

* Corresponding Author's Email: abhinavsinghal41@gmail.com.

In: Phyto-Nanomedicine
Editors: Hitesh Chopra, Vinod Kumar Gauttam, Ajmer Singh Grewal et al.
ISBN: 979-8-89530-317-7

Keywords: nanophytoherbals, safety, regulatory considerations, preclinical assessment, standardization, global perspectives

Abbreviations

FDA	Food and Drug Administration
DNA	Deoxyribonucleic acid
EU	European Union
EMEA	European Medicines Agency
ALL	Acute lymphoblastic leukemia
R&D	Research & Development
TCM	Traditional Chinese Medicine

Introduction

Encasing vital ingredients from medicinal plants to treat ailments like diabetes and cancer is known as "nanophytomedicine," a rapidly developing field in medicine. Identifying potentially active ingredients and encapsulating them is essential for treating illnesses without major negative impacts. With the advent of nanophytomedicine, medicinal compounds that were previously insoluble in various combinatorial drug formulations have become more bioavailable. Research indicates that phyto-bioactive substances offer enhanced benefits in the treatment of several diseases (Cheng & Zhen, 2004). However, their low concentrations often limit bioavailability, stability, and dissolution at specific brain regions due to the blood–brain barrier, as demonstrated by *in vivo* studies. Controlled-size nanomedicine, ranging from 1 to 100 nm, has been employed to circumvent these challenges. Nanotechnology presents a promising solution to the limitations of conventional herbal remedies, and advancements in nanophytomedicine have made significant strides in the treatment of various diseases. This approach addresses biopharmaceutical challenges inherent in herbal medicine, making it a reliable and safer alternative to synthetic drugs (Newman et al., 2007). Galen, a Greek pharmacist who lived from 129 to 200 AD, was the first to recognize the medicinal potential of herbal therapy. Natural products are essential in the search for lead compounds that can be used to treat a variety of illnesses; in fact, natural products serve as the source of 60% of the pharmaceuticals currently on the market. Furthermore, phytodrugs provide primary healthcare to 80% of the population in Asian and African nations. The use of phytomedicines has increased due to their high efficacy and lower side effects compared to allopathic treatments (Anagnostaki et al., 2012). Despite their benefits, the use of phytomedicines in treating and preventing various diseases is limited due to low bioavailability and poor solubility in water. To overcome these challenges, the field of material nanoscience has developed nanophytomedicine, which addresses issues of toxicity, solubility, degradation, absorption, and biological responses associated with phytomedicine. Nanophytomedicines are typically prepared from standardized extracts or active phytoconstituents, exhibiting improved biological and therapeutic activities compared to their traditional counterparts. Recent developments in nanotechnology illustrate significant growth in this field, with increasing R&D expenditures worldwide (Newman, 2008).

Nanotechnology finds extensive applications across various industries, including communication, information technology, electronics, telecommunications, medicine, and the food business. However, while nanotechnology presents opportunities for human advancement, it also poses serious risks to the environment, human health, and life. As a relatively new topic, the effects of nanomaterials on the human body and the environment remain poorly understood (Khare, 2004). Due to their rapid membrane penetration, nanomaterials can enhance the biological activity of loaded pharmaceuticals and elicit reactions from large molecular weight biological macromolecules, such as DNA, miRNAs, and proteins. Consequently, nanoparticles may pose hazards to humans and animals due to their toxic qualities. The lack of oversight in nanotechnology complicates monitoring the presence and impacts of nanoparticles and nanomaterials in the environment (Rasonaivo et al., 2011). Currently, there is no sui generis law, despite the European Union's (EU) adoption of regulations regarding nanotechnology in 2004. Through EU legislation, the public is intended to benefit from cutting-edge nanotechnology while ensuring privacy, health, and environmental protection. Historically, plants have been recognized and utilized as herbal medicinal products for sustenance and illness treatment in many cultures. Scientific advancements have transformed drug availability, increasing the strength of active ingredients and enabling the reinstatement of compounds previously excluded due to formulation failures (Javed et al., 2019; Javed et al., 2018). The pharmaceutical industry has shown growing interest in nanotechnological advancements for their potential to create novel formulations that were previously unattainable regarding multiple active constituent aspects and modified release schemes. While many treatments benefit from breakthroughs in nanotechnology, it is essential to acknowledge certain disadvantages, including exorbitant costs and scalability issues. Inhaling simple nanoparticles could result in serious lung conditions and other illnesses that disrupt homeostasis or even cause death (Ghosh et al., 2013).

Phytomedicine Historical Perspective

Around 60,000 years ago, plants and plant components were utilized as medicines, according to reports from ancient Babylon. Evidence of phytomedicine dates back approximately 5,000 years in Egypt and China, while records from Asia Minor and Greece trace back nearly 2,500 years. A wide range of techniques, ideologies, herbal therapeutic systems, and herbal-based practices has been documented, each significantly influenced by the geographical region in which it originated. In China, herbal remedies have evolved from Sheng-Nong's Herbal Book, published around 3000 B.C., to a present-day list of 11,146 species of plants and herbs used in Traditional Chinese Medicine (Rajendran et al., 2013). Additionally, "The Divine Farmer's Classic of Herbalism," compiled in China about 2,000 years ago, is the oldest known book on herbal medicine. This work, along with various compiled evidence and statistics on herbs and plants, has led to the production of numerous monographs on specific herbs and herbal pharmacopoeias. In the first century A.D., Dioscorides authored "De Materia Medica," an influential list of phytomedicines (Alam et al., 2017). During the Middle Ages, Catholic monks preserved the knowledge of ancient phytomedicine, even as general practitioners operated outside established frameworks. Western herbal medicine was further influenced by the research and practices of Arab physicians in the eighth century A.D., who conducted extensive studies on therapeutic herbs from Europe, India, Persia, and the Far East. Until the nineteenth century, medicinal plants remained the primary source of substances necessary for maintaining health. Ayurveda, an authentic Indian traditional medical system developed by ancient Hindu physicians and saints, has been practiced for over 5,000 years in various parts of India and its neighboring regions (Hasnain et al., 2019). Its associated compilation, materia medica, offers a comprehensive description of over 10,000 formulas and 1,500 plants. Recognized by the Indian government as a holistic healthcare system that complements Western medical techniques, Ayurveda continues to thrive. Moreover, around 148 formulas of Kampo medicine, a Japanese herbal remedy with roots extending back 1,500 years, have also been documented (Sharma et al., 2019).

Regulatory Concerns and Ethical Questions in Nanophytomedicine

Similar ethical criteria should be applied to clinical research involving nanophytomedicines, in accordance with national and international ethical regulations and guidelines for product development. The methodology and research strategy must adhere to established ethical standards. All ethical concerns should be thoroughly discussed, identified, and addressed in line with these standards, particularly those relevant to the nature and implications of nanophytomedicine. Despite advancements in nanotechnology research and the significant marketing of this field, numerous ethical issues remain to be addressed. Many of these dilemmas are analogous to those faced by most emerging technologies. Furthermore, ethical questions concerning the development of phytomedicine have arisen even before the technology itself has been fully realized (Mishra et al., 2019). This ongoing dialogue emphasizes the profound impact these issues have on individuals' daily lives. At times, scientific advancements can outpace ethical considerations, leading to situations where ethical confusion arises. The interplay between ethical and regulatory perspectives is crucial in medical practice, and this is equally true for nanophytomedicine. The FDA is currently working on clear regulations that will apply to biotechnological products. Addressing every ethical dilemma associated with emerging technologies, such as nanophytomedicine, is a complex task; however, it would be beneficial to proactively resolve many of these issues. Common ethical concerns related to nanophytomedicines include particle size, impacts on human health, environmental safety, unforeseen side effects, and potential harm from their use. In response, universities in the U.S. have received federal funding to study the ethical, legal, and societal challenges associated with the use of nanotechnology (Dorocki et al., 2015; Potto et al., 2019).

Effects of Nanophytomedicines on Society

Historically, the introduction of any new scientific technique has been accompanied by ethical dilemmas, particularly concerning containment and control. Technologies with significant influence are expected to give rise to even more ethical quandaries. Nanophytomedicines, due to their multidisciplinary nature and ability to treat a wide range of illnesses, have the potential to impact society profoundly. The unique properties of small-sized active ingredients in phytomedicine offer numerous advantages; however, these same properties can also present specific challenges. The minuscule size of nanoparticles makes them difficult to remove using existing filtration methods, which hampers the effective distribution of the untapped potential of nanophytomedicine. Additionally, these tiny particles are undetectable to the human eye, raising critical questions about their containment (Nigar et al., 2016; Potto et al., 2019). Public caution persists, especially in light of recent environmental disasters such as Love Canal and Three Mile Island, which underscore the importance of these outstanding concerns in nanophytomedicine. Workers involved in the manufacturing of nanophytomedicines face the risk of exposure through skin penetration, inhalation, or ingestion, potentially leading to increased exposure levels. Unpredictably toxic, nanoparticles may pose greater risks than their larger counterparts (Potto et al., 2019).

Ethics in Nanophytomedicine

Nanobiotechnology, like other emerging technologies, is subject to ethical scrutiny, though it has not introduced entirely new ethical concerns. As this technology develops and is applied in medicine, it is crucial to address both the tangible and abstract issues it raises to mitigate potential negative impacts on the environment and human health, and to prevent public dissent. Challenges in nanomedicine include interpreting ethical constraints as part of a fair risk assessment and addressing the complex issues that arise from the interplay of technology and human nature (Ferreira et al., 2010). In 2006, the National Science Foundation supported the Nanoethics Group at Cal Poly State University to explore the moral implications of nanotechnology, particularly concerning enhancements such as hormone therapy or cosmetic surgery, as well as the potential creation of sophisticated cybernetic organs or brain implants, which pose significant ethical dilemmas (Phillopson, 2001). In 2007, the Nanoethics Group published several articles addressing a wide range of issues, including the benefits and risks of nanotechnology, its environmental and human health impacts, and ethical concerns related to human enhancement, privacy, and potential future developments such as space travel and extended life expectancy (Mainardes et al., 2006). Current ethical concerns in nanomedicine involve assessing the risks of nanomaterials, differentiating between germline and somatic cell therapies, investigating the enhancement of human capabilities, managing the adverse effects of engineered nanomaterials, and understanding the toxicity of nanoparticles. For example, researchers are studying the in vitro toxicity of various nanoparticles using cell lines that mimic spermatogonial stem cells to assess their impact on human germline stem cells (Grill et al., 2009).

Regulatory Aspects of Nanotechnology-Based Phytomedicines

Given the nascent stage of nanobiotechnology, it is not surprising that legal uncertainties abound. Currently, there is no specific legislation governing nanotechnology, raising concerns about potential future conflicts related to the safety of nanoparticles in healthcare, the environment, and the workplace. Therefore, adhering to existing regulations that govern medications and therapies is imperative. However, as nanotechnology introduces unprecedented challenges, establishing clear regulations is crucial. The primary goal should be to ensure human safety through comprehensive legislative measures (Chorilli, 2007). There is some apprehension that the European Union's REACH (Registration, Evaluation, Authorization, & Restriction of Chemicals) policy could be applied to nanotechnology, potentially shifting the burden of proof for safety from the government to manufacturers (Bonifacio et al., 2014). Recent publications have reviewed current and upcoming EU regulations on nanotechnology, providing a comparative analysis of regulatory frameworks in the US and EU. In response to advancements in nanotechnology-phytomedicines, the European Medicines Agency (EMEA) has broadened the scope of phytomedicines incorporating nanotechnology for human use (Barkat et al., 2019). Nanotechnology is a rapidly growing field with diverse applications and is expected to enhance illness detection and treatment. Both the EU and US have approved products using nanoparticles under existing regulatory systems. However, the FDA does not have a specific definition for nanotechnology and oversees a broad range of products, including foods, cosmetics, medications, electronics, and veterinary supplies, that may incorporate nanomaterials. Navigating the regulatory approval process for nanotechnology-based products can be challenging (Sofias et al., 2017; Bernabeu et al., 2017). To address these challenges, the FDA has established an internal task force on nanotechnology to develop regulatory strategies aimed at facilitating the development of novel, safe, and effective products incorporating nanotechnology materials. The fusion of traditional herbal treatments with nanotechnology has led to the creation of nanophytoherbs, presenting unique safety and regulatory issues (Harshita et al., 2019).

- *Toxicity:* Nanomaterials can exhibit different toxicological profiles compared to their bulk counterparts. Safety assessments must consider the potential toxicity of the nanomaterials used in the formulation and any interactions with the phytochemicals present in the herbal extracts.
- *Bioavailability:* Nanophytoherbs are designed to enhance the bioavailability and efficacy of herbal compounds by improving their solubility, stability, and targeted delivery. However, this increased bioavailability may lead to unintended side effects or interactions with other drugs (Kundu et al., 2012).
- *Regulatory Approval*: Regulatory agencies such as the FDA in the United States and the EMA in Europe have specific guidelines for approving nanomedicines. Nanophytoherbs may require additional safety and efficacy data compared to conventional herbal medicines or standalone nanomedicines.
- *Characterization:* Accurate characterization of nanophytoherbal formulations is essential to ensure their safety and efficacy. This includes assessing particle size, shape, surface charge, and stability, as well as understanding how these properties may change over time or under different conditions.
- *Quality Control*: Implementing quality control measures is vital to ensure the consistency and reproducibility of nanophytoherbal formulations. This involves standardized manufacturing processes, rigorous testing for contaminants or impurities, and batch-to-batch consistency (Li et al., 2012).
- *Labelling and Packaging:* Clear labeling of nanophytoherbal products is crucial to inform consumers about their composition, intended use, and potential risks or precautions. Special packaging may be required to ensure stability and prevent degradation of nanoparticles or herbal extracts.
- *Long-term Effects*: Long-term studies are needed to assess the safety of nanoparticles over extended periods of use, including the potential accumulation of nanoparticles in the body and any associated health risks (Shi et al., 2012).

- *Ethical Considerations*: Ethical issues related to the use of nanotechnology in traditional medicine, the potential exploitation of indigenous knowledge, and equitable access to nanophytoherbal therapies should also be addressed.
- *Safety and regulatory*: These considerations involve addressing the unique characteristics of nanophytoherbal formulations while ensuring their efficacy and safety for human use.

Challenges Encountered in Nanophytomedicine Product Development

Although there are currently no established guidelines for evaluating the efficacy of nanoparticle-based drugs, ongoing efforts aim to develop a diverse range of therapeutic agents. Despite significant advancements in nanotechnology and the increasing number of commercial products utilizing nanoparticles, new challenges persist in nanoscience and technology. Recent interest in nanophytomedicine focuses on reducing side effects and achieving precise drug delivery. Phytomedicines, or herbal medicines, have been used for millennia in ancient medical systems and are now recognized as adjunctive therapeutic alternatives to conventional medicine (Deepa et al., 2012). They are also employed as functional foods and nutraceuticals. Innovations in drug delivery technologies have created opportunities to develop phytomedicines that are both less toxic and more effective. Nanophytomedicine aims to leverage nanotechnology to deliver phytomedicines precisely to targeted areas, enhancing therapeutic benefits while minimizing drug toxicity. However, key challenges include the screening, isolation, and identification of active components from plants, which can be scarce and vary due to internal and external factors. These variations can lead to delays in obtaining sufficient quantities for preclinical research. The nanoparticle preparation process seeks to deliver phytomedicines to specific targets without affecting other body parts. *In vitro* experiments assess efficacy, while future studies should involve *in vivo* animal models to further understand the effects of phytomedicines (Han et al., 2012). Improving nanomaterial production for nanoparticle synthesis is crucial, with challenges including controlling nanoparticle size and ensuring batch consistency. Biosurfactant molecules are beneficial for scaling up production and advancing technological processes (Chang et al., 2011). Characterizing nanomaterials remains challenging due to their unique physical and chemical properties. Current methods, such as fluorescence-based assays and cytotoxicity studies, require improvement. Future research should focus on enhancing drug loading efficiency, reducing dosage disposal, and investigating the immunotoxicity of nanoformulations due to potential immune responses (Hu et al., 2010; Sutthanut et al., 2009). Additionally, future studies should aim to formulate and fabricate nanophytomedicine systems for diverse biological and therapeutic applications, emphasizing *in vivo* composition analysis. While traditional characterization methods are often employed, they can be costly compared to newer techniques that offer enhanced safety.

Conclusion

This study examines the safety and regulatory issues related to nanophytoherbal therapeutics. It explores the regulatory framework governing the creation and marketing of nanophytoherbal products, with a particular focus on international perspectives and disparities. The research aims to assess the safety profiles of nanophytoherbal formulations using preclinical models, scrutinize existing regulations and guidelines relevant to these therapies, propose suggestions for standardizing safety evaluations in nanophytoherbal research, and explain the implications of safety findings on the approval process. The study employs a systematic literature review, incorporating data from preclinical studies, clinical trials, and regulatory documents. Comparisons are made to identify commonalities and variations in safety assessments for different nanophytoherbal formulations. The findings highlight the diverse safety profiles among nanophytoherbals, emphasizing the need for standardized evaluation methods. Additionally, the research reveals the dynamic nature of guidelines across regions, stressing the importance of a nuanced approach to compliance. Key findings suggest potential improvements in current safety assessment protocols, which could enhance the quality and reliability of nanophytoherbal therapies. In conclusion, this study underscores the significance of standardized safety assessments to ensure the credibility of research outcomes and advocates for regulatory harmonization. This has important implications for both the scientific community and regulatory bodies, facilitating a safer and more streamlined development process for nanophytoherbal therapeutics.

References

Alam, M. S., Garg, A., Pottoo, F. H., Saifullah, M. K., Tareq, A. I., Manzoor, O., Mohsin, M., & Javed, M. N. (2017). Gum Ghatti mediated, one pot green synthesis of optimized gold nanoparticles: Investigation of process-variables impact using Box-Behnken based statistical design. *International Journal of Biological Macromolecules, 104*(A), 758–767.

Alam, M. S., Javed, M. N., Pottoo, F. H., Waziri, A., Almalki, F. A., Hasnain, M. S., Garg, A., & Saifullah, M. K. (2019). QbD approached comparison of reaction mechanism in microwave synthesized gold nanoparticles and their superior catalytic role against hazardous nitro-dye. *Applied Organometallic Chemistry, 33*(9), e5071.

Anagnostaki, E. E., & Zografos, A. L. (2012). 'Common synthetic scaffolds' in the synthesis of structurally diverse natural products. *Chemical Society Reviews, 41*(17), 5613–5625.

Barkat, M. A., Beg, S., Pottoo, F. H., & Ahmad, F. J. (2019). Nanopaclitaxel therapy: An evidence-based review on the battle for next-generation formulation challenges. *Nanomedicine, 14*(10), 1323–1341.

Bernabeu, E., Cagel, M., Lagomarsino, E., Moretton, M., & Chiappetta, D. A. (2017). Paclitaxel: What has been done and the challenges remain ahead. *International Journal of Pharmaceutics, 526*(1–2), 474–495.

Bonifácio, B. V., Silva, P. B., Santos Ramos, M. A. D., Silveira Negri, K. M., Bauab, T. M., & Chorilli, M. (2014). Nanotechnology-based drug delivery systems and herbal medicines: A review. *International Journal of Nanomedicine, 9*, 1–15.

Chang, L. C., Wu, C. L. W., Liu, C. W., Chuo, W. H., Li, P. C., & Tsai, T. R. (2011). Preparation, characterization and cytotoxicity evaluation of tanshinone IIA nanoemulsions. *Journal of Biomedical Nanotechnology, 7*(4), 558–567.

Cheng, Z., & Zhen, C. (2004). *The Cheng Zhi-Fan Collectanea of Medical History*. Beijing: Peking University Medical Press.

Chorilli, M., Brizante, A. C., Rodrigues, C. A., & Salgado, H. R. N. (2007). Aspectos gerais em sistemas transdérmicos de liberação de fármacos. *Revista Brasileira de Farmácia, 88*(1), 7–13.

Deepa, V., Sridhar, R., Goparaju, A., Reddy, P. N., & Murthy, P. B. (2012). Nanoemulsified ethanolic extract of *Pyllanthus amarus* Schum and Thonn ameliorates CCl4 induced hepatotoxicity in Wistar rats. *Indian Journal of Experimental Biology, 50*(11), 785–794.

Dorocki, S., & Kula, A. (2015). Przestrzenne zróżnicowanie rozwoju nanotechnologii w Europie. *Prace Komisji Geografii Przemysłu Polskiego Towarzystwa Geograficznego, 1*(29), 27–41.

Ferreira, V. F., & Pinto, A. C. (2010). A fitoterapia no mundo atual. *Química Nova, 33*(9), 1829–1838.

Ghosh, V., Saranya, S., Mukherjee, A., & Chandrasekaran, N. (2013). Antibacterial microemulsion prevents sepsis and triggers healing of wound in Wistar rats. *Colloids & Surfaces B: Biointerfaces, 105*, 152–157.

Grill, A. E., Johnston, N. W., Sadhukha, T., & Panyam, J. (2009). A review of select recent patents on novel nanocarriers. *Recent Patents on Drug Delivery & Formulation, 3*(2), 137–142.

Han, L., Fu, Y., Cole, A. J., Liu, J., & Wang, J. (2012). Co-encapsulation and sustained-release of four components in ginkgo terpenes from inject PELGE nanoparticles. *Fitoterapia, 83*(4), 721–731.

Harshita, M. A., Barkat, M. A., Rizwanullah, M., Beg, S., Pottoo, F. H., Siddiqui, S., & Ahmad, F. J. (2019). Paclitaxel-loaded nanolipidic carriers with improved oral bioavailability and anticancer activity against human liver carcinoma. *AAPS PharmSciTech, 20*(2), 87.

Hasnain, M. S., Javed, M. N., Alam, M. S., Rishishwar, P., Rishishwar, S., Ali, S., Nayak, A. K., & Beg, S. (2019). Purple heart plant leaves extract-mediated silver nanoparticle synthesis: Optimization by Box-Behnken design. *Materials Science and Engineering: C, 99*, 1105–1114.

Hu, L. D., Xing, Q., Meng, J., & Shang, C. (2010). Preparation and enhanced oral bioavailability of cryptotanshinone-loaded solid lipid nanoparticles. *AAPS PharmSciTech, 11*(2), 582–587.

Javed, M. N., Alam, M. S., Waziri, A., Pottoo, F. H., Yadav, A. K., Hasnain, M. S., & Almalki, F. A. (2019). QbD applications for the development of nanopharmaceutical products. In *Pharmaceutical Quality by Design* (pp. 229–253). New York: Academic Press.

Javed, M. N., Kohli, K., & Amin, S. (2018). Risk assessment integrated QbD approach for development of optimized bicontinuous mucoadhesive limicubes for oral delivery of rosuvastatin. *AAPS PharmSciTech, 19*(3), 1377–1391.

Khare, C. P. (2004). *Indian herbal remedies: Rational Western therapy, Ayurvedic, and other traditional usage*. New York: Springer.

Kundu, P., Mohanty, C., & Sahoo, S. K. (2012). Antiglioma activity of curcumin-loaded lipid nanoparticles and its enhanced bioavailability in brain tissue for effective glioblastoma therapy. *Acta Biomaterialia, 8*(7), 2670–2687.

Li, Z., Wu, X., Li, J., Yao, L., Sun, L., Shi, Y., Zhang, W., Lin, J., Liang, D., & Li, Y. (2012). Antitumor activity of celastrol nanoparticles in a xenograft retinoblastoma tumor model. *International Journal of Nanomedicine, 7*, 2389–2398.

Mainardes, R. M., Urban, M. C. C., Cinto, P. O., Chaud, M. V., Evangelista, R. C., & Gremião, M. P. D. (2006). Liposomes and micro/nanoparticles as colloidal carriers for nasal drug delivery. *Current Drug Delivery, 3*(3), 275–285.

Mishra, S., Sharma, S., Javed, M. N., Pottoo, F. H., Barkat, M. A., Harshita, M. S., Alam, M. S., Amir, M., & Sarafroz, M. (2019). Bioinspired nanocomposites: Applications in disease diagnosis and treatment. *Pharmaceutical Nanotechnology, 7*(3), 206–219.

Newman, D. J. (2008). Natural products as leads to potential drugs: An old process or the new hope for drug discovery? *Journal of Medicinal Chemistry, 51*(9), 2589–2599.

Newman, D. J., & Cragg, G. M. (2007). Natural products as sources of new drugs over the last 25 years. *Journal of Natural Products, 70*(3), 461–477.

Nigar, S., Pottoo, F. H., Tabassum, N., Verma, S. K., & Javed, M. N. (2016). Molecular insights into the role of inflammation and oxidative stress in epilepsy. *Journal of Advances in Medical & Pharmaceutical Sciences, 10*(1), 1–9.

Phillipson, J. D. (2001). Phytochemistry and medicinal plants. *Phytochemistry, 56*(3), 237–243.

Pottoo, F. H., Barkat, M. A., Ansari, M. A., Javed, M. N., Jamal, Q. M., & Kamal, M. A. (2019). Nanotechnological based miRNA intervention in the therapeutic management of neuroblastoma. *Seminars in Cancer Biology*.

Pottoo, F. H., Javed, M. N., Barkat, M. A., Alam, M. S., Nowshehri, J. A., Alshayban, D. M., & Ansari, M. A. (2019). Estrogen and serotonin: Complexity of interactions and implications for epileptic seizures and epileptogenesis. *Current Neuropharmacology, 17*(3), 214–231.

Pottoo, F. H., Tabassum, N., Javed, M. N., Nigar, S., Rasheed, R., Khan, A., Barkat, M. A., Alam, M. S., Maqbool, A., Ansari, M. A., Barreto, G. E., & Ashraf, G. M. (2019). The synergistic effect of raloxifene, fluoxetine, and bromocriptine protects against pilocarpine-induced status epilepticus and temporal lobe epilepsy. *Molecular Neurobiology, 56*(2), 1233–1247.

Pottoo, F. H., Tabassum, N., Javed, M. N., Nigar, S., Sharma, S., Barkat, M. A., Harshita, M. S., Alam, M. S., Ansari, M. A., Barreto, G. E., & Ashraf, G. M. (2020). Raloxifene potentiates the effect of fluoxetine against maximal electroshock induced seizures in mice. *European Journal of Pharmaceutical Sciences, 146*, 105261.

Rajendran, R., Radhai, R., Kotresh, T. M., & Csiszar, E. (2013). Development of antimicrobial cotton fabrics using herb loaded nanoparticles. *Carbohydrate Polymers, 91*(2), 613–617.

Rasoanaivo, P., Wright, C. W., Willcox, M. L., & Gilbert, B. (2011). Whole plant extracts versus single compounds for the treatment of malaria: Synergy and positive interactions. *Malaria Journal, 10*(1 Suppl.), S4.

Sharma, S., Javed, M. N., Pottoo, F. H., Rabbani, S. A., Barkat, M. A., Harshita, M., Sarafroz, M., & Amir, M. (2019). Bioresponse inspired nanomaterials for targeted drug and gene delivery. *Pharmaceutical Nanotechnology, 7*(3), 220–233.

Shi, F., Zhao, J. H., Liu, Y., Wang, Z., Zhang, Y. T., & Feng, N. P. (2012). Preparation and characterization of solid lipid nanoparticles loaded with frankincense and myrrh oil. *International Journal of Nanomedicine, 7*, 2033–2043.

Sofias, A. M., Dunne, M., Storm, G., & Allen, C. (2017). The battle of 'nano' paclitaxel. *Advanced Drug Delivery Reviews, 122*, 20–30.

Sutthanut, K., Lu, X., Jay, M., & Sripanidkulchai, B. (2009). Solid lipid nanoparticles for topical administration of *Kaempferia parviflora* extracts. *Journal of Biomedical Nanotechnology, 5*(2), 224–232.

List of Contributors

Abhinav Singhal
Guru Gobind Singh College of Pharmacy, Yamuna Nagar, Haryana, India

Abhishek Marwari
M.M. College of Pharmacy, Maharishi Markandeshwar (Deemed to be University), Mullana, Ambala, 133207, Haryana, India

Aiman Usmani
Amity Institute of Pharmacy, Amity University, Noida, 201301, Uttar Pradesh, India

Ajmer Singh Grewal
Guru Gobind Singh College of Pharmacy, Yamuna Nagar, Haryana, India

Akash Jain
M.M. College of Pharmacy, Maharishi Markandeshwar (Deemed to be University), Mullana, Ambala, 133207, Haryana, India

Anchal Sharma
Shiva Institute of Pharmacy, Chandpur, Bilaspur, Himachal Pradesh, India

Anshika Chaudhary
Amity Institute of Pharmacy, Amity University, Noida, Uttar Pradesh, India

Anuj Malik
M.M. College of Pharmacy, Maharishi Markandeshwar (Deemed to be University), Mullana, 133207, Ambala, Haryana, India

Arushi
Shiva Institute of Pharmacy, Chandpur, Bilaspur, Himachal Pradesh, India

Astha Singh
Amity Institute of Pharmacy, Amity University, Noida, 201301, Uttar Pradesh, India

Bhumika Thakur
Shiva Institute of Pharmacy, Chandpur, Bilaspur, Himachal Pradesh, India

Chaitanya Vinayak Narayan
I.T.S. College of Pharmacy, Delhi-Meerut Road, Ghaziabad, Uttar Pradesh, India

Chander Parkash
Chitkara College of Pharmacy, Chitkara University, Punjab, India

Davinder Kumar
College of Pharmacy, PGIMS, Pt. B.D. Sharma University of Health Sciences, Rohtak, Haryana, India

Dhrubajyoti Sarkar
Faculty of Pharmaceutical Science, Assam Down Town University, Sankar Madhab Path, Gandhinagar, Panikhaiti, Guwahati, Assam, India

Dinesh Kumar
School of Pharmacy, Deshbhagat University, Mandi Gobindgarh, Fathehgarh Sahib, 147301, Punjab, India

Gagandeep Kaur
Chitkara University School of Pharmacy, Chitkara University, Himachal Pradesh, India

Garima Kapoor
KIET School of Pharmacy, KIET Group of Institutions, Ghaziabad, Uttar Pradesh, India

Himanshi Tanwar
Department of Pharmacy, Banasthali Vidyapith, Banasthali, Jaipur, Rajasthan, India; Department of Pharmaceutical Sciences, Guru Jambheshwar University of Science & Technology, Hisar, Haryana, India

Hitesh Chopra
Department of Biosciences, Saveetha School of Engineering, Saveetha Institute of Medical and Technical Sciences, Chennai, Tamil Nadu, India

Indu Singh
Amity Institute of Pharmacy, Amity University, Noida, 201301, Uttar Pradesh, India

Isha Chawla
M.M. College of Pharmacy, Maharishi Markandeshwar (Deemed to be University), Mullana, Ambala, 133207, Haryana, India

Jasmine Chaudhary
M.M. College of Pharmacy, Maharishi Markandeshwar (Deemed to be University), Mullana, Ambala, 133207, Haryana, India

Jyoti Uikey
I.E.S. Institute of Pharmacy, I.E.S. University, Bhopal, Madhya Pradesh, 462044, India

Jyotiram Arjun Sawale
Krishna Institute of Pharmacy, Krishna Vishwa Vidyapeeth (Deemed to be University), Karad, Maharashtra, India

Karan Goel
M.M. College of Pharmacy, Maharishi Markandeshwar (Deemed to be University), Mullana, Ambala, 133207, Haryana, India

Kavita Munjal
Amity Institute of Pharmacy, Amity University, Noida, Uttar Pradesh, India

Kirti Goel
M.M. College of Pharmacy, Maharishi Markandeshwar (Deemed to be University), Mullana, Ambala, 133207, Haryana, India

Kumar Guarve
Guru Gobind Singh College of Pharmacy, Yamuna Nagar, Haryana, India

Lakshmi Maurya
KIET School of Pharmacy, KIET Group of Institutions, Ghaziabad, Uttar Pradesh, India

Lovish Sharma
Chitkara University School of Pharmacy, Chitkara University, Himachal Pradesh, India

Manasvi Saini
College of Pharmacy, Shivalik Campus, Dehradun, Uttrakhand, India

Manisha Bhatia
M. M. College of Pharmacy, Maharishi Markandeshwar (Deemed to be University), Mullana, Ambala, Haryana, India

Manu Sharma
Department of Pharmacy, Banasthali Vidyapith, Banasthali, Jaipur, Rajasthan, India

Monika Saini
M.M. College of Pharmacy, Maharishi Markandeshwar (Deemed to be University), Mullana, Ambala, Haryana, India

Munish Ahuja
Department of Pharmaceutical Sciences, Guru Jambheshwar University of Science & Technology, Hisar, Haryana, India

Narinderpal Kaur
Chitkara University School of Pharmacy, Chitkara University, Himachal Pradesh, India

Navidha Aggarwal
M.M. College of Pharmacy, Maharishi Markandeshwar (Deemed to be University), Mullana, Ambala- 133207, Haryana, India

Neelam Singh
Noida Institute of Engineering and Technology (Pharmacy Institute), Greater Noida, Uttar Pradesh, India

Nitika Garg
Chitkara College of Pharmacy, Chitkara University, Punjab, India

Nitin Jangra
Chitkara University School of Pharmacy, Chitkara University, Himachal Pradesh, India

Pallavi Bassi
Chitkara College of Pharmacy, Chitkara University, Punjab, India

Parul Gupta
Guru Gobind Singh College of Pharmacy, Yamuna Nagar, Haryana, India

Parul Sood
Chitkara University School of Pharmacy, Chitkara University, Himachal Pradesh, India

Preeti
Gurugram Global College of Pharmacy, Farruknagar, Gurugram, Haryana, India

Prinsy Rana
M.M. College of Pharmacy, Maharishi Markandeshwar (Deemed to be University), Mullana, Ambala, 133207, Haryana, India

Priyanka Rathore
Sagar Institute of Research Technology and Science, Pharmacy, Bhopal, Madhya Pradesh, India

Purav Gupta
M.M. College of Pharmacy, Maharishi Markandeshwar (Deemed to be University), Mullana, Ambala, 133207, Haryana, India

Raman Kumari
M.M. College of Pharmacy, Maharishi Markandeshwar (Deemed to be University), Mullana, 133207, Ambala, Haryana, India

Ravi Berwal
Department of Pharmaceutical Sciences, Guru Jambheshwar University of Science & Technology, Hisar, Haryana, India

Rohan Nagpal
Amity Institute of Pharmacy, Amity University, Noida, Uttar Pradesh, India

Rohit Kamboj
Guru Gobind Singh College of Pharmacy, Yamuna Nagar, Haryana, India

Rubina Bhutani
School of Medical and Allied Sciences, GD Goenka University, Gurgaon, Haryana, India

Samrat Chauhan
Chitkara College of Pharmacy, Chitkara University, Punjab, India

Sanchit Dhankhar
Chitkara College of Pharmacy, Chitkara University, Punjab, India

Shikha Baghel Chauhan
Amity Institute of Pharmacy, Amity University, Noida, 201301, Uttar Pradesh, India

Shikha Kamboj
Guru Gobind Singh College of Pharmacy, Yamuna Nagar, Haryana, India

Shiv Kumar
Shiva Institute of Pharmacy, Chandpur, Bilaspur, Himachal Pradesh, India

Shiva Tushir
Department of Pharmacy, Panipat Institute of Engineering & Technology, Panipat, Haryana, India

Shiwali Sharma
Chitkara University School of Pharmacy, Chitkara University, Himachal Pradesh, India

Shreya Kaul
Amity Institute of Pharmacy, Amity University, Noida, Uttar Pradesh, India

Shuchi Dave
Guru Ramdas Khalsa Institute of Science and Technology (Pharmacy), Jabalpur, Madhya Pradesh, India

Simran
M.M. College of Pharmacy, Maharishi Markandeshwar (Deemed to be University), Mullana, Ambala, 133207, Haryana, India

Somia Chauhan
Amity Institute of Pharmacy, Amity University, Noida, Uttar Pradesh, India

Suhas P. Padmane
Gurunanak College of Pharmacy, Mauza-Nari, Nagpur, Maharashtra, India

Sumnit Wadhwa
M.M. College of Pharmacy, Maharishi Markandeshwar (Deemed to be University), Mullana, Ambala, 133207, Haryana, India

Sunayna Choudhary
M.M. College of Pharmacy, Maharishi Markandeshwar (Deemed to be University), Mullana, Ambala, 133207, Haryana, India

Swati Verma
I.T.S. College of Pharmacy, Delhi-Meerut Road, Ghaziabad, Uttar Pradesh, India

Sweta Kamboj
Guru Gobind Singh College of Pharmacy, Yamuna Nagar, Haryana, India

Teena Vishwakarma
I.E.S. Institute of Pharmacy, I.E.S. University, Bhopal, Madhya Pradesh, India

Umesh Patil
Department of Pharmaceutical Sciences, Dr. Harisingh Gour Vishwavidyalaya, Sagar, Madhya Pradesh, India

Uttam Singh Baghel
Gurukul Pharmacy College, Ranpur, Kota, Rajasthan, India

Vaibhav Jaiswal
I.E.S. Institute of Pharmacy, I.E.S. University, Bhopal, Madhya Pradesh, 462044, India

Vinod Kumar Gauttam
Shiva Institute of Pharmacy, Bilaspur, Himachal Pradesh, India

Vishnu Mittal
Guru Gobind Singh College of Pharmacy, Yamuna Nagar, Haryana, India

Vivek Chourasia
I.E.S. Institute of Pharmacy, I.E.S. University, Bhopal, Madhya Pradesh, India

About the Editors

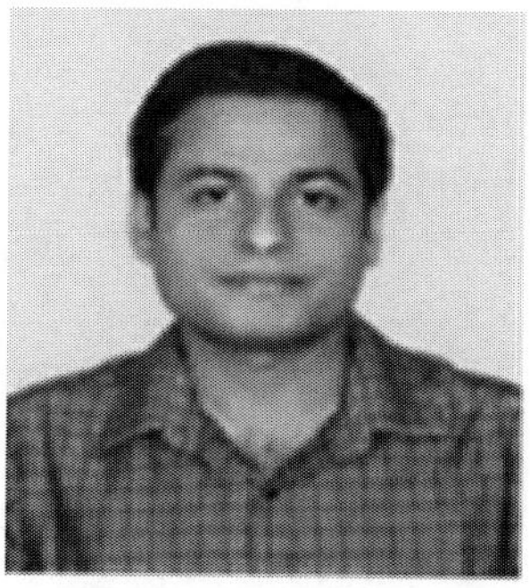

Dr. Hitesh Chopra, PhD, is a distinguished researcher with expertise in nanoformulations, natural polymers, cancer therapy, wound healing, and metabolic disorders. His prolific contributions to the scientific community include numerous publications in high-impact journals, collectively boasting a total impact factor of over 1000. His work is recognized for advancing the field of nanomedicine and its applications in treating complex medical conditions.

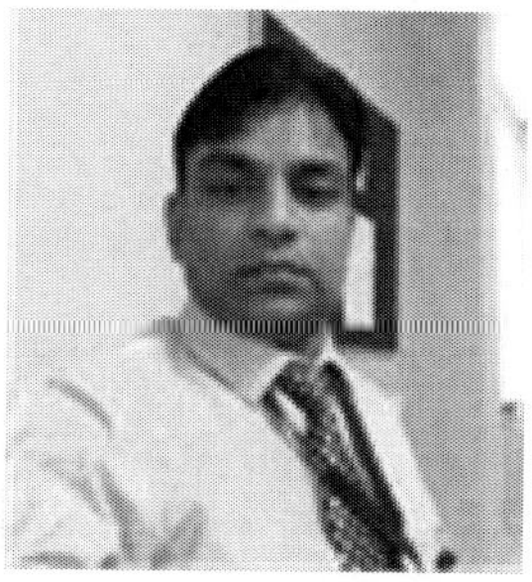

Dr. Vinod Kumar Gauttam, Professor (Pharmacognosy & Phytochemistry), Shiva Institute of Pharmacy, Bilaspur (Himachal Pradesh) is an academician researcher with more than 20 years of experience in the field of natural product chemistry. His prior areas of research include natural product chemistry, formulation development of herbals, analytical method development, drug design, etc. He is a recipient of Eminent Principal Award, IPA, MP state branch and best Researcher Award by CEGR, New Delhi. Dr. Gauttam has almost 45 publications in peer reviewed and scopus indexed journals, 02 books, 15 book chapters and 5 patents. He has presented his research in several International and National conferences and fetched Dr. PD Sethi Best Paper Award 2020. He is a reviewer in peer reviewed journals.

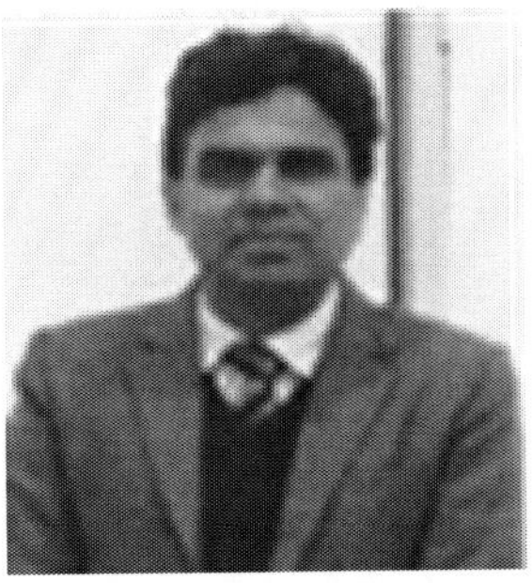

Dr. Ajmer Singh Grewal, Professor (Pharmaceutical Chemistry), Guru Gobind Singh College of Pharmacy, Yamuna Nagar, Haryana (India), is having academic and research experience of 12+ years in medicinal chemistry. His present areas of research include structure-based drug design and medicinal chemistry of MMP2 and MMP9 inhibitors as anticancer agents, antibacterial drug resistance (NDM-1), GK activators as anti-diabetic agents, AR inhibitors for diabetic complications, PPAR agonists for metabolic syndrome, multi-potent anti-Alzheimer's agents, selective PDE-4 & -7 inhibitors as anti-inflammatory agents and environmental chemistry. He owns to his credit more than 100 publications in national and international journals of repute, 20 book chapters, 14 books, and 6 patents (3 granted). He is a life member of the Indian Society for Technical Education (ISTE) and APTI.

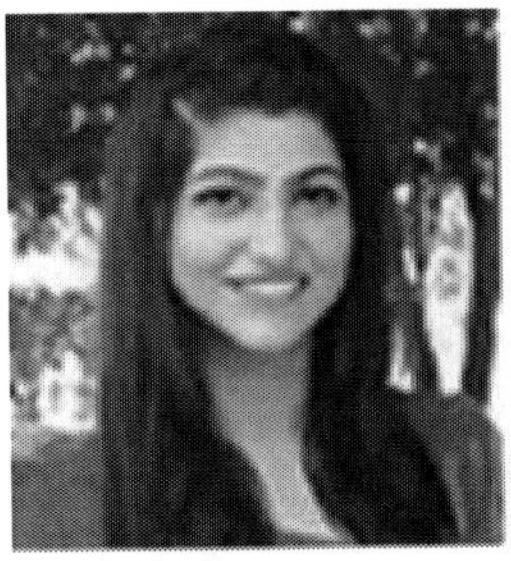

Dr. Kavita Munjal, Assistant Professor (Pharmacognosy & Phytochemistry), Amity Institute of Pharmacy, Amity University, Noida (Uttar Pradesh) is an academician researcher with more than 10 years of experience in the field of natural product chemistry. Her prior areas of research include isolation of natural products, formulation and drug design etc. Dr. Kavita has qualified the GPAT test with a very high percentile score. She also qualified for the National Eligibility Test (NET) in 2019. She is a recipient of Senior Research Fellowship from ICMR, Delhi and Research Grant Award from BIRAC-SRISTI, Ahmedabad. Dr. Kavita has almost 35 publications in peer reviewed and SCOPUS indexed journals with four major research publications in Lancet, 12 book chapters and 3 patents. She has presented her research in several International and National conferences and fetched Best paper Award in ICRMR Malaysia 2018, Best Oral Presentation Award 2019, Dr. PD Sethi Best Paper Award 2020, etc.

Index

A

B

C

D

E

F

G

H

O

P

Z

B